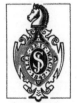

Werner Glinz

Chest Trauma
Diagnosis and Management

With 133 Figures

Springer-Verlag
Berlin Heidelberg New York 1981

Priv.-Doz. Dr. WERNER GLINZ
Universitätsspital Zürich
Chirurgische Klinik B
Rämistraße 100, CH-8091 Zürich

Translators:

G. H. MUNDINGER, Sr.
1170-A Monroe Drive, Boulder, Colorado 80303/USA

G. H. MUNDINGER, Jr.
6724 Glenkirk Road, Baltimore, Maryland 21239/USA

Title of the German Edition: Werner Glinz, Thoraxverletzungen
© Springer-Verlag Berlin Heidelberg 1978 and 1979

ISBN-13: 978-3-642-67859-2   e-ISBN-13: 978-3-642-67857-8
DOI: 10.1007/978-3-642-67857-8

Library of Congress Cataloging in Publication Data. Glinz, Werner. Chest trauma. Translation of Thoraxverletzungen. Bibliography: p. Includes index. 1. Chest-Wounds and injuries. I. Title. [DNLM: 1. Thoracic injuries–Diagnosis. 2. Thoracic injuries–Surgery. WF985 G56lt] RD536.G5913 617'.54059 80-25209

This work is subject to copyright. All rights are reserved, whether the whole or part of the material is concerned, specifically those of translation, reprinting, re-use of illustrations, broadcasting, reproduction by photocopying machine or similar means, and storage in data banks.
Under § 54 of the German Copyright Law where copies are made for other than private use a fee is payable to "Verwertungsgesellschaft Wort", Munich.
© by Springer-Verlag Berlin · Heidelberg 1981
Softcover reprint of the hardcover 1st edition 1981

The use of registered names, trademarks, etc. in this publication does not imply, even in the absence of a specific statement, that such names are exempt from the relevant protective laws and regulations and therefore free for general use.

2124/3130-543210

Preface to the German Edition

Expanded knowledge about the pathophysiologic effects of severe injuries, advancements in the intensive care of victims of multiple injuries, and the treatment made possible by modern cardiovascular surgery make it appear sensible to combine the assessment and therapy of thoracic injuries into a synthesis of various branches of medicine.

This monograph, therefore, is intended not only for the specialist in thoracic or cardiac surgery but also primarily for the person who is the first to be confronted by thoracic injuries, namely, the general surgeon or the traumatologist.

It reflects my own personal experience as chief surgeon of an emergency surgery ward of a university hospital and as head of an intensive care unit for the severely wounded, which treats well over 100 patients with severe thoracic injuries annually, and is based on an analysis of these cases. My experience as a military surgeon in Vietnam was also taken into consideration.

Many wounds in the area of the thorax can be successfully treated with simple, conservative procedures, though by "conservative" I do not mean to imply "inactive." An aggressive conservatism is needed, which must pay attention to small details. In given cases, however, it requires the quick decision-making capability of the competent surgeon. For this reason, considerable space is devoted to questions of evaluation and practical procedures.

In most instances, thoracic wounds are accompanied by other wounds. Among our patients, more than 75% of all patients hospitalized with blunt thoracic injuries were wounded in other parts of the body. My respected chief and teacher, Professor H. U. BUFF, frequently called attention to the fact that the severely injured patient belongs in the care of a facility that accepts responsibility for the treatment of all of his wounds and that he may not be parceled out to a multiplicity of specialists on the basis of his injured organs. This principle was put into practice in the Surgical Department B of the University Hospital in Zürich. The spirit of that approach, I hope, finds expression also in the text of this book; precisely in the chapters of the first section an attempt is made to present thoracic trauma within the framework of the patient's other wounds along with their mutual consequences.

Zürich, Spring 1978　　　　　　　　　　　　　　　　　　　　Werner GLINZ

Acknowledgments. I am especially indebted to Professor Å. SENNING, my teacher, in whose clinic I was able to work for many years where I had the opportunity to learn the most modern techniques of cardiac and thoracic surgery. I am grateful for his permission to use the case histories of the Surgical Clinic A at the University of Zürich. All of the roentgenograms pertain to my own patients and were prepared at the Central Institute for Radiology of the University Clinic in Zürich. The autopsy preparations were performed at the Institute for Pathology of the University of Zürich. I would like to thank Professors J. WELLAUER and CH. HEDINGER for their consent to use these pictures.

Many of the ideas and concepts for treatment of thoracic injuries that are presented in this book have been influenced by daily discussions held with my colleagues in the hospital of whom I would particularly like to mention Doctors G. HALDEMANN and K. REIST of the Institute for Anesthesiology and Dr. P. C. BAUMANN, head of the Intensive Care Unit of the Department of Internal Medicine.

The care of seriously injured patients would be impossible without the untiring devotion of the nursing personnel in the intensive care unit and the emergency ward. I wish to express my appreciation to all of them for their assistance.

I am very grateful to the following for their active support in the preparation of this book: to Mrs. A. JUNG and her colleagues in the central photography laboratory who worked on all the figures in this book, to Mr. B. STRUCHEN who did the sketches, and to Miss B. SCHÜTZ, my loyal and industrious secretary.

Contents

Part I General Considerations for the Assessment and Treatment of Thoracic Injuries

Chapter 1 Initial Considerations in the Management of Severe Thoracic Injury 3

    I. The Ten Vital Questions in the Initial Evaluation of Severe Thoracic Injuries 4
    II. Evaluation After Initial Management 7

Chapter 2 The Patient with Additional Injuries in Other Parts of the Body 11

    I. Craniocerebral Injuries 12
    II. Intra-abdominal Injuries 13
    III. Injuries of the Extremities 14
    IV. Maxillofacial Injuries 14
    V. Injuries to the Vertebral Column and Spinal Cord 15

Chapter 3 Interpretation of the Chest Roentgenogram . . 16

    I. Basic Considerations 16
    II. Opacities 20
    III. Accumulation of Air 22
    IV. The "Widened Mediastinum" 24

Chapter 4 Respiratory Insufficiency 29

    I. Basic Considerations 29
    II. Assessment of Respiration in Patients with Thoracic Injuries 29
    III. Respiratory Insufficiency Caused by the Thoracic Injury Itself 37

IV.	Aspiration	38
V.	Adult Respiratory Distress Syndrome (ARDS)	40
VI.	Fat Embolism	47
VII.	Other Forms of Respiratory Insufficiency Among the Injured	49
VIII.	Lung Damage Caused by Therapeutic Measures	50
IX.	Conclusions and Consequences for Prophylaxis and Therapy	55

Chapter 5 Indications for Operation in Blunt Thoracic Trauma — 57

I.	Indications for Immediate or Early Operation	57
II.	Indications for Subsequent Operations	59
III.	Contraindications to Operative Intervention	60

Chapter 6 Operative Approaches — 61

I.	Anterolateral Thoracotomy	61
II.	Posterolateral Thoracotomy	64
III.	Median Sternotomy	66
IV.	Approach to the Great Vessels of the Superior Thoracic Aperture	66
V.	Thoracoabdominal Approach	69

Chapter 7 Special Considerations in Penetrating Chest Injuries — 70

I.	Causes of Injury and Intrathoracic Injuries	70
II.	Evaluation and Therapeutic Procedure	72
III.	Prognosis	76

Chapter 8 Aspects of Intensive Care of Patients with Thoracic Injuries — 78

I.	Basic Considerations	78
II.	Monitoring and Evaluating the Patient with Thoracic Injuries in Intensive Care	79
III.	Mechanical Ventilation	81
IV.	Principles for the Infusion of Fluids	81
V.	Subsequent Pulmonary Complications	83

Chapter 9 Physiotherapy of Patients with Thoracic Injuries — 91

    I. Basic Considerations 91
    II. General Measures 92
    III. Forced Expiration 93
    IV. CO_2-Induced Increase in Ventilation 94
    V. Intermittent Positive Pressure Breathing (IPPB) . 95
    VI. Maximal Voluntary Inspiration 96

Part II Diagnosis, Clinical Significance, and Treatment of Specific Injuries

Chapter 10 Rib and Sternum Fractures 101

    I. General Considerations 101
    II. Specific Types of Fractures 104
    III. Diagnosis 108
    IV. General Considerations for Therapy in Rib and Sternal Fractures 110
    V. Pain Control 113
    VI. Therapy of Flail Chest 115

Chapter 11 Pneumothorax and Hemothorax 122

    I. Pneumothorax 122
    II. Tension Pneumothorax 126
    III. Open Pneumothorax 130
    IV. Hemothorax 131
    V. Clotted Hemothorax, Fibrothorax 133
    VI. Thoracentesis 135
    VII. Intercostal Tube Drainage 136

Chapter 12 Traumatic Emphysema 149

    I. Subcutaneous Emphysema 149
    II. Mediastinal Emphysema 152

Chapter 13 Lung Injuries from Blunt Trauma 155

    I. General Considerations 155
    II. Lung Laceration, Lung Rupture 157

III.	Intrapulmonary Hematoma	159
IV.	Traumatic Lung Pseudocysts (Pneumatoceles)	160
V.	Lung Contusion	161
VI.	Blast Injuries	165

Chapter 14 Tracheal and Bronchial Injuries 167

I.	Injuries to Trachea and Bronchi Caused by Blunt Trauma	167
II.	Old Bronchial Ruptures	171
III.	Penetrating Injuries to Trachea and Bronchi	172

Chapter 15 Injuries to the Esophagus 174

I.	Rupture of the Esophagus, Penetrating and Iatrogenic Esophageal Injuries	174
II.	Traumatic Esophagotracheal Fistula	178

Chapter 16 Injuries to the Heart by Blunt Trauma 180

I.	Basic Considerations	180
II.	Pericardial Injuries, Luxation of the Heart	182
III.	Hemopericardium, Cardiac Tamponade	184
IV.	Posttraumatic Pericarditis	189
V.	Cardiac Contusion	191
VI.	Heart Wall Ruptures	204
VII.	Traumatic Septal Defects	205
VIII.	Heart Valve Injuries	205
IX.	Injuries of the Coronary Arteries	206
X.	Traumatic Cardiac Aneurysm	207

Chapter 17 Penetrating Wounds of the Heart 208

I.	Penetrating Cardiac Injuries	208
II.	Late Sequelae of Penetrating Cardiac Injuries	217
III.	Foreign Bodies in the Heart	219

Chapter 18 Injuries of the Great Intrathoracic Vessels . . . 222

I.	Rupture of the Aorta	222
II.	Penetrating Injuries of the Aorta	236
III.	Closed Injuries of the Supra-aortic Arteries	238

IV. Injuries of the Great Veins and Pulmonary Vessels 239
V. Penetrating Injuries of the Vessels of the Superior Thoracic Aperture 240
VI. Posttraumatic Late Sequelae in the Great Vessels 242

Chapter 19 Injuries of the Diaphragm 246

I. Diaphragmatic Ruptures 246
II. Penetrating Diaphragmatic Injuries 256

Chapter 20 Other Injury Patterns and Consequences of Injury in Thoracic Trauma 258

I. Traumatic Asphyxia 258
II. Injuries of the Thoracic Duct, Chylothorax . . 261
III. Cholothorax 264
IV. Traumatically Induced Hernias of the Chest Wall 265
V. Arterial Air Embolism 266

Bibliography 270

Subject Index 295

Part I

General Considerations for the Assessment and Treatment of Thoracic Injuries

Part 1

Chapter 1
Initial Considerations in the Management of Severe Thoracic Injury

The evaluation of thoracic injuries is only one aspect of the **total assessment** of a severely injured patient. Even though each patient represents a unique case with its own peculiarities and special problems, there is nevertheless a **logical sequence** of diagnostic and therapeutic procedures. Both **diagnosis and therapy go hand in hand.** As in the care and management of every severely injured patient, the basic principle of elective surgery — "first investigate and make the diagnosis, then treat the illness" — is a dangerous illusion. The most threatening situations and injuries must first be correctly recognized and then treated, even if only symptomatically.

Often the most important question is not **whether** a certain procedure is to be carried out, but rather **when.** The performance of a certain diagnostic or therapeutic precautionary procedure may delay others, which under certain circumstances may be lifesaving.

Some Examples:

1. If a tension pneumothorax has been recognized on the basis of clinical examination, taking roentgenograms of the thorax will only serve to delay the prompt insertion of a lifesaving chest tube.

2. Intubation and mechanical ventilation applied in a tension pneumothorax without drainage only makes matters worse.

3. In a case of obvious respiratory insufficiency, a blood gas analysis will only delay the necessary intubation and mechanical ventilation.

4. Severe penetrating cardiac injuries or heart wall ruptures can be treated successfully by immediate operative intervention, even if cardiac arrest has occurred, if no time is lost in additional diagnostic procedures.

5. An attempt to perform aortography on a patient in severe shock with a ruptured aorta that has perforated into the thoracic cavity causing a left-sided hemothorax usually gambles away any chance of operating in time.

6. An emergency tracheostomy keeps the surgeon occupied for a valuable period of time; it is indicated primarily only if the patient cannot be intubated.

Even in severe thoracic injuries, there are only a few situations in which there is an **immediate** threat to life; many of them can be detected and treated by simple means.

I. The Ten Vital Questions in the Initial Evaluation of Severe Thoracic Injuries

The first step is to make a **rough estimate of the status of the circulatory and respiratory systems.** This provides the first diagnostic clues and often determines which therapeutic action is to be taken. **Specific questions** are then posed pertaining to individual injuries or their consequences (Table 1).

Table 1. Ten questions to be asked in the initial assessment of severe blunt thoracic injuries

1. Hypovolemia?	
2. Respiratory insufficiency?	Immediately life-threatening; diagnosis and
3. Tension pneumothorax?	therapy before taking roentgenograms
4. Cardiac tamponade?	

5. Multiple rib fractures? (paradoxical respiration?)
6. Pneumothorax? (subcutaneous emphysema? mediastinal emphysema?)
7. Hemothorax?
8. Diaphragmatic rupture?
9. Aortic rupture?
10. Cardiac contusion?

1. Hypovolemia?

If there are clinical signs of hypovolemic shock, **volume replacement** is begun immediately after the establishment of venous access and is continued throughout the remainder of the examination.

Measurement of the **central venous pressure** is essential in every case of severe thoracic injury. This makes it possible to differentiate between hypotension caused by loss of blood and a drop in blood pressure caused by cardiac tamponade or cardiac insufficiency. The measurement also serves as a guide in managing volume replacement. It must be pointed out emphatically, however, that the monitoring of central venous pressure does not help to detect lung-damaging overinfusion with electrolyte solutions.

Massive blood losses resulting from thoracic trauma manifest themselves in the form of a hemothorax or mediastinal hemorrhage. The analysis of 200 patients with blunt thoracic injuries who had an arterial blood pressure below 100 mmHg upon admission to the emergency ward revealed, however, that in half of all the cases (98 patients) an intra-abdominal injury was partially or fully responsible for the hemorrhagic shock. In 53 of these patients, the spleen had been ruptured.

2. Respiratory Insufficiency?

Initial evaluation of ventilation is provided by an examination of the patient's breathing and thoracic movements, auscultation of the chest, and testing of the expiratory airflow by holding the hand in front of the mouth and nose. Even in severe respiratory insufficiency, **cyanosis** does not necessarily occur; with massive blood loss, the necessary 5 g% of reduced hemoglobin are often not attained.

If there is a pneumothorax, it is drained. In all other forms of respiratory insufficiency, an open airway is maintained by endotracheal intubation, and mechanical ventilation is provided if necessary. In addition to facilitating ventilation, intubation makes effective and repeated endotracheal suctioning possible and prevents aspiration.

3. Open Pneumothorax? Tension Pneumothorax?

A **pneumothorax that is open to the outside** can usually be recognized immediately by the characteristic sound of air flowing into and out of the wound ("sucking wound"); however, its danger is often underestimated. Emergency treatment consists of sealing the thoracic wound by applying a compression bandage or by temporarily closing it with the flat of the hand protected by a sterile glove. Under clinical conditions, however, intubation and mechanical ventilation is usually the preferred alternative.

A life-threatening **tension pneumothorax** caused by blunt thoracic trauma is occasionally overlooked even though clinical diagnosis is usually easy. It may be revealed by the appearance of subcutaneous emphysema in the area of the chest or neck or auscultatory evidence of mediastinal emphysema. The immediate relief of pressure by external drainage is lifesaving. Under hospital conditions, no time should be wasted on attempts at needle aspiration, which is inadequate anyway. Instead, a chest tube is inserted immediately. It is no more time-consuming, and sterile chest tubes, available for immediate use, should be part of the basic equipment of every emergency room.

4. Cardiac Tamponade?

In penetrating thoracic injuries, the localization of a wound in the precordial area itself will indicate the possibility of cardiac tamponade. The classic triad (high venous pressure, arterial hypotension, diminished heart sounds) is found in only 35% – 40% of trauma patients with such injury [507, 508]. The prominent sign is that of venous

Table 2. Elevated central venous pressure in thoracic injuries

Warning: straining and coughing may also cause elevated central venous pressure
Cardiac tamponade
Tension pneumothorax
Massive undrained hemothorax (after volume replacement)
Possibly mediastinal emphysema
Cardiac insufficiency
Overtransfusion

congestion: distended neck veins and elevated central venous pressure. A paradoxical pulse (see p. 186) will also raise suspicion of cardiac tamponade.

Raised venous pressure (Table 2) is, of course, not pathognomonic of tamponade but can also indicate a tension pneumothorax, a massive undrained hemothorax, mediastinal emphysema, cardiac insufficiency, and overtransfusion. Elevated central venous pressure may also be erroneously measured in patients who are straining and coughing.

Pericardiocentesis (see Chap. 16 for technique) can and should be employed as a diagnostic aid. It is also the first, though not definitive, therapeutic measure. If acute cardiac tamponade is diagnosed, operation is usually indicated for control of the injury.

* * *

Not until the emergency measures occasioned by these first four questions have been carried out should time be taken for **radiologic examinations.** The thoracic roentgenogram is the basic tool for the diagnosis and evaluation of other thoracic injuries, which as a rule do not pose an immediate threat to life.

This does not mean, however, that the patient is to be sent to the radiology department. A severely injured person is X-rayed in the emergency room with portable equipment so as not to interrupt monitoring and treatment.

According to a study by Key [6], the average time required for a roentgenogram of the thorax under optimal conditions is 14 min, assuming the work is done in the radiology department.

* * *

5. Rib Fractures? (Paradoxical Respiration?)

Rib fractures are often not visible on a roentgenogram even if they are located in the bony part of the rib. **Clinical findings,** therefore, play an important role in diagnosis.

If the patient demonstrates guarded breathing and is not breathing deeply, it is often difficult to detect **paradoxical respiration.** This clinical diagnosis is facilitated if the patient can be induced to breathe as deeply as possible. Intubation and mechanical ventilation are indicated only if there is respiratory insufficiency.

6. Pneumothorax? (Subcutaneous Emphysema?) (Mediastinal Emphysema?)

If there is no tension pneumothorax, the drainage of a clinically suspected **pneumothorax** should be postponed until the thoracic roentgenogram is obtained since if the diaphragm is ruptured, gas-filled abdominal organs (stomach, colon) displaced into the thoracic cavity can simulate a pneumothorax. **Subcutaneous emphysema,** by itself, is not significant. **Mediastinal emphysema** is more important since it may herald a tracheobronchial or esophageal rupture. It can often be diagnosed by a characteristic finding upon auscultation of the heart (see p. 152) before it becomes visible on the roentgenogram and before subcutaneous air accumulates in the cervical area.

7. Hemothorax?

Only a massive hemothorax results in a restriction of ventilation that is clinically detectable. Clinical diagnosis is sometimes difficult since percussion findings may be misleading if there is a simultaneous pneumothorax.

8. Diaphragmatic Rupture?

This is recognized clinically only when bowel sounds are audible in the thoracic area. In general, the diagnosis is made radiologically. False diagnosis of a hemothorax is not uncommon. Initially, a rupture of the diaphragm often follows an undramatic course, but the increasing displacement of intra-abdominal organs into the thoracic cavity progressively leads to respiratory insufficiency.

9. Rupture of the Aorta?

In addition to clinical symptoms of a pseudocoarctation syndrome, i. e., weakened pulses in the lower extremities, an occasional systolic murmur, and signs of compression in the upper mediastinum, the radiologic finding of a **widened mediastinum** (see Chap. 3) is the chief indicator of this injury. Further verification requires the use of aortography. If the patient already has a left-sided hemothorax and is in a state of uncontrollable shock, emergency operative intervention is performed without preceding angiography.

10. Cardiac Contusion?

This injury occurs much more frequently than is commonly supposed. Contusion of the heart is to be suspected following any accident involving compression of the sternum against the spinal column. The changing picture makes diagnosis difficult. The most common findings are variations in the ECG (mainly disturbances in repolarization and heart rhythm); however, the ECG can be normal initially, and in rare instances remain normal. The cardiac enzymes (see p. 194) are always elevated. The clinical significance of this injury lies in the danger of life-threatening disturbances of cardiac rhythm and acute cardiac insufficiency.

II. Evaluation After Initial Management

During the initial phase of diagnostic and therapeutic procedures, the condition of the patient will have to be checked at regular intervals. The early course of development, especially the success of shock therapy, is often of greater significance than the nature of the injury itself in determining the need for operative intervention.

Table 3. Injuries frequently overlooked or diagnosed late

	Frequency
1. Cardiac contusion 2. Paradoxical respiration 3. Diaphragmatic rupture 4. Aortic rupture 5. Bronchial rupture 6. Esophageal rupture	▽

Table 4. Synopsis of initial assessment of the most important thoracic injuries

	Suspected if there is	Additional examination required	Initial therapeutic measures
Tension pneumothorax	Inflated hemithorax with reduced mobility of thorax Hypersonorous auscultation Weakened breath sounds Venous congestion; increasing elevation of central venous pressure	None →	Immediate thoracic drainage
Open pneumothorax	Thoracic wounds with sounds of air rushing in and out ("sucking wound")	None →	1. Tight bandage or 2. Intubation, mechanical ventilation
Cardiac tamponade	Location of wound in the precordium or corresponding tract of the bullet or knife	None →	Pericardiocentesis Operation
Rib fractures	Local tenderness Compression pain Possibly crepitation on auscultation Inspection: possibly paradoxical respiration	Chest roentgenogram	Relief of pain Intubation and mechanical ventilation when respiratory insufficiency occurs
Pneumothorax	Hyperresonance Diminished breath sounds	Chest roentgenogram	Thoracic drainage
Hemothorax	Dullness to percussion	Chest roentgenogram	Thoracic drainage
Subcutaneous emphysema	Subcutaneous crepitus on palpation	Chest roentgenogram	–

Table 4. Continued

	Suspected if there is	Additional examination required	Initial therapeutic measures

Mediastinal emphysema	Characteristic crunching sound above the heart, synchronous with the heart beat (Hamman's sign)	Chest roentgenogram
		Central venous pressure
		Determination of possible cause by means of:
		  Bronchoscopy
		  Esophagography
			Cervical mediastinotomy only when there is significant venous congestion and no rupture of bronchus or esophagus

Diaphragmatic rupture	Percussion: dampened or hypersonorous percussion sounds	Roentgenogram of thorax with possible use of nasogastric tube and/or contrast media	Operation
Rupture of bronchus	Mediastinal emphysema Pneumothorax or tension pneumothorax No expansion of lung during thoracic drainage Total atelectasis	Bronchoscopy	Operation
Rupture of esophagus	Mediastinal emphysema	Esophagography	Operation

Rupture of aorta	Possibly pseudocoarctation syndrome
	Possibly compression syndrome in the upper mediastinum
	Possibly systolic murmur
	Roentgenogram:
	  Wide mediastinum
	  Tracheal displacement to the right
	  Displacement of the left bronchus downward
	  Possible left-sided hemothorax
		Aortography	Operation

Cardiac contusion	ECG:
	  Irregularities in repolarization
	  Disturbances in rhythm and conduction
	  Infarct pattern
		Cardiac enzymes	ECG monitoring
			Drug treatment of rhythm irregularities and of possible cardiac insufficiency

The ongoing surveillance of the patient includes **monitoring of arterial blood pressure, central venous pressure,** and **respiration. Arterial blood gas analyses** are absolutely essential in the treatment of severe injuries. They provide the only means for correctly determining the need for mechanical ventilation in all cases where the degree of respiratory insufficiency cannot be clearly judged clinically. The hourly **urine output** is a good measure of the tissue perfusion.

It is especially important to closely follow the progress of **thoracic drainage.** The total amount of drainage and, even more so, the rate of additional blood loss provide valuable indicators as to whether bleeding can be stopped by conservative measures or whether operative intervention is necessary. Similarly, the presence and rate of an air leak provides important diagnostic information.

In every case of severe thoracic trauma, a **12-lead ECG** should be recorded in the early stages, which can then also serve as a basis of comparison for evaluating subsequent variations. As a rule, continuous **ECG monitoring** is done. This is essential if cardiac injury is suspected since only ECG monitoring enables the timely detection and treatment of cardiac arrhythmias.

The **indications for an operative intervention** are described in Chap. 5.

In blunt thoracic trauma, there are six types of injury that are **frequently overlooked** or **belatedly detected.** Analysis of our case records clearly showed that diagnosis of these injuries, which are listed in Table 3, was often delayed when compared to other lesions in the thoracic area. The injuries involved are by no means rare ones. Blair et al. [2] came to similar conclusions. Knowledge of diagnostic difficulties associated with these types of injury can help significantly in reducing the instances in which they are either overlooked or diagnosis is delayed.

This is illustrated impressively in the cases of cardiac contusion. In 1971 only two patients were diagnosed clinically as having a cardiac contusion. Five years later, among a comparable number of patients with thoracic injuries, there were 31 cases.

Chapter 2

The Patient with Additional Injuries in Other Parts of the Body

The force of impact to which a person is subjected in an accident does not respect anatomic boundaries. Whereas a majority of gunshot and stab wounds are restricted to organs of the chest, blunt trauma usually involves multiple injuries.

In our case records, more than three-quarters of all patients hospitalized with blunt thoracic injuries had companion injuries in other parts of the body.* 55% of the patients with thoracic injuries caused by blunt trauma also suffered craniocerebral trauma (including concussion), 20% had significant abdominal injuries, and 38% fractures of the extremities.

At this point we shall refer only to those factors that are of special diagnostic and therapeutic significance when thoracic trauma is accompanied by injuries to other organ systems. Interrelationships and reciprocal influences will be noted.

In the treatment of blunt thoracic injuries, operative intervention is rarely necessary. After the insertion of chest tubes, intubation, and mechanical ventilation, none of which are very time-consuming, even severe thoracic injuries are usually sufficiently taken care of to allow for urgent surgical procedures, such as a laparotomy for intra-abdominal bleeding or a craniotomy for intracranial hematoma. If the thoracic injury also requires immediate operative intervention, it may be necessary for two surgical teams to operate simultaneously.

It is a tried and tested rule that a **prophylactic chest tube** should be inserted in every patient with multiple rib fractures who is to undergo an operation under general anesthesia even when there is neither evidence of a hemothorax nor of a pneumothorax. Otherwise, during ventilation, a life-threatening tension pneumothorax can quickly develop, the prompt recognition of which is by no means assured if the anesthesiologist is fully occupied with volume replacement and other problems and if the thoracic area is, in addition, covered with surgical drapes.

The chances of **adult respiratory distress syndrome (ARDS)** occurring are directly proportionate to the severity of the general injuries and the number of blood transfusions (see Chap. 4) [4]. Positive end-expiratory pressure (PEEP) should always be applied to a severely injured patient during an emergency operation unless there are cardiovascular contraindications. Craniocerebral injuries are an exception to this (see below). After the operation, ventilation with PEEP is continued until repeated blood gas analyses have shown that there is no significant intrapulmonary right-to-left shunt [13].

---

* The proportion of patients with multiple injuries admitted to the University of Zurich Surgical Clinic B is probably higher than that of other hospitals since many patients with especially severe injuries are referred to it from other hospitals.

I. Craniocerebral Injuries

The combination of a thoracic and a craniocerebral injury is not only very common, but the two injuries have a high degree of reciprocal influence on each other, both in diagnostic and therapeutic terms.

1. A pure thoracic injury can produce the **clinical symptoms of a cerebral injury or an intracranial hematoma.** This is especially true in the case of a severe **hypoxia.** A coma and fixed dilated pupils can be caused by hypoxia alone or in combination with a state of shock. It is therefore absolutely essential that a normal supply of oxygen be provided to the brain by restoration of circulation and adequate mechanical ventilation before the final evaluation of a patient with head injuries is made.

Example: A 6-year-old patient was admitted to the hospital with left-sided multiple comminuted rib fractures and suspected intracranial hemorrhage. On the way to the hospital, ventilatory assistance was necessary because spontaneous breathing was inadequate. Upon admission, the patient was comatose, had a wide, dilated left pupil, and did not react to painful stimuli. There was a tension pneumothorax. Following insertion of a chest tube, the patient recovered consciousness and the left pupil contracted. There was slight residual difference in pupil size caused by direct trauma to the bulb of the eye.

In some cases, cerebral dysfunction is also part of the clinical picture of **traumatic asphyxia** (see Chap. 20). This syndrome is the result of a massive thoracic compression that produces a sudden rise of venous pressure in the head and neck, which in turn causes multiple small hemorrhages and, in some cases, severe neurologic deficit and even coma. The characteristic clinical features (bluish-violaceous discoloration of head and neck, cutaneous petechiae, and subconjunctival hemorrhages) reveal the diagnosis at a glance. In general, the prognosis is good.

Fat embolism should also be mentioned in this context. It is usually not caused by thoracic trauma; nevertheless, the pulmonary damage is of essential importance for diagnosis and because of its effect on oxygenation. Disturbances of consciousness may be caused directly by fat embolization in the brain or by hypoxia caused by the pulmonary involvement.

Example: A 20-year-old patient suffered a fracture of the lower leg. One day after the accident, he was admitted to the hospital in a comatose state. During the administration of oxygen by mask prior to the anticipated intubation, the patient regained consciousness, and when the oxygen supply was interrupted, the patient again lapsed into unconsciousness. Petechiae, a characteristic roentgenogram, the blood gas analysis, and the EEG left no doubt as to the diagnosis of a fat embolism with cerebral involvement. The patient recovered completely without residual effects after 10 days of mechanical ventilation.

2. Conversely, a craniocerebral injury tends to have an adverse effect on every patient with thoracic injury. **Impairment of breathing,** secondary to central nervous system damage, and the **inability of the patient to perform breathing exercises** and to **expectorate secretions** require in many cases intubation and mechanical ventilation, which could be avoided in conscious patients with identical thoracic injuries. **Primary aspiration** of blood or stomach contents by the unconscious patient also plays an important role in this context.

3. Not only an inadequate perfusion resulting from the decreased cardiac output associated with shock or heart failure but also an **impairment of venous return** to the

heart promotes the formation of **cerebral edema** in brain injuries. Special attention should therefore be paid to central venous pressure when treating combined thoracic and cerebral injuries. An increase in venous pressure caused by mediastinal emphysema, mediastinal hematoma, pericardial effusion, or cardiac insufficiency may not go untreated in patients with craniocerebral injuries.

4. **Therapeutic conclusions:** because of the danger of cerebral edema in cerebral hypoxia, **adequate oxygenation** is of even greater importance in craniocerebral injuries than in other types of trauma. In these cases, we require a minimal arterial PO_2 of 80 mmHg. This value is higher than that required of other patients (see Chap. 4). If this minimal level of PO_2 is not attained by administration of oxygen, mechanical ventilation is indicated.

Special care must be exercised in calculating the **amount of blood** to be transfused. At the "ideal hematocrit" of 32% to 35%, the beneficial flow properties of blood in this range allow optimal oxygenation of the tissues [11], provided there has been a compensatory increase of cardiac output. In elderly persons and patients with cardiac disease, this compensatory mechanism is limited, and in such cases one should aim for a higher hematocrit. Overtransfusion should always be avoided.

A **high central venous pressure** is detrimental. In addition to keeping the head raised, appropriate measures for reducing the elevated central venous pressure should be taken, namely, aggressive treatment of cardiac insufficiency, broader indication for a cervical mediastinotomy for treatment of mediastinal emphysema, etc. For the same reasons, positive end-expiratory pressure (PEEP), which is otherwise applied generously in ventilating severely injured patients, is to be reserved for cases for which no adequate oxygenation can be attained by other means.

II. Intra-abdominal Injuries

In the diagnosis of **lower rib fractures,** their frequent combination with spleen and liver injuries should always be kept in mind. **Diaphragmatic ruptures** are often accompanied by fractures of the pelvis. Since these are usually caused by a heavy, broad-surfaced impact upon the abdomen and thorax, there are often intra-abdominal companion injuries. In the majority of cases, this means a rupture of the spleen. In gunshot and stab wounds in which a perforated diaphragm is suspected because of the external point of entry or internal path (as in the case of a bullet), an exploratory abdominal operation is indicated.

If the roentgenogram does not reveal a significant hemothorax or widening of the mediastinum, an intrathoracic hemorrhage can usually be ruled out as the cause of hypovolemic shock. It should then be remembered that internal hemorrhages are most often caused by **injuries to intra-abdominal organs.** Among our cases, 30% of the patients with multiple rib fractures also had intra-abdominal injuries.

The clinical assessment of the abdomen can be difficult with associated severe thoracic injuries, particularly in the unconscious patient. For such cases, **peritoneal lavage** has become an indispensable diagnostic aid.

III. Injuries of the Extremities

In minor thoracic injuries presenting neither diagnostic nor therapeutic problems, there is no contraindication to the immediate operative treatment of fractures and ligamentous injuries.

The **timing of internal fixation** of fractures in severe thoracic and multiple injuries is presently under debate. Every operative intervention adds additional trauma, particularly if it has to do with operations on the femur and pelvis, which usually involve considerable blood loss [1, 3, 16, 17, 144]. Furthermore, it interferes with subsequent assessment of the severely wounded (e. g., determining the state of consciousness) and hinders further diagnostic procedures that may be necessary.

Experiences with an aggressive program of mechanical ventilation and continuation of PEEP ventilation after the operation [13], however, clearly show that they significantly reduce the frequency of pulmonary complications (ARDS, fat embolism), which are occasionally observed after a primary internal fixation of the major long bones [16, 17, 144].

In agreement with other authors [12, 14, 15], in treating the severely injured we always perform **primary internal fixation** on fractures with concomitant vascular injuries, open injuries to joints and other wide, open fractures, or dislocations that cannot be reset or cases in which surgical intervention is unlikely to impose an additional burden on the patient. In severely injured patients, ventilation with PEEP is also continued postoperatively.

If primary internal fixation is waived on the day of the accident, then **early internal fixation** is performed a few days after the accident provided that the patient's general condition and skin permit operation. If possible, we try to avoid a longer delay for the following two reasons:

1. When treating patients with severe thoracic injuries and patients receiving mechanical ventilation, it is important to provide changing **lateral positions** for the patient to avoid pulmonary complications. Skeletal traction not only prevents the patient from being turned but also makes the general care of the patient more difficult. Distal fractures can be immobilized temporarily in a plaster cast, but for a femoral fracture, internal fixation is necessary if the patient is to be turned in bed.

2. The longer a patient remains in intensive care before internal fixation of a fracture is performed, the greater the **danger of infection** with highly pathogenic organisms.

IV. Maxillofacial Injuries

Fractures of the skeletal bones of the face are accorded a low priority. Combined with thoracic trauma, they occasionally pose two problems:

1. **Immediate aspiration** of blood frequently occurs. Also after the accident, continued hemorrhaging from the nose and throat can cause repeated minor aspiration of blood, which the patient then coughs up. This is often misinterpreted as hemoptysis.

2. **Subcutaneous emphysema** can also occur locally in the facial area, in which case it is caused not by thoracic injury but by a maxillofacial fracture with sinus involvement.

V. Injuries to the Vertebral Column and Spinal Cord

Fractures of the thoracic vertebrae not only result in the formation of a mediastinal hematoma but also cause hemothorax and, in rare instances, hemopericardium (especially fractures of T-9) or a reactive pericardial effusion [293].
Transverse lesions in the upper thoracic area or in the lower cervical spinal cord cause paralysis of the intercostal musculature. If the damage is below C-4, such patients are usually able to breathe adequately with the innervation of the diaphragm intact. However, if there is a significant paralysis of the intercostal musculature, even a minor thoracic injury can cause severe respiratory insufficiency. Furthermore, pulmonary complications, such as the formation of atelectasis and pneumonia, are extremely frequent in such cases. If spontaneous breathing is adequate, such complications may be prevented by the immediate institution of specific pulmonary therapy, particularly intermittent positive pressure breathing (IPPB).

Chapter 3
Interpretation of the Chest Roentgenogram

I. Basic Considerations

The thoracic roentgenogram is the most important diagnostic tool in the assessment of thoracic injuries. It is not the intent of this chapter to review the radiodiagnostic features of individual injuries. For the most part, these are well-known and are discussed in the separate chapters in the special section of this book as well as in comprehensive radiologic texts [19]. Rather, the following paragraphs are intended to call attention to the **difficulties and errors** that are associated with the interpretation of chest roentgenograms taken after trauma and to summarize the **indications for special radiologic examinations.**

Taking Roentgenograms of Recumbent Patients

The evaluation of the thoracic roentgenogram is much easier if it is taken in an **upright position;** however, it is usually impossible to take the desired roentgenogram of a severely injured patient in a standing or sitting position. It is senseless and only a waste of time to attempt a roentgenogram of the seated patient in such cases. It is much better in the evaluation of thoracic roentgenograms taken in a **recumbent position** to pay attention to the special characteristics and possible sources of error. In a recumbent patient, the **domes of the diaphragm are elevated. Accumulations of fluid** in the thoracic cavity are distributed throughout that cavity and the shadow it causes becomes more diffuse. Even a slight cloudiness signifies an accumulation of several hundred milliliters of blood or other fluid (Fig. 1). The classic picture of an effusion with an elevated fluid level against the lateral thoracic wall never appears on this roentgenogram. A **pneumothorax** appears just the same on the roentgenogram of a recumbent person as that of an erect person: the border of the lung is brought into relief from the wall of the thorax and can hardly be overlooked if the roentgenogram is examined carefully. If there is significant hemothorax at the same time, however, a pneumothorax will occasionally remain undetected because of the opacity of the entire part of the thorax. This is of no clinical significance since treatment consists of insertion of a chest tube with suction in any case. Later roentgenograms taken after evacuation of blood from the thoracic cavity will show whether the lung is fully expanded.
Only if a roentgenogram of the chest is taken with the patient in an upright position will a pneumohemothorax be revealed by the horizontal **fluid level.** The latter invari-

Basic Considerations

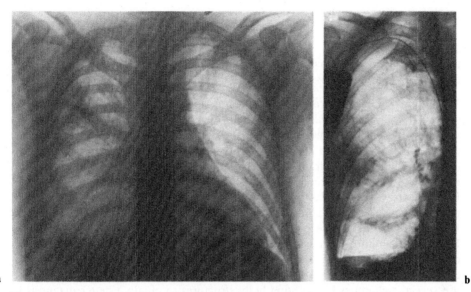

Fig. 1 a, b. With the patient in a **recumbent** position, a hemothorax is distributed throughout the entire half of the thorax; even a significant accumulation of blood may produce only a mild cloudiness (thoracic drainage = 1 liter of blood)

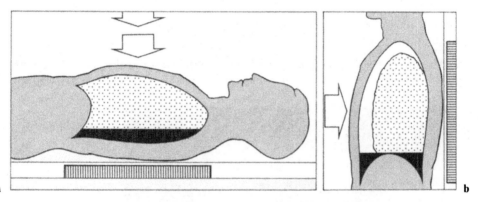

Fig. 2 a, b. Roentgenograms in **standing or sitting** positions make it possible to identify even small accumulations of fluid; in each case a horizontal fluid level confirms the presence of a pneumothorax

ably indicates the presence of free air in the thoracic cavity even if the contour of the lung, set off in relief from the wall of the thoracic cavity, is either not visible at all or shows up very unclearly (Fig. 2).

The assessment of the **mediastinum** in a roentgenogram of the thorax of a recumbent patient can present special problems. The false picture of a "widened mediastinum" can appear. We shall discuss the great practical significance of this problem later on.

What the Chest Roentgenogram "Cannot Do"

The inexperienced person usually expects the roentgenogram to furnish information that it cannot possibly provide. This can result in errors of interpretation and attendant serious consequences:

1. **Multiple rib fractures are usually more numerous than the roentgenogram demonstrates.** It is understandable that rib fractures in the cartilaginous part of the ribs will not be visible, but even fractures of the bony part, unless the ribs are dislocated, will often not show up in roentgenograms taken immediately after the accident (Fig. 3). Additional rib fractures are frequently discovered on follow-up chest roentgenograms taken during the course of hospitalization.

In an autopsy analysis of 30 patients with multiple rib fractures, we found almost twice as many sites of rib fracture as had been revealed by the roentgenograms. Fractures of the first and second ribs were the ones most often overlooked.

However, the number of fracture sites is usually irrelevant clinically in the diagnosis of rib fractures. Of much greater importance are their functional effects and the presence of intrathoracic companion injuries. One should therefore not be tempted to use special techniques highlighting bony structures to obtain a better diagnosis of rib fractures at the expense of a poorer assessment of the pleura and lungs.

When diagnosing rib fractures, one should bear in mind the large number of **rib anomalies** that exist. According to Köhler and Zimmer [24], such rib anomalies occur in 0.15% – 0.3% of all thoracic roentgenograms. These include cervical ribs, missing or underdeveloped first ribs, bony fusion of the two uppermost ribs (Srb's anomaly), lumbar ribs, bifurcation (Luschka's bifurcated rib), splitting of ribs, and synostoses.

2. **The thoracic roentgenogram will not reveal a possible impairment of lung function.** This is typically the case in adult respiratory distress syndrome (ARDS), in

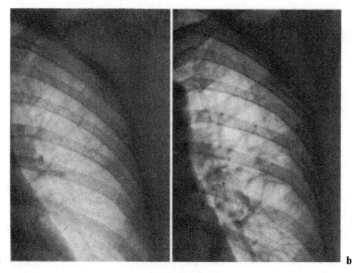

Fig. 3 a, b. Rib fractures often cannot be detected radiologically. **a** Day of accident; **b** 5 days after the accident

which initially there are no radiologic changes or only very slight ones, while at the same time the pulmonary function is seriously impaired (see Chap. 4). While the minimal pulmonary findings on the roentgenogram often generate a false sense of security, it is the arterial blood gas analysis that provides the diagnosis of such life-threatening conditions.

3. In **acute cardiac tamponade** resulting from a hemopericardium, there is virtually never a tent-shaped widening of the heart shadow, as is characteristic of chronic pericardial effusion. In the acute stage, the accumulation of 150 ml in the inelastic pericardium suffices to threaten the life of the patient. Acute cardiac tamponade too is a clinical, not a radiologic, diagnosis.

The Roentgenogram Is Always a Momentary Picture

The apparently self-evident fact that the chest roentgenogram only records the condition at a particular moment does not seem to be taken sufficiently into consideration. Even if the initial roentgenogram appears to be normal, in the further course of development there may be findings that allow the correct diagnosis to be made. This is of practical significance in the case of **lung contusion** (whose radiologic signs continue to increase during the first few days after trauma because of further hematoma and edema formation), in the case of **diaphragmatic rupture** (in which diagnosis cannot be made until the abdominal viscera have herniated into the thoracic cavity), and in the case of **aortic rupture** (which occasionally goes unsuspected until attention is called to it by the growing hematoma formation in the upper mediastinum). Obviously, a **hemothorax** or **pneumothorax** can increase in volume or may even appear for the first time after the initial assessment. **Repeated follow-up radiologic examinations are therefore indispensable in the management of every thoracic injury.**

Indications for Special Radiologic Examination

1. Lateral Thoracic Roentgenograms

In an acute stage of severe thoracic trauma, a lateral thoracic roentgenogram is seldom helpful. In exceptional cases, it may provide the outline of the aortic arch or localization of circumscribed accumulations of blood. During **subsequent stages,** a lateral roentgenogram may occasionally be helpful in determining the exact location of the chest tube, especially if circumscribed effusions of blood or accumulations of air are not draining properly. A lateral roentgenogram may also be needed to pinpoint localized atelectasis or traumatic pulmonary pseudocysts.

2. Lateral Roentgenograms of the Sternum

The diagnosis of a **sternal fracture** cannot be made with an anteroposterior roentgenogram. A lateral roentgenogram of the sternum is the method of choice if an injury of this type is suspected.

3. Tomograms

There has never been a case in our records where a tomogram was indicated in the acute phase. In **later stages,** tomograms may become necessary to differentiate between a posttraumatic intrapulmonary hematoma and a preexisting carcinoma, or to localize posttraumatic pseudocysts and delineate them from postpneumonic liquefaction or tuberculous caverns. Occasionally, **fractures of the sternum** can be exhibited only by means of tomography.

4. Esophagography

If an **esophageal injury** is suspected, esophagography with a water-soluble contrast medium [meglucamine diatrizoate (Gastrografin)] is the examination method of choice. The indication for this simple procedure with its low level of complications should be viewed as broadly as possible. Every penetrating injury of the posterior mediastinum and all unexplained mediastinal emphysema should be investigated to exclude the possibility of an esophageal lesion.

5. Bronchography

There is **no** indication for bronchography in acute trauma. The diagnosis of an injury of the bronchus is made by means of bronchoscopy. The only conditions in which bronchography has meaningful application is in posttraumatic sequelae, i.e. in suspected stenosis or occlusion of the bronchus.

6. Aortography

The indications for this investigation are discussed in detail later on (see "widened mediastinum").

II. Opacities

The fact that most of the intrapleural opacities after thoracic trauma are caused by a **hemothorax** occasionally results in missed diagnoses with serious consequences. If the opacity is caused by an intrapleural effusion of some other origin, e. g., a preexisting pleural effusion with cardiac insufficiency, a differential diagnosis is neither possible nor necessary since examination of the thoracic drainage material will provide the correct diagnosis.
There are two principal differential diagnoses in which the insertion of a chest tube is contraindicated, and in both cases serious damage may result if such placement is attempted. They are diaphragmatic rupture and atelectasis.

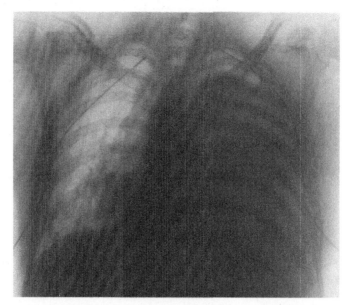

Fig. 4. Diaphragmatic rupture on the left side. Misinterpretation of this roentgenogram as a hemothorax led to an attempt at a thoracic drainage in which stomach contents were evacuated

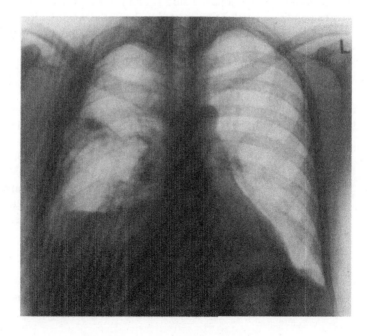

Fig. 5. Right middle lobe atelectasis

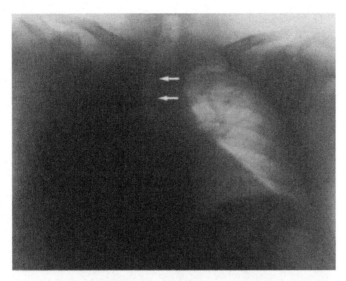

Fig. 6. Total atelectasis of the right lung. In contrast to a hemothorax, the mediastinum is drawn toward the shaded side. Note the deviation of the lower trachea to the right.

Diaphragmatic Rupture

Opacities in the thoracic area that are **sharply defined,** as well as opacities with **areas of increased translucence** corresponding to air in the displaced magenblase or intestinal loops, suggest a rupture of the diaphragm (Fig. 4). The **displacement of the mediastinum** to the opposite side is often more pronounced in these cases than in corresponding opacification caused by hemothorax. It happens again and again that the stomach or the intestinal loops are injured in the attempt to drain what is thought to be a hemothorax.

Atelectasis

Atelectasis seldom occurs immediately after trauma. However, when it does occur and is wrongly diagnosed as a hemothorax, the attempt to drain the pleural cavity usually results in injury to the lungs.
Segmental and lobar atelectasis is differentiated from hemothorax by the **sharply defined borders** (Fig. 5). The most distinguishing feature in every atelectatic formation is the **displacement of the mediastinum,** especially the heart and trachea **toward the opacified side** (Fig. 6). All other causes of opacification in the thoracic area leave the mediastinum in the middle or push it over to the opposite side.

III. Accumulation of Air

Problems arise here particularly when there is **subcutaneous emphysema,** but not because of its diagnosis, which, clinically and radiologically, is the simplest in the

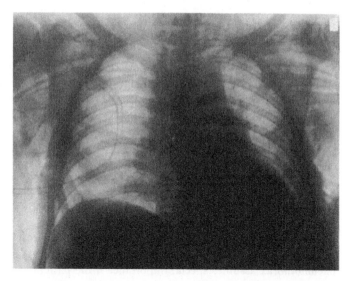

Fig. 7. An instructive roentgenogram: 1. The massive subcutaneous emphysema prevents an assessment of intrathoracic conditions. Only the displacement of the mediastinum to the left reveals the presence of a tension pneumothorax on the right side. 2. The proper insertion of a chest tube can be made difficult by massive subcutaneous emphysema; the tube, inserted on the basis of clinical diagnosis, lies outside the thorax. It drains air from the subcutaneous tissues

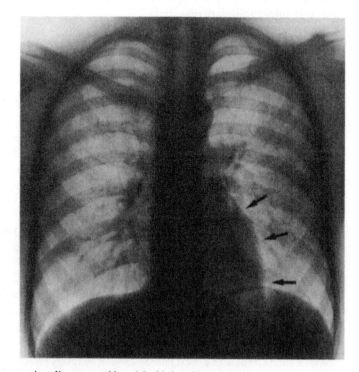

Fig. 8. Simulated pneumopericardium caused by a Mach's band (see text)

whole of thoracic traumatology. However, an extended area of subcutaneous emphysema prevents the correct evaluation of the underlying pleural cavity and lungs in the roentgenogram. Its hazy radiologic picture, permeated with small fields of radiolucency and opacities, may overlay large areas of the lungs. Under these circumstances, a pneumothorax is hardly detectable (Fig. 7). Since the extensive subcutaneous emphysema also prevents clinical diagnosis of a pneumothorax and since the latter is frequently the cause of the emphysema, a chest tube is inserted in doubtful cases even though the diagnosis has not been verified.

The difficulty in identifying significant intrapulmonary lesions and evaluating their course is also clinically important. This applies to pulmonary contusions, pulmonary edema, and particularly to the diagnosis of aspiration. Missed diagnoses or mistakenly interpreted intrapulmonary shadows are frequent in this situation.

Mediastinal emphysema can often be detected clinically by a characteristic auscultation of the heart before the radiologic evidence (double contour of the heart silhouette on the left, appearance of more air in the mediastinum) is available.

Because of the danger of a tension pneumothorax, the diagnosis of even a minimal **pneumothorax** assumes special importance if the patient requires ventilation for either an operation or treatment of respiratory insufficiency. In the case of diaphragmatic rupture, an air-filled stomach that herniates into the thoracic cavity can simulate a pneumothorax or even a tension pneumothorax [25].

Traumatic **pneumopericardium** is extremely rare. Sometimes the diagnosis is made erroneously: either there is nothing more than mediastinal emphysema or a pneumopericardium is simulated by a Mach's band* (Fig. 8) (this is particularly true in cases with intrapulmonary opacities).

IV. The "Widened Mediastinum"

Special significance is attached to a widened mediastinum when diagnosis of an aortic rupture is involved. In my experience, an aortic rupture will not be overlooked if the widened mediastinum is recognized. If in this situation the decision is made to forego aortography, this should be done for well-founded reasons after thorough consideration. In all cases in which an aortic rupture was overlooked, the widening of the mediastinum was not detected, although it was almost always visible upon retrospective study of the chest roentgenograms.

A widening of the mediastinum can also occur for purely **technical reasons.** The thoracic roentgenogram of a severely injured person is usually taken with the patient lying down, in expiration, often with an elevated diaphragm, and in an anteroposterior direction. All these factors may make the mediastinum appear to be widened [18]. It is particularly the picture taken with **portable** X-ray equipment, with its **short distance beetween tube and plate** and with anteroposterior direction of its rays, that exhibits a widened mediastinum [18, 31] (Fig. 9).

---

* Mach's band (1866) is an optical phenomenon: a relatively bright or dark band perceived in a zone where the brightness increases or decreases rapidly.

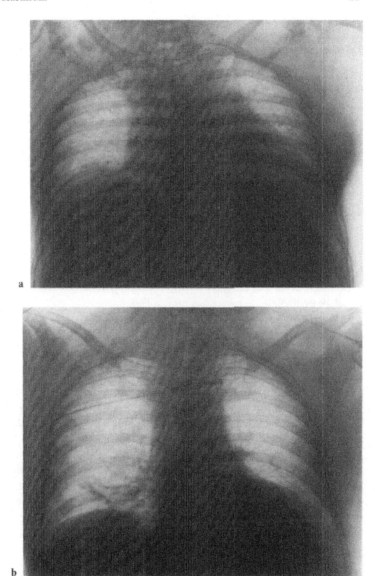

Fig. 9 a, b. Apparent widening of the mediastinum resulting from the radiologic technique. **a** Roentgenogram taken upon admission to emergency room; **b** 12 h later

However, even when the mediastinum is actually widened, the cause can be traced to aortic rupture in only a minority of the cases. Of 64 patients whose first roentgenograms taken after emergency admission showed a widened upper mediastinum, **only 11** were subsequently found to have **ruptured aortas**. The numerous other causes are summarized in Table 5. The most common are **hematomas in the mediastinum** caused by spinal fractures, sternal fractures, or multiple dorsal paravertebral rib fractures. Equally frequent are **hemorrhages into the mediastinum from the small-**

Table 5. Causes of widening of the mediastinum

1. Technical cause	Short distance between X-ray tube and plate Anteroposterior direction of roentgenogram Patient in horizontal position
2. Fracture hematoma	Sternal fracture Vertebral fracture Paravertebral multiple rib fractures
3. Aortic rupture, avulsion or laceration of supra-aortic branches	
4. Other arterial hemorrhage into the mediastinum	Internal thoracic artery Intercostal arteries
5. Venous bleeding	Small veins (mediastinal veins, internal thoracic veins, thyroid veins, branches of the subclavian vein) Rupture of the vena cava or brachiocephalic vein
6. Iatrogenic causes	Hematoma after carotid angiography
7. Dilatation of aorta or change in its position	Preexisting aortic aneurysm (also syphilitic mesoaortitis) Extensive aortic sclerosis Poststenotic dilatation of aorta Pectus excavatum

er venous vessels. In such cases, the source of the bleeding is not identified. **Arterial bleeding** from an internal mammary artery or an intercostal artery is less common.

In each of three patients, a mediastinal hematoma was caused, respectively, by a **tear in the superior vena cava,** a **rupture of the right ventricle,** and by an **iatrogenic hematoma following carotid angiography.** We also found one case of mediastinal widening caused by a **poststenotic dilatation connected with aortic stenosis** (77-year-old female patient), one case of **syphilitic mesoaortitis,** one case of **aortic dilatation caused by arteriosclerosis** in a 78-year-old male patient, and one case of **dislocation of the aorta by pectus excavatum.**

Indications for Aortography

Successful recognition of an aortic rupture depends upon the conscious allowance for negative aortographies. The wide mediastinum associated with an aortic rupture is not always caused by bleeding from the rupture site on the aorta. A mediastinal hematoma caused by tearing of small vessels in the vicinity of the aorta may point toward injury of the aorta itself (see p. 227). **In case of doubt, an angiogram should always be performed.** Since this examination of the severely injured often represents a considerable expenditure of time and effort, several additional considerations and hints may be helpful in deciding whether aortography is indicated.

1. The widening of the mediastinum is often not the only sign of an aortic rupture. In addition to clinical signs (see Chap. 18), there are **other radiologic findings** that while not diagnostic in themselves do corroborate the suspicion:

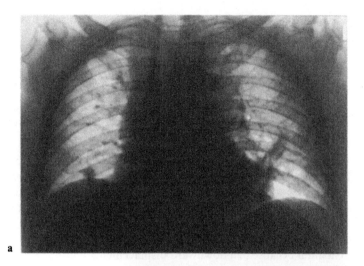

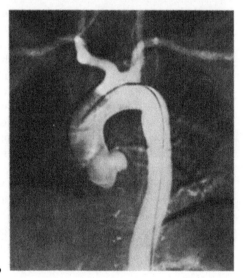

Fig. 10. a Widened mediastinum caused by mediastinal hematoma in fracture of thoracic vertebrae 7, 8, and 11. **b** Aortography excludes the presence of an aortic rupture

— **Displacement of the trachea to the right** is an important sign less commonly associated with other causes of mediastinal hematoma [23]
— **Downward displacement of the left main bronchus**
— **Abnormal aortic contour** or **fuzzy delineation of the aortic arch on the left**
— Association with a **left-sided hemothorax**

Aortography becomes imperative if one of these additional radiologic findings is present.

2. In almost all clinically significant cases, the aortic rupture is located in the area of the isthmus. By taking the **roentgenogram with the left side of the thorax turned for-**

ward at an angle of 30°, the descending aorta can be turned further away from the mediastinal shadow and thus be evaluated more accurately.

3. A vertebral fracture or multiple paravertebral rib fractures help to explain the cause of a mediastinal hematoma, but they should not serve to exclude the possibility of an aortic rupture. Particularly left-sided dorsal paravertebral rib fractures can be associated with an aortic rupture, as was the case in one of our patients. If there is any suspicion, aortography should be performed also in these cases (Fig. 10).

4. If, because of only minor mediastinal widening, the decision is made to dispense with aortography, roentgenograms should be used to check the **subsequent course** of development. On the day of the accident, it is advisable to repeat the chest roentgenogram after 4 h. If the mediastinum has grown in width, aortography is imperative. If the widening can no longer be demonstrated, the first finding may have resulted from faulty technique. However, Greenway [21] and Sandor [28] observed that in aortic ruptures the mediastinal hematoma may no longer be detectable in the roentgenogram because of a downward displacement.

It should be pointed out that even a **normal chest roentgenogram does not exclude the possibility of an aortic rupture.** In the autopsy of two of our patients, we found aortic ruptures that were not accompanied by any significant hematoma formation. They were not, however, the cause of death. Retrospective examination of the roentgenograms of these patients also revealed no abnormalities. Flaherty [20] described the case of an aortic rupture in which there was no mediastinal widening but in which the trachea was pushed to the right in the roentgenogram.

If aortography is indicated, **every further delay** of this examination (scheduling aortography on the following day as part of hospital routine) represents an **unnecessary risk.** It should be postponed only in favor of other, more life-threatening injuries that demand immediate attention.

Immediate operation on the aortic rupture without aortography may be necessary if the rupture shows signs of incipient perforation into the left hemothorax. However, if time permits, it is preferable to perform aortography before proceeding with the operation. Although an aortic rupture can be overlooked even in a radiologic examination with contrast medium [29], its diagnostic reliability is greater than that of surgical exploration of the aorta [529].

Chapter 4
Respiratory Insufficiency

I. Basic Considerations

Respiratory insufficiency in severely injured patients is often a multifactorial event in which the part played by individual causal components is difficult to estimate. For this reason, there appears to be a resigned tendency in the more recent literature to group such respiratory disturbances together under a common term (e. g., "adult respiratory distress syndrome" or "shock lung"). Unless these expressions are used very restrictively, there is a danger of lumping a number of diseases with varying clinical significance together under a single label.

In the care of severely injured patients, I regard it of decisive importance to strictly dissociate respiratory disturbances, which can be **delineated and defined etiologically,** from a collective term of the above type. They are incomparably more frequent and differ with respect to treatment and prognosis. The pathologic condition that remains is quite rare among cases given optimal initial treatment and can no longer be defined etiologically but is characterized precisely with respect to its clinical features and functional effects. In this book, I use the most current expression "adult respiratory distress syndrome" (ARDS) for this condition.

Admittedly, in individual cases this differentiation can be difficult; however, there are a series of special investigations available for this purpose.

Some of the **therapeutic procedures** undertaken in the treatment of the severely injured may, alone or in combination with other factors, be responsible for impaired pulmonary function. It is essential that cognizance be taken of them in the treatment of thoracic injuries, and it is certainly justifiable to summarize them in a special section.

II. Assessment of Respiration in Patients with Thoracic Injuries

1. Clinical Assessment

Let us keep in mind right from the beginning that, **by itself,** a clinical assessment of respiration of a severely injured patient is not sufficient. Thoracic roentgenograms and, above all, an arterial blood gas analysis are absolutely essential. Nevertheless, a clinical examination is of decisive importance, particularly in cases of thoracic injury; it is senseless, for example, to diagnose or to document a tension pneumothorax with the aid of blood gas analysis. Every respiratory problem that is clearly life-threatening demands immediate treatment, which, apart from the insertion of a chest tube, usually consists of immediate intubation and mechanical ventilation. Subsequent diagnostic procedures are then carried out with the patient stabilized on a respirator.

2. Chest Roentgenograms

This examination, which is conducted as a matter of course on every patient with thoracic injuries, often produces diagnostic hints as to injuries and the effects of injuries of the thorax; however, it says nothing about functional impairment of respiration. It is quite typical that in ARDS the initial appearance of the lung is normal or nearly normal on the roentgenogram despite already existing severe functional respiratory disturbance (Fig. 11). Conversely, massive lesions shown on the roentgenogram (hemothorax, pneumothorax, aspiration, pneumonia) often cause only minor functional disturbances.

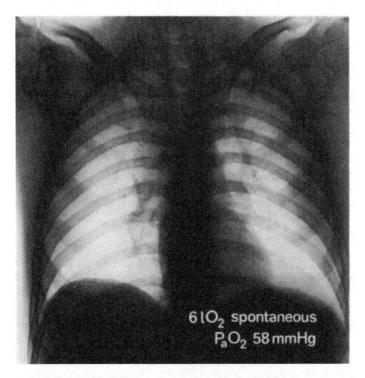

Fig. 11. Typical of ARDS: in an almost normal roentgenogram of the thorax, there is already a significant functional impairment: spontaneous breathing on 6 liters O_2, $P_aO_2 = 58$ mmHg; after 12 h of ventilation ($F_iO_2 = 1.0$) $P_aO_2 = 63$ mmHg. The patient died from the lung damage

3. Arterial Blood Gas Analysis

1. If conditions permit, the blood gas analysis is carried out at first with the patient spontaneously breathing **room air.** In this way **a regional hypoventilation ("uneven ventilation")** can be recognized. If one part of the pulmonary parenchyma is ventilated to a lesser degree, this results in a decrease in the partial pressure of the oxygen in the affected alveoli. The oxygen content at the end of the capillaries of the affected pulmonary area is thereby lowered. This is a characteristic finding in patients with rib fractures. If oxygen is administered, the partial pressure of the oxygen in the affected alveoli is raised so high that this abnormality may no longer be detectable (see example in Table 6).

2. **Blood gas analysis during administration of a known quantity of oxygen** helps to answer the question of whether sufficient oxygenation is being attained and, above all, provides a means for monitoring further developments.

3. Significant diagnostic information is provided by blood gas analysis after 20 min of **respiration or mechanical ventilation with pure oxygen,** i. e., the **oxygenation test.** It is used to evaluate the degree of the intrapulmonary right-to-left shunt that occurs in ARDS or in the formation of atelectasis. The arterial PO_2 remains at a low level (see example in Table 6). With this type of respiratory insufficiency, this test can also be helpful in the daily monitoring of the patient's course.

Table 6. Differentiation between regional hypoventilation (uneven ventilation) and intrapulmonary right-to-left shunt: two typical examples

	Spontaneous breathing: P_aO_2			Therapy
	Ambient air ($F_I O_2 = 0.21$)	6 liters O_2	Pure O_2 ($F_I O_2 = 1.0$)	
Regional hypoventilation M.W., ♂, 20 yrs old: Multiple comminuted fractures of ribs V–IX on the left side with paradoxical respiration, fractured clavicle, cardiac contusion, rupture of spleen, fracture of pelvis, torn knee ligaments	59 mmHg	154 mmHg	353 mmHg!	O_2 administered nasally Analgesics Breathing exercises
Right-to-left shunt R.C., ♂, 34 yrs old: Multiple fractures of ribs I–IV on the right side, compression fracture of thoracic vertebra IX **ARDS**	60 mmHg	79 mmHg	125 mmHg!	Ventilation (PEEP) Steroids

Fig. 12. The three basic types of severe disturbances in ventilation-perfusion distribution (see text)

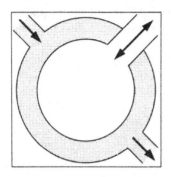
Normal

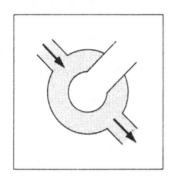
Collapsed alveoli with perfusion – **shunt**

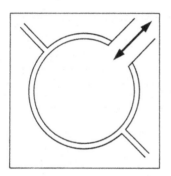
No perfusion with ventilated alveoli – **dead space**

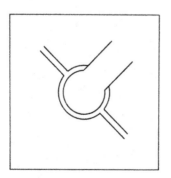
No ventilation and no perfusion – **silent unit**

4. Disturbances in the Ventilation-Perfusion Ratio ($\dot{V}_A/\dot{Q}$)

Of the three basic types of disturbances in the ratio between alveolar ventilation ($\dot{V}_A$) and perfusion ($\dot{Q}$) (Fig. 12), the intrapulmonary right-to-left shunt as well as the increase of dead space ventilation after thoracic injury and general trauma are of vast clinical importance. Specific and somewhat demanding measurement techniques make it possible to accurately calculate their extent. In daily practice, however, it is permissible to use simplified examination procedures that provide sufficiently accurate estimates of functional disturbance.

Intrapulmonary Right-to-Left Shunt

Under normal conditions, approximately 3% of the cardiac output is not available for gas exchange because it flows through **anatomic shunts** from the right to the left side of the heart via bronchial and pleural veins and via the thebesian veins. If nonventilated alveoli are perfused, there will be an additional **capillary shunt**. The **total shunt volume** (unfortunately also misleadingly referred to as "physiologic shunt") is composed of an **anatomic shunt** and a **capillary shunt**.
In every severely injured patient, there will be a modest increase in this total shunt volume. A right-to-left shunt of 12% – 15% can be observed in almost all patients with multiple injuries [188].
A **considerable increase** in the right-to-left shunt is a characteristic feature of the **pulmonary disturbances in ARDS and in atelectasis.** The flow of venous blood from the right side of the circulation system to the left side of the heart, not coming into contact with any ventilated alveoli and hence not participating in the gas exchange, results in a mixing of venous blood with arterial blood and thereby causing **arterial hypoxia.** An **increase in the oxygen concentration of the inspired air** naturally has no effect upon the oxygen content of this venous blood admixture. This circumstance can be used to differentiate it from other forms of arterial hypoxia.
The **total shunt volume compared to the volume of cardiac output** ("shunt fraction" $\dot{Q}_S/\dot{Q}_T$) can be calculated during inhalation of pure oxygen according to the following formula [40, 92], in which the measured arterial (C_a) and mixed venous ($C_{\bar{v}}$) oxygen content are compared with the maximal oxygen content theoretically attainable at the end of the pulmonary capillaries (C_c):

$$\frac{\dot{Q}_S}{\dot{Q}_T} = \frac{C_c - C_a}{C_c - C_{\bar{v}}}$$

In which
$C_c = Hb \cdot 1.39 + P_AO_2 \cdot 0.003$
$P_AO_2 = P_B - P_AH_2O - P_ACO_2$
P_B: actual barometric pressure; P_ACO_2: see p. 34
P_AH_2O: water vapor pressure; at 37° C = 47 mmHg
$C_a = Hb \cdot 1.39 \cdot S_a + P_a \cdot 0.003$
$C_{\bar{v}} = Hb \cdot 1.39 \cdot S_{\bar{v}} + P_{\bar{v}} * \cdot 0.003 *$

The oxygen content of the blood corresponds essentially to the hemoglobin-bound oxygen (hemoglobin content × 1.39 × oxygen saturation of the hemoglobin; it is assumed that the hemoglobin is totally saturated at the end of the capillaries, hence is equal to 1.0) and to the physically dissolved oxygen ($PO_2 \times 0.003$), which is so minimal that the corresponding term in the equation (marked with asterisks) can be ignored in actual practice.

Simplified formulas for the calculation of shunt [38] proceed on the assumption that there is an O_2 saturation of 100% in the arterial blood. In a large shunt (i.e., a very low P_aO_2), this can lead to errors in calculation. When P_aO_2 values exceed 150 mm Hg, however, the $\dot{Q}_S/\dot{Q}_T$ can be calculated as follows:

$$\frac{\dot{Q}_S}{\dot{Q}_T} = \frac{(P_A - P_a) \cdot 0.003}{(C_a - C_{\bar{v}}) + (P_A - P_a) \cdot 0.003}$$

However, the exact calculation of the shunt fraction is based on the determination of the oxygen saturation of mixed venous blood. If the blood used is taken from the superior vena cava or from the right atrium, serious errors in calculation may result. The only blood that is genuinely mixed venous is that **taken from the pulmonary artery** [113, 121]. Because a pulmonary catheter must be inserted (e.g., Swan-Ganz catheter), the practical application of the shunt measurement is restricted.

From a clinical point of view, there is no reason to doubt the significance of a diagnosis of right-to-left shunt; however, when interpreting the calculated values, it is well to remember that an alveolar **oxygen content of 100%** promotes the **formation of microatelectasis,** and because of that, a shunt fraction is created that is higher than that obtained during inhalation of a mixture of oxygen and air. In fact, this effect has been observed after only 5 min of ventilation with pure oxygen [91].

Oxygenation Test, Alveolar-Arterial Oxygen Gradient

There are two clinical measurements, both of which are easier but considerably less precise, that can be used to identify an intrapulmonary right-to-left shunt, namely, the determination of arterial PO_2 during ventilation with pure oxygen or the calculation of the alveolar-arterial oxygen gradient. In the process, the patient inhales pure oxygen for 20 min through a three-way air valve.

The partial pressure of the **alveolar oxygen** ($P_A O_2$) is equal to the barometric pressure (P_B) minus the two partial pressures remaining in the alveoli after the nitrogen has been completely washed out, namely, the partial pressures of P_ACO_2 and water vapor (PH_2O). Because CO_2 diffuses so well, it can be assumed that the alveolar and arterial CO_2 partial pressures are identical.

Alveolar-arterial oxygen gradient:

$$A - a\ DO_2 = (P_B - P_ACO_2 - PH_2O) - P_aO_2$$
$$[P_ACO_2 = P_aCO_2]$$

The use of the alveolar-arterial oxygen gradient as a standard of measurement for the intrapulmonary right-to-left shunt, however, is subject to several significant and very restrictive assumptions. The following values must remain unchanged during repeated investigations: (1) hemoglobin content, (2) cardiac output, and (3) position of the hemoglobin dissociation curve. Only when these conditions are met can there be a direct relationship between A – a DO_2 and the shunt. Since these values do not remain constant over a prolonged period of time, however, there are considerable possibilities for error.

The determination of the arterial PO_2 after inhalation of pure oxygen serves as a quick method of orientation, not only in emergency situations but also in the routine hospital setting. In unequivocal cases, it effectively differentiates pathologic conditions with a distinct intrapulmonary right-to-left shunt from arterial hypoxia caused by regional hypoventilation (see example in Table 6). The same restrictions apply here as in the calculation of the alveolar-arterial oxygen gradient.

For **clinical purposes,** an arterial PO_2 of over 300 mmHg ($F_IO_2 = 1.0$) can be taken as a sign that there is no life-threatening right-to-left shunt present. Values below 250 mmHg ($F_IO_2 = 1.0$) indicate the presence of a distinct right-to-left shunt and, in my judgment, require aggressive therapy.

The P_aO_2 values measured **under clinical conditions** are always **lower** than those arrived at theoretically. This is caused by technical difficulties associated with the measurement of PO_2 at high partial pressures of oxygen. It is of special importance that there be no delay in making the blood gas analysis since oxygen escapes into the ambient air and blood itself uses up oxygen. To a lesser degree, there is also an oxygen loss at the electrodes [73]. Obviously, the same problem also exists in calculating the shunt. In actual practice, the examination should be carried out as soon as possible after the blood sample has been taken, and if the analysis cannot be performed in the vicinity of the patient, the blood samples should be covered with ice while being taken to the laboratory.

This dependence of arterial PO_2 upon the magnitude of the intrapulmonary right-to-left shunt and on the alveolar oxygen tension can be illustrated by computed curves (Fig. 13). They show that the detection of a marked right-to-left shunt is much easier if the patient is inhaling concentrated oxygen rather than ambient air.

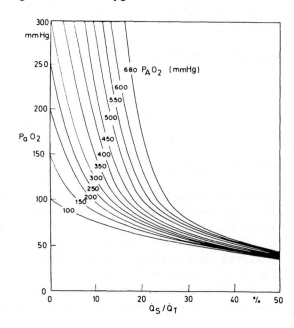

Fig. 13. Calculated values of the arterial partial oxygen pressure (P_aO_2) related to alveolar partial oxygen pressure (P_AO_2) and to pulmonary right-to-left shunt quotients ($\dot{Q}_S/\dot{Q}_T$). Assumptions: hemoglobin 15 g%, arterial pH 7.40, arteriovenous oxygen difference 6 ml/100 ml, standard hemoglobin dissociation curve. Pontoppidan et al. [108]

Increase in Dead Space

Dead space is defined as that portion of the inhaled volume of air that does not participate in the carbon dioxide exchange. In adults, the volume of anatomic dead space amounts to approximately 150 ml. The alveolar dead space, which is the ventilated volume of nonperfused alveoli, is practically zero under normal conditions of rest.

Dead space to tidal volume ratio (V_D/V_T)

$$\frac{V_D}{V_T} = \frac{P_A CO_2 - P_E CO_2}{P_a CO_2}$$

$P_E CO_2 = PCO_2$ of expired air collected in a container for 3 min.

Normal value: $\frac{150}{450} = 0.3$.

No doubt this determination is of considerable theoretical importance, but its application in actual practice is not obligatory since the arterial PCO_2 value obtained via the blood gas analysis will quickly indicate whether the necessary increase in ventilation minute volume required to compensate for the increased fraction of dead space has in fact occurred.

There is always an increase of dead space ventilation in every severe thoracic injury, during hypovolemic shock, and in every significant increase of the intrapulmonary right-to-left shunt. This increase in dead space also causes an increase in the work of breathing. Compensation can usually be made for V_D/V_T values of up to 0.6, but when the ratio exceeds 0.7, adequate spontaneous breathing is no longer possible because at this level of V_D/V_T the increased CO_2 production, generated by the necessary increase in the work of breathing, exceeds the ability of such effort to eliminate the additional CO_2.

5. Disturbance in Diffusion

Acute respiratory insufficiency is doubtlessly often accompanied by a disturbance in diffusion. However, severe disturbances in diffusion occur in ARDS only in advanced stages, particularly of course after formation of hyaline membranes [185].

6. Cardiac Output

Cardiac output usually **increases** if there is a significant intrapulmonary right-to-left shunt. This process is a thoroughly sensible compensatory mechanism that attempts to guarantee an adequate supply of oxygen to the vital organs despite a low arterial PO_2. (If the right-to-left shunt reaches 50%, there are 2.5 liters/min of oxygenated blood available for perfusion of organs at a cardiac output of 5 liters/min; however, if the cardiac output is 10 liters/min, there are 5 liters/min of oxygenated blood available.) The calculation of the shunt fraction by itself provides only a superficial assessment of the overall situation and of the prognosis of the patient.

The increased burden upon the heart, however, entails the danger of cardiac failure. The situation becomes critical if the pulmonary conditions remain poor and cardiac output decreases. Only by measurement of cardiac output can such a decrease be detected in time.

The cardiac output in turn has an effect upon the **size of the shunt** in that a rise in cardiac output not only brings about a corresponding increase in the amount of venous blood being mixed with arterial blood, but it also increases the shunt fraction (QS/QT) of the total cardiac output [74, 119].

III. Respiratory Insufficiency Caused by the Thoracic Injury Itself

The impairment of ventilation caused by **pneumothorax** and **hemothorax** is easily eliminated by immediate drainage. In **rib fractures, pain** and **mechanical restrictions upon breathing** usually lead to a regional hypoventilation. The corresponding lowering of arterial PO_2 that this causes can almost always be compensated for by administration of oxygen. If there is no craniocerebral injury and if the oxygenation test provides no evidence of ARDS, a more conservative attitude toward providing mechanical ventilation is justified. In such cases, we would tolerate spontaneous respiration as long as, with the administration of oxygen, the P_aO_2 does not fall below 60 mmHg. In our case records, 30% of the patients with multiple rib fractures had to receive ventilatory assistance, often necessitated by a combination of thoracic injury with other severe lesions, especially simultaneous brain injuries.

The restriction on breathing caused by pain or mechanical factors is also accompanied by **inadequate expectoration.** The accumulation of secretions can lead to formation of atelectasis or infection. These deleterious consequences, which often cause a secondary respiratory insufficiency, can be prevented by adequate analgesia and above all by **intensive breathing exercises,** which are begun on the day of the accident.

By itself, **paradoxical respiration** involving a free fragment of chest wall resulting from multiple double rib fractures is not an indication for ventilatory assistance. Only with evidence of respiratory failure is long-term mechanical ventilation unavoidable, unless it is one of the rare cases where surgical stabilization of the thoracic wall promises to be successful. Three-quarters of our patients with paradoxical respiration required mechanical ventilation.

Even a satisfactory blood gas analysis does not take away from the fact that in multiple rib fractures the **function of the lungs is restricted to a considerable degree.** In the first few days after the accident, the **vital capacity** is reduced an average of 40% of normal (Fig. 14). Of the 23 patients with multiple rib fractures whom we tested daily during one full week for lung function, there were 3 patients with a forced vital capacity below 20% of normal (13%, 16%, and 19%, respectively). In their cases adequate spontaneous respiration was possible.

The vital capacity continues to drop slightly in the first 2 days after injury, then begins to slowly but steadily rise; as a rule, significant respiratory insufficiency seldom occurs after the critical 4-day period following the accident. Even with a normal

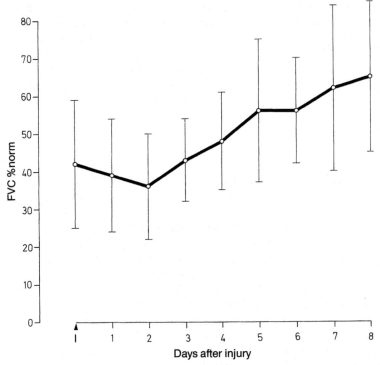

Fig. 14. Restriction of forced vital capacity (FVC) in patients with multiple rib fractures during the first 8 days after the accident (n = 23; normal values according to Anderhub et al. [33])

PCO_2, the dead space ventilation is elevated in proportion to the total ventilation (V_D/V_T). The consequence of this is an increase in the work of breathing, which during the critical period can lead to symptoms of fatigue.

Patients with thoracic injuries are especially sensitive to **excessive infusion of fluids.** This is particularly true of the pathologic picture of **pulmonary contusion,** which is harmless in most cases, yet occasionally can develop into a form analogous to ARDS. There can be no doubt that shock treatment and fluid resuscitation are particularly significant in these instances. If on the basis of the blood gas analysis done during the oxygenation test, a pulmonary contusion with respiratory insufficiency is diagnosed, the treatment indicated is ventilation with positive end-expiratory pressure (PEEP) and accompanying therapy as with ARDS.

IV. Aspiration

Primary aspiration is common in the case of **injuries to the nose-throat area,** in **fractures of the upper jaw,** in the **unconscious patient,** and in **severe injuries to the lungs.** What is aspirated is a crucial question. **Aspirated foreign bodies,** such as teeth or

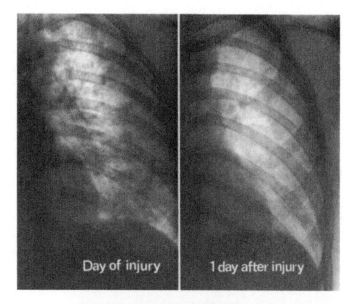

Fig. 15. Progress of aspiration of blood as revealed by roentgenograms on the day of the accident and 1 day later

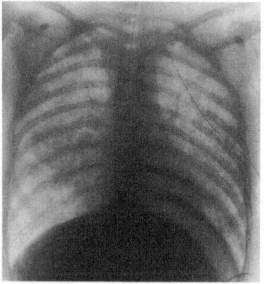

Fig. 16. Toxic lung edema after aspiration of gastric contents (Mendelson syndrome)

broken dentures, must be removed by bronchoscopy. Aspiration of **blood** produces a striking thoracic roentgenogram, in most cases showing relatively little functional impairment. The radiologic findings return to normal as a rule very quickly (Fig. 15). Pneumonia developing after **aspiration of emesis** usually responds well to treatment.

A special form presents itself in the **aspiration of acidic gastric fluids (Mendelson's syndrome)** [94]. This life-threatening acute condition coupled with severe hemorrhagic edema of the lungs (Fig. 16) demands immediate, aggressive treatment: ventilation with positive end-expiratory pressure and administration of steroids. If this therapy is applied promptly, the prognosis is good [50, 114].

We must also call attention to the imperceptible, "silent" aspiration of material passing the cuff in patients with a tracheotomy or with an endotracheal tube. It is not clear whether this repeated aspiration of small amounts of saliva is deleterious or not; however, it may play an essential role in the formation of pulmonary infections [51].

V. Adult Respiratory Distress Syndrome (ARDS)

The term "adult respiratory distress syndrome" (ARDS) should be used in a restrictive sense for a well-defined posttraumatic pathologic condition. It is characterized by a **substantial intrapulmonary right-to-left shunt, a decreased functional residual capacity,** and an **interstitial lung edema** (Fig. 17). Characteristic findings in early stages are listed in Table 7.

Table 7. Characteristic findings in the early stages of ARDS

Arterial PO_2 ↓
Arterial PCO_2 normal (in rare cases ↓: hyperventilation)
Cardiac output ↑
Right-to-left shunt ↑
Functional residual capacity ↓
Interstitial lung edema

The pathologic condition is defined by its functional consequences, **not by its etiology.** The concept "shock lung" is misleading to the extent that in most cases the shock is not the most important, let alone the sole cause of respiratory insufficiency [95]. It must be regarded as established fact that this pathologic condition also occurs without a preceding state of shock. Instead of "shock lung," I use the expression "adult respiratory distress syndrome" (ARDS). In the literature there are over 40 terms for this one pathologic condition [45], for example:

— Posttraumatic pulmonary insufficiency (Moore et al. [98])
— Congestive atelectasis (Jenkins [80])
— Wet lung (Burford and Burbank [47])
— Progressive pulmonary insufficiency (Collins [52])
— Capillary leak syndrome (Derks and Peters [57])
— Progressive pulmonary consolidation (Safar [118])
— Respiratory distress syndrome (Ashbaugh [34], Petty and Ashbaugh [107])

In optimal treatment of patients with multiple injuries, ARDS is **relatively rare.** In general, it occurs more frequently the more severely the patient is injured.

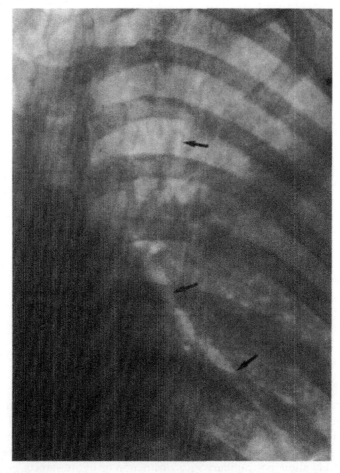

Fig. 17. Severe interstitial lung edema. Lobular and segmental bronchi show up only in advanced cases (air bronchogram)

Pathophysiologic Mechanisms

The purpose of this brief overview is to summarize the results of the more recent clinical and experimental investigations (Fig. 18). No final judgment is as yet possible regarding the importance and significance of the individual factors.

1. Capillary Permeability

The central feature of this event is the damage done to the capillary wall along with an increase in capillary permeability. In electron-microscopic investigations of lung biopsies, Wegmann and I [68] were able to demonstrate that edematous swelling of the capillary endothelium is an early change. Sodium ions and proteins [130] cross over into the interstitial tissue and bind there a corresponding amount of water,

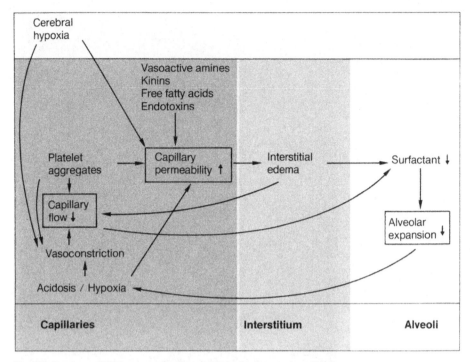

Fig. 18. Reciprocal influences of pathophysiologic changes in ARDS

which results in **interstitial edema.** This can be demonstrated by means of electron microscopy [103] and with the use of tracer substances [71]. The capillary wall is damaged either **directly** by hypoxia, catecholamines, kinins, histamine, free fatty acids in fat embolism, and by endotoxins, or **indirectly** via a precapillary and presumably also a postcapillary vasoconstriction or by substances produced by platelet aggregates (see below).

2. Vasoconstriction of Terminal Vessels

In contrast to the periphery, hypoxia leads to vasoconstriction of the small vessels in the lung (von Euler-Liljestrand effect [134]). What is involved in this is a significant adjustment of circulation to ventilation. An acidosis has the same effect [61]. Circulating catecholamines, histamine, and other substances set free by the platelet aggregates likewise result in vasoconstriction. Accordingly, this gives rise to an increase of resistance in the vascular system of the lungs.

3. Surfactant

Surfactant, a phospholipid, reduces the surface tension as a means of lining the alveoli and in so doing keeps the alveoli open. The type II alveolar epithelial cells, which synthesize surfactant, are damaged in the state of shock [75]. The reserve of surfactant lasts, however, for some 18 h. This may explain the frequently observed latency in the development of the pathologic picture. Moreover, surfactant is rendered inactive by transudate in the alveoli.

When the surfactant content is reduced, atelectasis forms, which produces a functional right-to-left shunt. This gives rise to a vicious cycle, which maintains arterial hypoxia.

4. Thrombocyte Aggregates, Disseminated Intravascular Coagulation

Thrombocyte aggregates in venous blood, which appear after soft tissue injury [39, 42], after local ischemia [85], and after hemorrhagic shock [86], are collected in the pulmonary capillaries [86]. This can cause a reduction in peripheral blood thrombocytes.

The increased resistance in pulmonary vessels, however, is not the result of mechanical blockade of the capillaries, which is impossible for quantitative reasons [112]. Rather, from the local thrombocyte aggregates certain substances are liberated that cause vasoconstriction: **histamine, catecholamines, and serotonin.** Except for histamine, these in turn lead to the further aggregation of platelets so that an additional vicious cycle takes place (Fig. 19). A second such vicious cycle consists of the liberation of ADP from the aggregated thrombocytes, which even in very small amounts produces the aggregation of platelets. Some of these substances also alter the permeability of the vessels [35, 36].

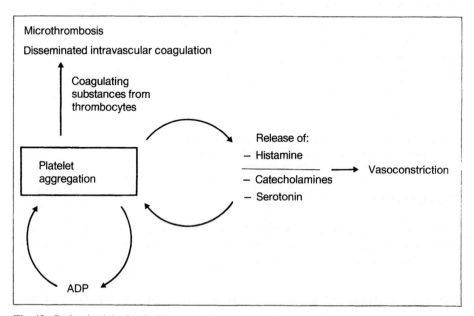

Fig. 19. Pathophysiologic significance of thrombocyte aggregates in the pulmonary microcirculation

The formation of such thrombocyte aggregates can be **fully reversible.** However, under the influence of clotting substances derived from the thrombocytes (platelet factors), a **microthrombosis** can result and if this development continues, it can lead to **disseminated intravascular coagulation,** which can be demonstrated to be consumption coagulopathy [112, 144]. In my experience, this has seldom been the case. Furthermore, I have seldom found such microthrombi in lung biopsies so that exclusive causal significance can hardly be ascribed to these thrombocyte aggregates. It is my judgment that the importance of this factor is frequently overrated.

Development and Prognosis

If these vicious cycles, which occur automatically in the lung the moment damage begins, cannot be interrupted by prompt and aggressive therapy, an increasing deterioration of the situation is unavoidable. The result of this is a continuing **reduction of lung compliance, development of hyaline membranes,** and finally **fibrosis of the lung.** The required minute ventilation volume and the concentration of inhaled oxygen must be increased. Respiration pressures increase. Tension pneumothoraces occur whereat the lung is unable to collapse. The conclusion of this development is the "hepatization" or "carnification" of the lung (Fig. 20).

As Wilson [139] has shown, the extent of the pulmonary right-to-left shunt allows **prognostical conclusions.** However, it must be related to the cardiac output. Moreover, it has been my experience that prognosis is rated as unfavorable if the shunt is not reduced when ventilation with positive end-expiratory pressure is applied (Table 8).

Table 8. Unfavorable prognosis of ARDS

Pulmonary right-to-left shunt over 50%
No reduction of right-to-left shunt during PEEP
Low cardiac output
Combination with renal failure

Table 9. Therapy for ARDS

I. Ventilation with positive end-expiratory pressure (PEEP)
II. Steroids (1 g methylprednisolone IV, repeat once after 6 h)

Therapy (Table 9)

It is decisive for the therapy of ARDS that treatment is instituted **early,** i. e., immediately after the diagnosis has been established. Every delay results in a progression of intrapulmonary abnormalities and conceals the danger of passing the point of no return.

1. Prompt ventilation with positive end-expiratory pressure (PEEP). This very decisive step in treatment is taken because it counteracts the reduction of functional residual capacity [111, 126]. Microatelectases are opened. A positive end-expiratory

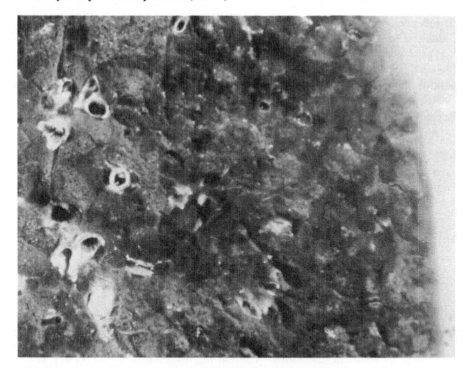

Fig. 20. Terminal stage of ARDS with extensive fibrosis of the lung ("hepatization")

pressure (PEEP) of +10 cm H_2O usually will not be detrimental to the function of the heart; in some instances, the cardiac output will even increase [e. g., 127].

2. Administration of high bolus dosages of corticosteroids, which directly affect the heightened permeability of the capillaries, according to more recent research [79, 82, 140] seems to be favorable. We administer 1 g methylprednisolone IV immediately and repeat this dosage once after 6 h. Simultaneous ventilation with positive end-expiratory pressure (PEEP) is maintained.

3. Maintenance of normal oncotic pressure in the intravascular area. According to Starling's law [123], the intravascular oncotic pressure is an essential factor in the return of fluid from the interstitial tissue to the capillaries. It is largely determined by the protein content of the serum and falls sharply in the presence of **hypoproteinemia.** (The relationship is shown in Table 10.)

Table 10. Calculated oncotic pressure dependent upon protein content of blood (Landis and Pappenheimer [84])

Serum protein	Calculated oncotic pressure[a]
7.5 g%	−28 mmHg
6.0 g%	−20 mmHg
5.0 g%	−15 mmHg

[a] According to the formula: $P = 2.1\,c + 0.16\,c^2 + 0.009\,c^3$ (c = plasma protein concentration)

Maintenance of a normal serum protein content by **restricted fluid supply** using **fresh blood** or **human albumin** as volume replacement can be significant during early therapy, as long as there is no severe damage to the pulmonary capillary wall.
The application of a concentrated albumin solution in manifest ARDS, however, is questionable and should be carefully considered in each individual case since even albumin can penetrate into the interstitium because of the increased permeability of the capillary wall for proteins [130].

The use of **heparin,** often recommended, is highly problematic and in the case of patients with multiple injuries is contraindicated. Besides, an indication would be given only if tests for coagulation provide evidence of a disseminated intravascular coagulation, something that in my experience is astonishingly seldom the case. A decrease in thrombocytes by itself is insufficient for this diagnosis; it occurs in every severely injured individual and especially after massive transfusions. Proof is lacking for the effectiveness of **proteinase inhibitors.**

Hypothermia

If despite optimal therapy the arterial PO_2 at an oxygen concentration of 0.6 at inspiration falls below 60 mmHg, the application of a hypothermia of 30°–32°C is recommended. This not only reduces the need for oxygen, it also decreases CO_2 production by reducing the entire metabolism; the necessarily increasing rise of the respiratory minute volume in such advanced cases can thereby be restricted. Because of the toxic effect of high oxygen concentrations at inspiration, I prefer to go this route rather than via the alternative of increasing the F_IO_2 beyond 0.6.

Extracorporeal Oxygenation

New perspectives in the treatment of severe advanced ARDS are suggested by the possibility of extended **extracorporeal oxygenation** with **membrane oxygenators.** If oxygenation can no longer be provided by the usual therapeutic measures, this procedure, which is slowly accomplishing the transition from experimental to clinical usage, can be considered. Because of the danger of severe bleeding, it must be restricted to those cases that undergo rapid and increasing deterioration despite optimal therapy.
On the other hand, the administration of long-term perfusion makes sense only before fibrosis of the lung has begun, i. e., in the first 10 days after the appearance and diagnosis of the syndrome. Even if there is a possibility of applying this therapy, the technical and personnel requirements are enormous.
There have been cases of patients with severe and otherwise unfavorable pulmonary insufficiency surviving long-term perfusion (up to 9½ days) [142]. According to the opinion of Hill [76], in cases of increasing deterioration, a P_aO_2 below 50 mmHg obtained with an F_IO_2 of 0.6 is an indication for this procedure.

VI. Fat Embolism

Is it justifiable to differentiate fat embolism from ARDS as a cause of respiratory insufficiency?

Fat embolism undoubtedly represents a **specific syndrome,** which due to the pulmonary changes it causes can indeed lead to ARDS. However, in addition to the prominent sign of respiratory insufficiency, it is usually accompanied by other symptoms that do not occur in ARDS. Of particular importance is **cerebral involvement** with disturbances in consciousness of every kind, which are by no means limited to hypoxia, but as a consequence of a specific pathologic event in the brain can also appear without arterial hypoxia [93]. The pure cerebral form of fat embolism without pulmonary involvement is well-known [37]. In addition, **petechiae of the skin** are characteristic of fat embolism (Fig. 21) and are observed in over 60% of the patients [37, 105]. They are not found in ARDS. The specific, though less frequently found changes in the retina [32] and kidneys [72] also suggest a unique and specific pathologic condition.

As far as the pulmonary situation is concerned, there is an important additional reason for separating it from ARDS: There are **two distinct forms** of **pulmonary fat embolism** that, completely independent of the findings of the chest roentgenogram, are distinguishable in their functional injury (Table 11). This differentiation is

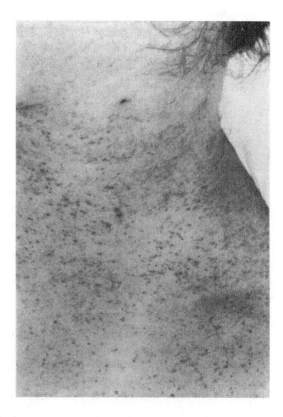

Fig. 21. Petechiae caused by fat embolism

Table 11. The two different forms of pulmonary fat embolism

	Type I	Type II
Characteristic	Insignificant intrapulmonary right-to-left shunt	Significant intrapulmonary right-to-left shunt
Diagnosis		
P_aO_2 air ($F_IO_2 = 0.21$)	Low or normal	Low
P_aO_2 ($F_IO_2 = 1.0$)	± Normal (over 300 mmHg)	Low (below 300 mmHg)
$A - a\ DO_2$	± Normal (below 350 mmHg)	Over 350 mmHg
Roentgenogram	Characteristic changes of fat embolism	
Prognosis	Good	Questionable, corresponding to ARDS
Therapy	Mechanical ventilation if necessary to guarantee sufficient P_aO_2	"Aggressive" as with ARDS: – PEEP – Maintenance of normal oncotic pressure – Steroids
Example	L. Ch., ♂, 26 yrs: Fragmented fracture of femur on the right Fracture of right lower leg Fracture of IVth lumbar vertebra Thoracic contusion	A.D., ♂, 29 yrs: Fracture of femur on the right Fracture of right lower leg Intra-abdominal bleeding Cerebral contusion
P_aO_2: Spontaneous breathing	48 mmHg (6 liters O_2)	69 mmHg (5 liters O_2)
P_aO_2: Mechanical ventilation (PEEP + 10)	128 mmHg ($F_IO_2 = 0.4$) 494 mmHg ($F_IO_2 = 1.0$)	72 mmHg ($F_IO_2 = 0.4$) 130 mmHg ($F_IO_2 = 1.0$)

based on the extent of the intrapulmonary right-to-left shunt and is probably rather arbitrary. However, it seems to me to be useful for clinical practice since it facilitates evaluation of the degree and further course of the pulmonary impairment and provides signs for the prognosis. Recovery from the severer form — type II — is not possible without treatment, and ventilation with PEEP is always necessary.

Type I Pulmonary Fat Embolism

In type I, there is an initial normal arterial PO_2 or arterial hypoxia, in which by spontaneous breathing or mechanical ventilation with pure oxygen a P_aO_2 corresponding to an F_IO_2 of 1.0 can be attained. In this form, there is **no significant right-to-left shunt**. The dead space quotient (V_D/V_T) is elevated. Because of arterial hypoxia, respirator treatment may be necessary, but adequate P_aO_2 values on the respirator should be attainable without difficulty. The prognosis of this first form of pulmonary fat embolism is good.

Type II Pulmonary Fat Embolism

In type II, arterial hypoxia is **caused by an essential functional intrapulmonary right-to-left shunt.** In breathing or mechanical ventilation with pure oxygen, the attainable P_aO_2 remains far below normal values. The alveolar-arterial oxygen gradient is greatly elevated. In its functional effects and prognosis, this form corresponds to ARDS.

In **both forms,** the **changes in the lungs as shown on the roentgenogram** are usually pronounced and characteristic (resembling "snow flurries" or a "fine-grained, miliary" picture of the lung). The functional limitation of respiration can, however, precede the pathologic X-ray picture by 1 or 2 days. The **thoracic roentgenogram therefore does not allow any conclusions to be drawn about which form of fat embolism is present.** The arterial blood gas analysis at room air is also inconclusive. Only examination of the blood gas on 100% O_2, during spontaneous breathing or, if need be with mechanical ventilation, can distinguish between the two forms.

Among our patients, we found almost twice as many with type I pulmonary fat embolism as with type II.

Differentiation between these two forms of pulmonary fat embolism appears to me to be important not only for prognosis but also for therapy. In the case of type II, it corresponds to the treatment for ARDS: aggressive mechanical ventilation with positive end-expiratory pressure (PEEP) and steroids in high dosage. In the case of type I, treatment can be restricted to guaranteeing an adequate supply of oxygen by means of mechanical ventilation. However, frequent monitoring of arterial blood gases is essential.

VII. Other Forms of Respiratory Insufficiency Among the Injured

Respiratory Disturbances in Craniocerebral Trauma

Severe cerebral injuries can result in a variety of respiratory disturbances, from **hyperventilation** to **various forms of hypoventilation** to **cessation of respiration** [124]. The **failure of deep breathing reflexes** and **inadequate expectoration** are also of significance. The treatment of the cerebral damage and of the brain edema naturally takes precedence. Intubation should be liberally employed to avoid aspiration and to allow endotracheal suction. Mechanical ventilation is also broadly indicated since under no circumstances should hypoxia be permitted to develop.

In addition to these basic respiratory disturbances, which have been known for a long time, it was the Moss group [101, 103, 104] that took note of mechanisms that give rise to **central lung edema.** (Attention must be called, however, to the fact that these investigations could not be confirmed by other authors.) Thus, a cerebral hypoxia leads to an increase in the permeability of the lung capillaries and thereby to a state that corresponds functionally to ARDS. In experiments with animals, such an interstitial lung edema could be produced by selective perfusion of the brain with oxygen-poor blood [101]. Medication with diphenylhydantoin produced a prophylactic effect. These lung changes were absent in denervation of the lung through autotransplantation [104].

Renal Failure

Posttraumatic failure of the kidneys has clearly become less frequent and is avoidable in most cases [56]. Adequate shock treatment, monitoring of kidney functions (urine production, osmolality, in certain cases creatinine clearance), appropriate, but not excessive administration of fluids, and correction of other extrarenal factors of kidney insufficiency (cardiac failure) as well as avoidance or correct dosage of potentially toxic substances (e. g., aminoglycoside antibiotics) will keep the number of dialyses needed to a minimum.

In many cases, renal failure is accompanied simultaneously by respiratory insufficiency. During the first few days after trauma, the latter might be occasioned by **overinfusion** inasmuch as the attempt is made by means of generous intravenous therapy to maintain adequate urinary output. What is important here is to recognize this danger early and to limit the amount of infusion drastically. In the case of obvious overinfusion, a timely dialysis with rigorous withdrawal of water can eliminate lung edema [143]. In such cases, one needs only minimal indication for the use of mechanical ventilation with positive end-expiratory pressure (PEEP). In the case of established ARDS accompanied by simultaneous anuresis, the lethality is extraordinarily high and survival is possible only in exceptional cases.

Lung changes caused by uremia conform largely to the image of ARDS. In an already damaged lung, a rise in urea and creatinine, which can be tolerated without difficulty by a person with healthy lungs, causes additional lung damage. The prognosis in such patients can only be improved by aggressive dialysis, which keeps the blood urea-nitrogen level below 90 mg% [53].

Smoke Inhalation

The inhalation of smoke or toxic gases generated by the combustion of modern synthetics, besides causing local damage to the larger respiratory passages, can in severe cases lead to changes in the lungs that correspond functionally to ARDS. Therapy would then follow the same principles. If treatment with a respirator is not considered necessary, intensive breathing exercises become decisively important. The early use of steroids in high dosages (two applications, each 1 g methylprednisolone IV) is helpful [58, 59, 125].

VIII. Lung Damage Caused by Therapeutic Measures

In the multifactorial event that leads to the progressive respiratory insufficiency of ARDS, the **damage to the lungs done by therapy** of the injured assumes major signif-

Table 12. Potential lung-damaging therapeutic measures and prophylaxis

	"Prophylaxis"
Blood transfusion	Freshest possible blood Special filters in massive transfusions Alternative: microaggregate-free blood components
Infusion of crystalloids in excess	Controlled fluid infusion
Oxygen	Oxygen on need basis $F_I O_2$ maximally 0.6
Supine position	Alternating side positions Early mobilization Breathing exercises

icance. Some measures that would be tolerated by an undamaged lung without bad effects will result in critical damage in the case of trauma or as a consequence of disturbed capillary permeability of the lung.

Knowledge of these various possibilities of damage caused by therapy is of great practical significance. Some severe injuries to the lungs could be avoided if in therapy of the severely injured, especially in primary shock treatment, more attention is paid to the lung (Table 12).

Excessive Use of Fluids

If blood loss is replaced with crystalloid solutions, multiple volumes will be necessary because noncolloidal solutions quickly disperse in intravascular and extravascular space in a ratio of 1:4 [97]. This fluid stays in the interstitial tissues. In a lung injury (e. g., lung contusion) or in otherwise damaged permeability of the lung capillaries, the lung retains this fluid to a far greater degree than other body tissues [88, 97, 131]. Furthermore, the plasma proteins are diluted by large amounts of crystalloids and concomitantly the oncotic pressure in the plasma is reduced (see Table 10). This also promotes the loss of water from the intravascular bed. In fact, in a severely injured individual, the levels of serum albumin and total proteins are lowered but this is not only caused by the infusion of salt solutions [54].

In a damaged lung, an excess infusion of crystalloids undoubtedly acquires decisive importance for further pulmonary developments.

However, this does not answer the question of whether primary shock treatment should be instituted with colloids or crystalloids. Colloids, especially the administration of albumin, can also exert deleterious effects on the lung. If the capillary permeability is impaired, proteins enter the interstitium, remain there, and are conducive to the formation of interstitial edema. This lung-damaging effect is probably more difficult to reverse than the edema alone.

I would once again like to call attention to the protective effect of prophylactic ventilation with PEEP for decreasing fluid retention in the lung.

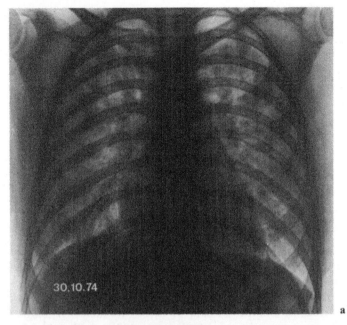

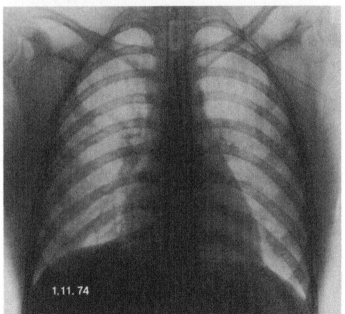

Fig. 22. a Severe allergic lung edema in a 20-year-old patient with facial lacerations after transfusion of one unit of blood. **b** Normalization of the lung condition 2 days after administration of steroids and ventilation with PEEP

Blood Transfusion

In stored whole blood, there are **thrombocyte and leukocyte aggregates** that are deposited in the lung during transfusion as microemboli, as Swank [128] pointed out for the first time in 1961. They consist of clumps of degenerated thrombocytes and leukocytes with a diameter of 15 – 200 µm and therefore pass through the normal blood filters that catch only particles over 170 µm in diameter.

The aggregate formation is dependent upon the length of preservation [128]. In preserved blood over 1 week old, this aggregate formation can reach 60 million in 400 ml of blood [100].

In massive transfusions, such microaggregates from stored blood share responsibility for the occurrence of ARDS. The damaging effect here most likely consists not in obstructing the capillaries of the lung but in liberating biologically active substances (serotonin, histamine, ADP) from the microaggregates.

Use of **micropore filters** can prevent the entry of such aggregate formations into the venous circulation. In massive transfusions, the early use of such special filters is required. However, their use in **transfusions of fresh blood** is not advisable since they also filter out an essential portion of functional platelets [77, 90]. In clinical usage, it is necessary that such special filters allow for an adequate filtering rate and do not clog too quickly.

An alternative to special filters would be the use of **microaggregate-free blood components,** such as fresh blood, fresh frozen plasma, and erythrocyte concentrates without a buffy coat [64]. It has been demonstrated experimentally that permeability disturbances of the pulmonary capillary wall caused by preserved blood do not occur when transfusions without platelets and without a buffy coat are administered [43].

Interstitial edema and the signs of ARDS can also develop on the **basis of an allergy.** In the literature, only a few cases are recorded [48, 135]. I have observed two such allergic reactions to blood transfusions resulting in interstitial lung edema and respiratory insufficiency, in one case after the transfusion of a single unit (Fig. 22). In both cases complete recovery resulted after respiratory treatment with positive end-expiratory pressure (PEEP) and steroids.

Oxygen Toxicity

Since the turn of the century, it has been known that laboratory animals that inhale pure oxygen longer than 3 or 4 days die of severe lung damage [122]. Oxygen in high concentrations is also deleterious to the human lung. Of decisive importance are the **partial pressure of the oxygen** being inhaled as well as the **time of exposure.**

In experiments on healthy persons who inhale 100% oxygen at a pressure of 1 atm, changes in the lungs appear after 24 h [49, 133]. At a pressure of 2 atm, lung damage is already detectable after 6 – 11 h [62].

Lower partial oxygen pressures are tolerated for a longer period of time without damage. Volunteers in the American space program inhaled oxygen at a PO_2 of 300 mmHg over a period of 3 days, and American astronauts breathed pure oxygen at 258 mmHg in the space capsules [116].

All of this applies to healthy persons with undamaged lungs. There is evidence to suggest that a **previously damaged lung** (e. g., by ARDS or after lung trauma) is more sensitive to the toxic effects of oxygen [120].

The clinical observation that **atelectasis** occurs more frequently even during a brief application of pure oxygen is easily explained by resorption. In actual oxygen toxicity, however, there is **direct tissue damage,** principally manifested by enzyme damage to the mitochondrial membranes [83] and interference of surfactant synthesis [99].

Based on these observations, **practical clinical conclusions** can be drawn:

Ventilation with pure oxygen is only justified in immediate emergencies, e. g., in cardiac arrest or during acute hypotension. In intensive care, the lowest suitable concentration of oxygen should be used for ventilation, i. e., oxygen should only be administered on the basis of "need." **An inspired oxygen concentration of more than 60% over an extended period of time is to be avoided at all costs!** If the intrapulmonary right-to-left shunt in ARDS is so extensive that no adequate arterial PO_2 can be attained with this oxygen concentration, then even an increase to 100% $F_I O_2$ will no longer produce any substantial gain, as can readily be seen in Fig. 13. In these cases, instead of raising the inspired oxygen concentration to toxic levels, the attempt should rather be made to lower **oxygen requirements** by means of **hypothermia.**

Supine Position

The distribution of ventilation and perfusion in individual sections of the lung depends upon the **position of the body.** In the lower parts of the lung, perfusion exceeds ventilation [137].

The **supine position** is the worst one for the patient because a large part of both lobes of the lung are poorly ventilated. The **functional residual capacity,** which is greatly reduced in ARDS, decreases 20% even in healthy lungs when the person is laid on his back [108]. Frequent changes of position are therefore extremely important for all patients who cannot be mobilized [115].

Sedatives and Narcotics

The suppression of deep breathing reflexes favors the formation of atelectasis. In addition, suppressing the cough reflex makes expectoration more difficult.

Long-term Ventilation

There is still discussion going on about the possibly damaging effect of long-term ventilation and its causes [138]. Persons with healthy lungs (e. g., poliomyelitis patients) were ventilated over a period of years without noticeable pulmonary damage. The question is academic since no long-term ventilation is undertaken without indication, and it is precisely in cases of interstitial lung edema that ventilation serves not for the maintenance of oxygenation but must be designated as actual therapy. If advancing pulmonary insufficiency nevertheless results, of all the possible damaging factors involved, mechanical ventilation is not primarily responsible. The expression "ventilator lung" is one of the worst that can be used for ARDS and implies a completely misleading causality that does not exist.

IX. Conclusions and Consequences for Prophylaxis and Therapy

1. Prophylaxis Against ARDS

— The **most effective prophylaxis against ARDS** in severely injured patients is **prophylactic ventilation with PEEP.** High-risk patients are intubated and ventilated for 1 – 3 days with PEEP at + 10 cm H_2O.
— Even if mechanical ventilation is instituted for other reasons (e. g., instability of the thoracic wall), **as a principle PEEP** is applied provided there are no contraindications present (e. g., brain injury).
— The amounts of **electrolyte solutions** should be carefully balanced against urinary output.
— **Microfilters** should be used in massive transfusions. This does not apply when **fresh blood** or **erythrocytes** are used.
— Avoid **excessive transfusion.**
— During volume infusion a **normal plasma protein content** (c. 7 g%) and concomitantly a **normal oncotic pressure** in the plasma should be maintained.

The infusion of **20% human albumin** is established practice in the primary volume replacement. Giving larger amounts of albumin in concentrations of 4 g% or 5 g% should be avoided as much as possible as it leads to dilution of protein.

2. Differential Diagnosis of Respiratory Insufficiency

— **Repeated arterial blood gas analyses** are indispensable.
— If there is arterial hypoxia, an **oxygenation test,** possibly during mechanical ventilation, is used to determine whether there is only a regional hypoventilation or a significant intrapulmonary right-to-left shunt involved, i. e., if atelectasis can be ruled out, whether the pathologic picture is that of ARDS or a functionally comparable disorder.

3. Adult Respiratory Distress Syndrome (ARDS)

— The diagnosis of ARDS or functionally equivalent disorders implies **intubation and ventilation with positive end-expiratory pressure (PEEP).**

— In this situation, consideration must be given to the fact that ventilation not only effects the maintenance of sufficient P_aO_2 but is also the most **essential therapeutic procedure** and is intended prophylactically to prevent deterioration of the disease.
— Administration of 1 g **methylprednisolone IV,** repeated once after 6 h.

4. Chest Drainage

— It is obvious that a **tension pneumothorax** must be recognized and drained before further diagnostic measures are taken.
— In all patients with multiple rib fractures who require mechanical ventilation for general anesthesia or because of respiratory insufficiency, a **prophylactic chest tube** is inserted.

Chapter 5
Indications for Operation in Blunt Thoracic Trauma

Operative intervention is **seldom** necessary in **blunt** thoracic injuries (in my experience, this occurred in only 8% of such hospitalized patients). There are **clearly defined indications** for surgery. The more experienced the surgeon is in the treatment of thoracic injuries, the less frequently (s)he will, as a rule, operate. This is especially true in pure lung injuries: the "lung suture" is for the most part unnecessary.

Conditions are similar in the case of **penetrating chest injuries.** The principles underlying their treatment and the special indications for operative intervention are discussed in Chap. 7.

There are situations in which an operation is **immediately** necessary, such as with heavy blood loss and in cardiac tamponade. In the majority of cases, however, an accurate diagnostic determination, e. g., by means of bronchoscopy, aortography, or esophagography, is possible. The operation then follows immediately upon **verification of the diagnosis** ("early operation") (Table 13).

Table 13. Indications for early operation in blunt chest injuries

1. Massive and persistent bleeding
2. Acute cardiac tamponade
3. Rupture of the aorta
4. Injury to the supra-aortic branches
5. Rupture of the trachea and bronchi
6. Rupture of the diaphragm
7. Rupture of the esophagus
8. Possibly operative stabilization of the thoracic wall

I. Indications for Immediate or Early Operation

1. Massive and Persistent Bleeding

After insertion of a chest tube, a frightening amount of blood is often lost. Most of the hemorrhaging from the chest wall or the lung parenchyma stops, however, after expansion of the lungs. It is a different story if the **internal thoracic artery,** an **intercostal artery, great vessels,** or the **heart** are injured.

There are no general, binding rules for operative indications in these instances. The amount of blood flowing out immediately after insertion of the chest tube is noted, but this provides no conclusive indication for proceeding with an operation. In general, surgical intervention is indicated when blood loss through the chest tubes continues to exceed 500 ml/h after 3 h or more than 150 ml/h after 6 h. Obviously, an operation is always indicated if a state of shock caused by intrathoracic bleeding or hemorrhaging into the mediastinum cannot be controlled despite volume substitution.

2. Acute Cardiac Tamponade

This situation, which occurs much less frequently in chest wounds through blunt force than through penetrating injuries, is caused by **heart wall ruptures, ruptures of the intrapericardial portion of the aorta,** or by **hemorrhage of the heart surface** or the **pericardium.** It constitutes an indication for immediate operative intervention. In acute cases, pericardiocentesis is never to be regarded as definitive therapy but only as a stopgap measure until the operation can be performed. An operation is also necessary in the exceedingly rare case of **luxation of the heart.**

3. Rupture of the Aorta

If intervention is not immediately necessary to treat acute hemorrhaging with left-sided hemothorax, a suspected rupture of the aorta should be confirmed preoperatively by means of **aortography.** After clarification of the diagnosis, the operation should not be delayed since lethal hemorrhaging could occur at any time.

4. Injuries to the Supra-aortic Branches

If there is no acute hemorrhage, the diagnosis of rupture of a supra-aortic artery or of intimal lesions with acute thrombosis should also be established preoperatively by means of angiography.

5. Ruptures of the Trachea and Major Bronchi

With a massive loss of air through the chest tube, especially where the lung cannot be reexpanded or if there is massive mediastinal emphysema, the diagnosis of a ruptured bronchus or injury to the trachea is verified by **bronchoscopy.** Confirmation of the diagnosis is an indication for surgery (see p. 170). Massive air leakage caused solely by injuries to the lung parenchyma do not represent an indication for operation if the lung can be fully expanded by the use of suction drainage.

6. Rupture of the Diaphragm

Early operation is always indicated.

7. Rupture of the Esophagus

This very rare injury is difficult to recognize and must be diagnosed and operated upon as early as possible. If there is any clinical doubt, the diagnosis can be clarified before the operation by means of **esophagography.**

8. Operative Stabilization of the Thoracic Wall

Operative stabilization of multiple rib fractures is justified only if the patient would have to be ventilated solely on account of the unstable thoracic wall. In general, this is the case only in multiple comminuted rib fractures with paradoxical respiration and resultant respiratory failure. There are further restricting factors involved in such an operation so that it should only be considered in a few exceptional cases. The problematic nature of the operative indications, which are not yet clarified by any means, is presented in greater detail in Chap. 10.

II. Indications for Subsequent Operations

1. Injuries to Intracardiac Structures

The operative correction of a traumatic septal defect or of valvular heart injuries calls for diagnostic clarification by means of heart catheterization and cineangiography. It goes without saying that the operation should be performed by the cardiac surgeon. An operative intervention in the acute posttraumatic phase is seldom indicated.

2. Clotted Hemothorax

If a large hemothorax cannot be adequately drained so that later functional disturbances are anticipated, the decision for a thoracotomy should be made early. One week after trauma the operation is still relatively simple and consists of a small thoracotomy with removal of hematoma; the operation several weeks after trauma, however, requires decortication of the lung.

3. Injuries to the Thoracic Duct

This rare lesion hardly presents an indication for an operation anymore since the leakage of chyle into the thoracic cavity generally stops by itself subsequent to chest suction drainage and parenteral nutrition. The operation, which consists of the ligature of the thoracic duct, should only be considered if healing fails to take place after 3 – 4 weeks of conservative management.

4. Traumatic Aneurysm of the Aorta

The diagnosis, once confirmed by aortography, provides the indication for an operation inasmuch as such an aneurysm can rupture at any time, even years after the trauma.

III. Contraindications to Operative Intervention

An operative intervention is contraindicated in **lung contusions, blast injuries of the lung, intrapulmonary hematomas,** and generally also in **lung lacerations.** Operative intervention is only indicated for lung lacerations when there is massive hemorrhaging or if the thoracic suction drainage cannot fully reexpand the lung. The healing tendency in parenchymal lung injuries is extraordinarily good [152]. All that an operation does is add to the morbidity and mortality.
In general, **hemoptysis** does not present any operative indication. The danger of aspiration is met by laying the patient on the injured side and in exceptional cases by use of a double-lumen endotracheal tube. With mechanical ventilation, traumatically induced hemoptysis is almost always brought to a halt. The value of an operation is therefore doubtful because the localization of hemorrhage in blunt trauma can be enormously difficult.
Operative intervention is naturally not indicated in cases of **cardiac contusion.** The only exception to this, a rare one, might be the occurrence of cardiac tamponade due to hemorrhaging from a contused myocardium.

Chapter 6
Operative Approaches

As with every surgical intervention, an adequate operative approach is decisive in injuries to intrathoracic structures. Since such interventions must occasionally be undertaken under great pressure of time, it is better in these situations to choose a simple approach that can be carried out quickly. Of special significance are the **possibilities for extension** since in contrast to elective cases, the amount of damage can often not be judged preoperatively. Although operative approaches must be accommodated to individual cases, it is generally possible to make standard incisions.

I. Anterolateral Thoracotomy

This approach to thoracic injuries is used most frequently and can be carried out most quickly. Since the incision is made through the front section of the chest wall, only very little musculature must be incised. Morbidity is minimal.

Indications

1. Cardiac injuries, cardiac tamponade, open heart massage
2. Removal of clotted hemothorax
3. Injuries to the thoracic wall (hemorrhaging from the internal thoracic artery or from intercostal vessels)
4. Severe lung injuries
5. Injuries to pulmonary vessels or to the vena cava
6. Injuries to the bronchus (fifth intercostal space)
7. Injuries to the intrathoracic trachea, unless a medial sternotomy is performed (right-sided thoracotomy)

Possibilities for Extension

1. The anterolateral thoracotomy can be extended in the direction of the posterolateral thoracotomy. In that case, there is a restriction only when the field of operation is limited posteriorly by the prior positioning of the patient. For this reason, when severe injury to the lung is suspected, a lateral position, as in a posterolateral thora-

cotomy, is advantageous. For the initial exploration, however, only the anterolateral incision is made.

2. An important possibility for extension is a transverse incision of the sternum enabling the surgeon to enter the other thoracic cavity.

Position

Oblique position (30°–40°) (Fig. 23) by bolsters under the hips and scapula.

Operative Procedure

The **skin incision** runs from the edge of the sternum in an arc approximately 5 cm below the nipple, in women along the breast crease. Posteriorly, the incision is again drawn more caudally (Fig. 23). If a posterior extension is necessary, it should run about 5 cm below the tip of the scapula.
In general, the thoracotomy takes place in the **fifth intercostal space.** The thoracic attachment of the major pectoral muscle is severed ventrally at the level of the fifth rib. Toward the side, corresponding to the course of the ribs, the anterior serratus muscle is spread apart in the direction of its fibers. The periosteum of the fifth rib is incised with an electrocautery close to the lower edge of the rib (Fig. 24 A).
The periosteum and bordering intercostal musculature are pushed back from the lower edge of the rib using a periosteum elevator (Fig. 24 B). The rib is lifted with a retractor, and the parietal pleura is incised with a scalpel and opened up with scissors in the direction of the course of the rib (Fig. 24 C). Near the sternal origin of the rib, the rib cartilage is cut; the next higher rib can be disarticulated at the sternocostal joint. If necessary, the internal thoracic artery is cut and ligated.

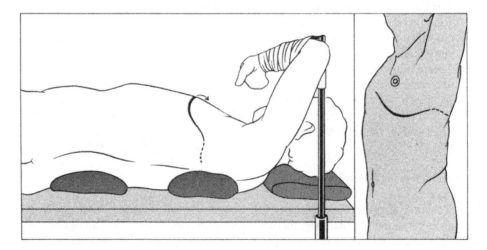

Fig. 23. Anterolateral thoracotomy: position and skin incision

Anterolateral Thoracotomy

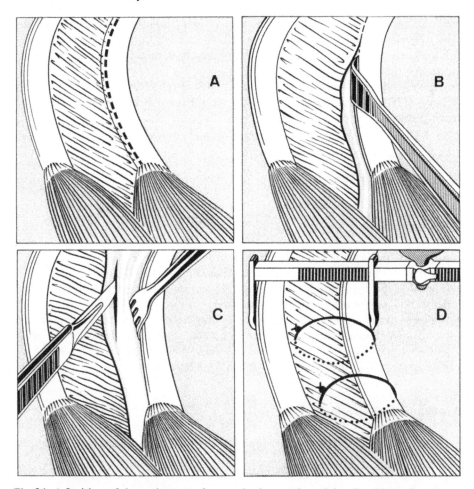

Fig. 24. A Incision of the periosteum close to the lower edge of the rib after cutting the attachments of the major pectoral muscle. Laterally, the anterior serratus muscle is spread apart in the direction of its fibers. **B** Pushing back the rib periosteum and the bordering intercostal musculature with its nerve and vessels by means of a periosteum elevator. **C** Raising the rib with a retractor and incising the parietal pleura. **D** Closure of thoracotomy: use of the rib approximator. The thick catgut sutures are placed; they encompass the upper rib and the intercostal soft tissues below the wound

Before closing up the thoracotomy, adequate **drainage** must be established; in injuries to the pericardium and the heart, a window is placed in the pericardium behind the phrenic nerve to allow drainage into the thoracic cavity. In general, two thoracic tubes are inserted intrathoracically: one anteriorly for the evacuation of air and one posteriorly running through the phrenicocostal sinus for the purpose of blood drainage. Bear in mind that the chest tube is not to be brought out too far posteriorly.

For the **closure of the thoracotomy,** Bailey's rib approximator is helpful. Thick catgut sutures (catgut No. 2) encompass the upper rib and the intercostal soft tissues inferior to the approach but not the rib below (Fig. 24 D). The closure should preserve the natural distance between the ribs and not cause the two ribs to override. Muscle layers that have been severed are sutured.

A rib resection is never necessary. The approach is made sufficiently large by means of a rib spreader.

Postoperatively, a 25 cm H_2O suction is usually attached to both chest tubes by means of a Y-connector. In pneumonectomies, only a very low suction (5 cm H_2O suction) should be applied.

II. Posterolateral Thoracotomy

Indications

1. Rupture of the aorta in classic location (fourth intercostal space)
2. Severe lung injuries, if the anterolateral thoracotomy is insufficient
3. Injuries to the intrathoracic esophagus (thoracotomy on the right side for the upper section, on the left for the lowest section)
4. Ruptures of the right diaphragm, old diaphragmatic injuries on the left, or also recent ones if simultaneous severe intrathoracic injuries are involved (in acute left-sided diaphragmatic ruptures without indications for an operation on the intrathoracic organs, the approach of choice is via laparotomy)

Possibilities for Extension

Continuation of the incision to the opposite side by cutting transversely across the sternum.

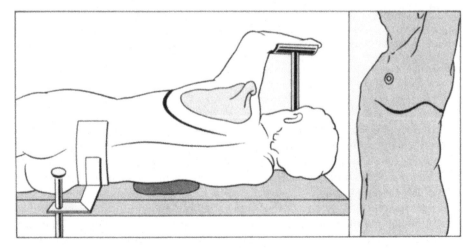

Fig. 25. Posterolateral thoracotomy: position and skin incision

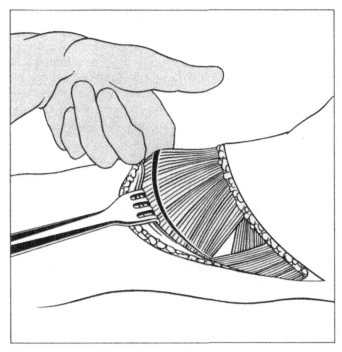

Fig. 26. Posterolateral thoracotomy: cutting the latissimus dorsi muscle as far distally as possible. Incising the trapezius and rhomboid muscles.

Positioning

Lateral position (Fig. 25). In severe injuries to the lung, the disadvantage in this position is that it is almost impossible to avoid aspiration of blood into the noninvolved lung. In these cases, a double-lumen endotracheal tube should be utilized.

Operative Procedure

In its anterior section, the skin incision corresponds to that of the anterolateral thoracotomy; it begins slightly anterior to the midclavicular line. Posteriorly, the incision runs in an arc 5 cm below the tip of the scapula and then goes cranially parallel to the spinal column, 5 cm lateral to the spinous processes, and proceeds to the level of the fifth thoracic vertebra (Fig. 25).

For the maintenance of better function, the latissimus dorsi muscle is severed as far distally as possible. Posteriorly, the trapezius and, if necessary, the rhomboid muscle lying underneath it are incised (Fig. 26). The anterior serratus muscle is also severed as far distally as possible; this muscle incision runs ventrally in the direction of the rib selected for access. The rest of the procedure, drainage, and closure correspond to the anterolateral thoracotomy.

III. Median Sternotomy

Splitting of the sternum, which is particularly applicable as a standard incision in heart surgery and whose special merits are its minimal impairment of pulmonary function and the fact that it does not require opening the pleural cavities, is hardly ever used in trauma cases. It takes more time, its extension possibilities are limited, and it is only in rare cases that we are faced with an injury in which there is convincing preoperative evidence that only the anterior mediastinum is affected.

Indications

1. Injuries to the ascending aorta
2. Possible injury to the intrathoracic trachea, provided preference is not given to a right-sided thoracotomy

Possibilities for Extension

Extended exposure of the vessel origins in the superior thoracic aperture can be gained by means of an oblique cervical incision.

Position

Supine position

Operative Procedure

The skin incision is made in the center line that begins from the suprasternal notch and extends caudally to the xyphoid. The periosteum is incised in the middle of the sternum using an electrocautery.
Using blunt finger dissection, the posterior aspect of the suprasternal notch and the xyphoid are freed. The sternum is then split longitudinally with an oscillating saw, and after pushing the pleura away from the posterior of the sternum, the spreader is inserted.
If, during the course of the operation the pericardium is opened, pericardial drainage is provided by insertion of a tube with a small catheter in its lumen, effecting a suction and flush drainage system.
Closure of the sternum is accomplished by means of a doubly laid and singly knotted suture through the sternum proper, using a thick, nonabsorbent material (e. g., nylon monofilament No. 3).

IV. Approach to the Great Vessels of the Superior Thoracic Aperture

In hemorrhaging injuries of the great vessels of the superior thoracic aperture, the choice of operative approach is of decisive significance. It must not only provide for the care of the lesion, but must also permit bringing the hemorrhage under control as quickly as possible. Before operative intervention, a clear picture of **operative tactics** must have been formed (see p. 241).

Approach to the Great Vessels of the Superior Thoracic Aperture

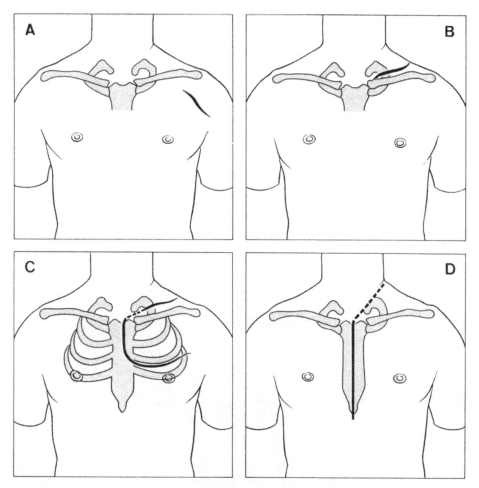

Fig. 27 A – D. Possible approaches to the vessels of the superior thoracic aperture: **A** Distal infraclavicular approach; **B** Supraclavicular approach, possibly with splitting of the clavicle; **C** Trapdoor approach: supraclavicular incision combined with an upper sternal split and a anterior thoracotomy in the third intercostal space; **D** Median sternotomy, possibly combined with cervical extension

1. Distal Infraclavicular Approach (Fig. 27 A)

This access comes into consideration only in injuries to the **axillary vessels.** The incision is made from the lower edge of the distal clavicle up to the area of the deltopectoral groove, where the cephalic vein runs. The major pectoral muscle is held away medially and downward. For an extension of the exposure, the insertion of the major pectoral muscle is severed at the humerus along with its fibers connected to the clavicle, and the insertion of the minor pectoral muscle is detached at the coracoid process. An additional supraclavicular approach to occlude the subclavian artery may become necessary.

2. Supraclavicular Approach (Fig. 27 B)

This is **the standard approach for injuries to the middle and distal section of the subclavian artery and vein.** In many cases, for purposes of better exposure of the distal vessel, there is an advantage in splitting the clavicle in the middle (e. g., with a Gigli saw) and subsequently restoring it by internal fixation. This approach can be expanded to a "trapdoor" type by a longitudinal cleavage of the sternum to the level of the third intercostal space.

3. "Trapdoor" Approach (Fig. 27 C)

By far the best exposure of the vessels of the superior thoracic aperture on a given side is gained by the trapdoor approach, which was publicized anew by Steenburg

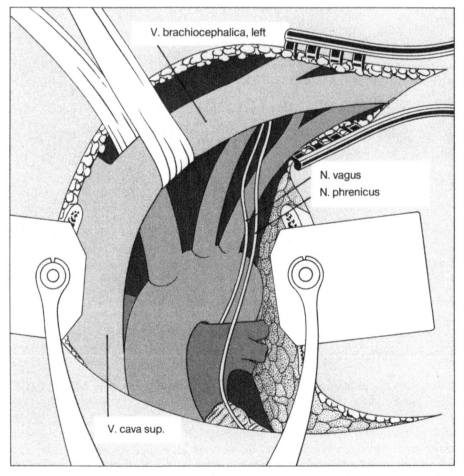

Fig. 28. The trapdoor approach permits a good exposure of the proximal supra-aortic branches, the brachiocephalic veins, and the proximal subclavian vein

and Ravitch [151] (Fig. 28). **It is the standard approach for injuries of the proximal portions of the subclavian artery and vein and of the brachiocephalic vessels.** It is a median sternotomy up to the level of the third intercostal space where, after cutting across the one side of the sternum, a small frontal thoracotomy is performed. In the upper section, the incision is made from the suprasternal notch supraclavicularly in a distal direction.

The incisions used in this procedure, which appear to be somewhat heroic, are tolerated astonishingly well and as a rule heal without complications.

4. Anterolateral Thoracotomy in the Third Intercostal Space

This approach permits a provisional **hemostasis** in hemorrhages into the thoracic cavity caused by injuries to vessels of the superior thoracic aperture. Its sole justification is as an emergency intervention for tamponade; the definitive treatment of the injury is usually not possible with this approach. The anterior thoracotomy can be extended to become a trapdoor approach.

5. Median Sternotomy, with Possible Cervical Extension (Fig. 27 D)

For injuries to the vessels near their origin at the aortic arch, especially on the right side, this approach offers an alternative to the trapdoor approach. It is associated with somewhat less morbidity. For injuries to vessels situated more distally, it is hardly suitable, however.

V. Thoracoabdominal Approach

For pure thoracic injuries, a thoracoabdominal approach is not indicated. In thoracoabdominal lesions, especially in gunshot and stab wounds, its application is also generally not advisable. If the operative opening of both body cavities is necessary, I prefer **separate approaches** by means of a midline laparotomy and a separate thoracotomy primarily because of the danger of infection.

A thoracoabdominal approach is accompanied by considerable morbidity. The pulmonary complication rate is higher, and the instability of the chest wall is not inconsiderable because of the incision through the rib cage. Above all, there is the danger of chondritis in the cartilaginous part of the rib.

However, there are some nonthoracic, specific abdominal injuries, especially severe liver ruptures, which in rare cases require a thoracoabdominal approach.

Chapter 7
Special Considerations in Penetrating Chest Injuries

Clinical procedures and treatment of penetrating injuries to individual thoracic structures and organs are described in the special chapters. Some general viewpoints are summarized separately here.

I. Causes of Injury and Intrathoracic Injuries

The circumstances surrounding gunshot and stab wounds to the thorax vary from country to country and region to region and reflect the mentality of the populace and the availability of individual weapons. Whereas in Finland, for example, virtually nothing but stab wounds necessitate clinical treatment [172, 179], in the southern parts of the United States gunshot wounds predominate [131]. Among 91 of our patients, nearly one-half (48%) of the penetrating injuries were caused by gunshot. Suicide attempts and criminal offences were about equally frequent.
Other are caused by impalement or by flying objects.

The degree of **destruction to tissue caused by a gunshot wound** depends upon two conditions:

1. The energy of the projectile (determined principally by its muzzle velocity and to a lesser extent by its mass) and its behavior during flight and at its target

2. The peculiar characteristics of the affected tissue

With a target velocity of less than 300 m/s, there is generally no tissue destruction to be expected essentially beyond the caliber of the bullet. Hand guns and machine pistols, with their relatively low muzzle velocity, do not attain this target speed. The tissue damage is therefore comparable to a stab wound.

It is a different story with the projectiles of modern flat-trajectory weapons (carbines, automatic rifles, machine guns). They have muzzle velocities of 750–850 m/s, the American M-16 automatic rifle even over 1000 m/s [153]. These high-velocity missiles not only create a tract corresponding to the size of the projectile as they slam through tissue, they also have an explosion-like effect with pressure-related laceration and contusion of the tissue **(cavitation)**.
The degree of this explosive effect is dependent upon the nature of the tissue, upon its elasticity, and its specific weight. Compact, parenchymous organs with high density, such as the liver, spleen, and kidneys, enhance this kind of tissue destruction. The same is true of the musculature and also of the thoracic wall.

Fig. 29. Machine rifle gunshot through the upper left lobe of the lung. Nearly complete disappearance of the parenchymal opacity within 1 week

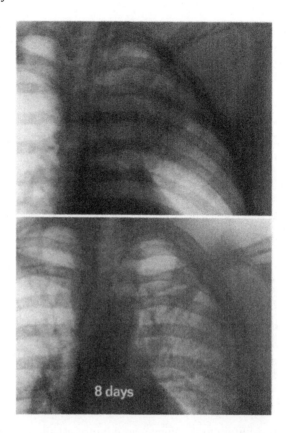

In this respect, **lung tissue** represents a special case compared to other body tissues. In contrast to the liver and muscles, which have a specific weight somewhat over 1, the specific weight of the lung is only 0.4 – 0.5 [153]. Furthermore, its high elasticity makes lung tissue more capable of resistance than other body structures. Amato [153] and Kolesov [168] have demonstrated experimentally that in gunshot wounds with high target velocity there is also a cavitation effect in the lung. This temporary cavitation, however, is much smaller than, for example, that of the muscles of the chest wall.

The resulting injury is a **mixture of lung laceration and lung contusion** (Fig. 29). In individual cases, a "lung contusion with respiratory insufficiency" may occur and is then characterized by a greatly reduced arterial PO_2, which is the result of the formation of an intrapulmonary right-to-left shunt [170].

It is remarkable that **tangential gunshot wounds of the thoracic wall** can cause greater lung damage than a shot through the lung itself. This is because the dense structure of the muscles of the chest wall and skeleton absorbs and transmits the shock of the projectile more intensively than the light and air-filled lung tissue [160, 161].

Example: In two of our patients with clean tangential gunshot wounds of the thoracic wall, we observed an extended opacity in the lung parenchyma corresponding to lung contusion, which gradually resolved [185] (Fig. 30).

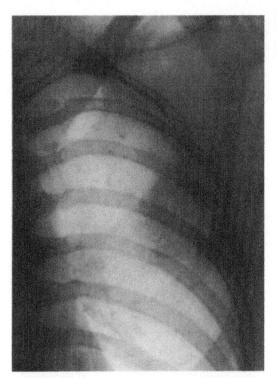

Fig. 30. Tangential gunshot wound of the thoracic wall without opening of the pleural cavity: contusion of lung tissue in the vicinity of the bullet tract

In addition to the lung, whose injury usually results in a **hemothorax** and/or **pneumothorax, all other intrathoracic structures** can obviously also be damaged. Injuries to the diaphragm (18% of our patients), the heart (16%), and the large vessels (12%) are relatively frequent. On the other hand, bronchial injuries brought to clinical attention are rare and even more so are lesions of the esophagus, intrathoracic trachea, aorta, and thoracic duct (among the 2811 cases reported from the Korean War by Valle [178], injuries to the four last-mentioned structures represented only 0.2% – 0.3% of all penetrating thoracic traumas).

II. Evaluation and Therapeutic Procedure

The difference in effect of a gunshot wound on lung tissue as compared to its effect on other tissues as well as the fact that hemostasis usually ensues spontaneously in an expanded lung as the result of the lower pressure in the pulmonary circulation makes it possible to **conservatively** treat the majority of cases. "Conservative" means, among other things, appropriate fluid therapy, chest tube drainage, and atelectasis prophylaxis. It does not mean being inactive. **Thoracotomy** is reserved for precisely defined indications. The demand occasionally raised that every penetrating thoracic wound to the chest cavity must be treated operatively [154, 175, 183] is not justified in view of the good results obtained when the decision to proceed surgically or conservatively is suited to each individual patient.

Experiences from Wartime Surgery

In Germany at the beginning of World War II, gunshot injuries to the thorax with a demonstrable lesion of the parenchyma were usually explored via thoracotomy [164, 167]. During the course of the war, however, a more conservative attitude asserted itself [159, 184]. People began to realize that the most essential problem was the management of the hemothorax. Besides thoracic puncture and prompt evacuation by means of thoracotomy, subsequent decortication of the lung also became general practice to prevent the later development of empyema and fibrothorax [165].
The experiences of the Korean and Vietnam Wars demonstrate unequivocally, however, that operative procedure should not be raised to the level of a rule and that decortication seldom becomes necessary, especially if there is ample early evacuation of air and blood from the pleural cavity [162, 181]. In contrast to the treatment by thoracentesis used principally in the Korean War [176, 178], with the introduction of the more effective chest tubes in the Vietnam War the results could again be improved and especially the frequency of empyema lowered [173, 174, 180].

Open Pneumothorax

Fortunately, in most cases of stab and gunshot wounds, as a consequence of spontaneous sealing of the wound tract by soft tissues of the chest wall, the dangerous situation of an open pneumothorax seldom develops. When it does, it is generally recognized immediately by the sucking sound of air entering the thorax. The acute threat is eliminated by **immediate airtight closure of the chest wound** or by immediate **intubation and mechanical ventilation** (see Chap. 11).

Treatment in the Absence of an Indication for Thoracotomy

If none of the indications for a thoracotomy listed below are present, stab wounds are sutered under **local anesthesia** and in gunshots, the wounds of entry and exit are surgically explored. Tissue that is contused and saturated with powder smoke is excised and the wound closed with suction drainage. Sources of more severe bleeding from the chest wall are either ligated or secured by suture. Smaller wounds are merely disinfected.
In cases of **hemothorax** and/or **pneumothorax**, a **chest tube** with 25 cm H_2O suction is applied. Upon insertion of the chest tube, up to 1500 ml of blood are usually evacuated. After expansion of the lungs, however, the bleeding almost always stops. The drainage must be efficient and must produce extensive evacuation of blood and complete reexpansion of the lungs. If need be, additional chest tubes are inserted.
Often the chest tube is removed **prematurely.** Gunshot wounds, in particular, cause considerable damage to the lung parenchyma and require several days, often up to 2 weeks, for sufficient sealing of the air leak. When a tube is removed prematurely, a recurrent pneumothorax is to be expected (Fig. 31).

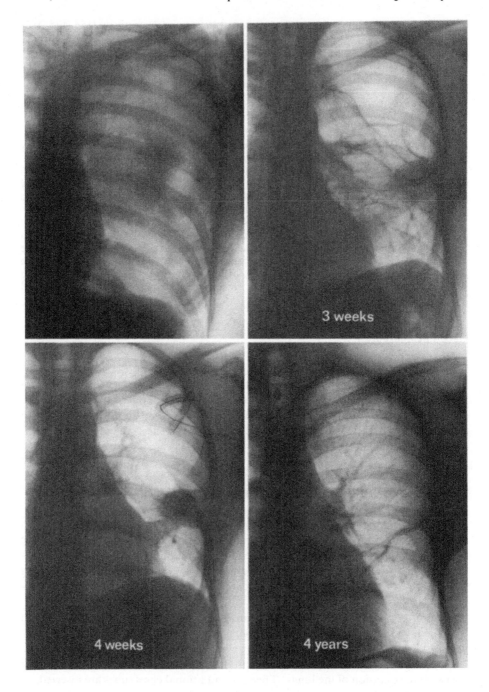

Fig. 31 a – d. Gunshot through the left side of lung caused by a revolver. **a** Upon admission, hemopneumothorax on the left side; **b** Thoracic drains removed prematurely: recurrence of pneumothorax in the left upper area; **c** Reexpansion after renewed suction drainage of the thorax; hematoma exists around the bullet tract; **d** Late appearance

Respiratory insufficiency and especially the appearance of adult respiratory distress syndrome in extensive lung contusions calls for respirator treatment. This is seldom the case in purely thoracic injuries.

A comprehensive **physical therapy program** is essential in every instance from the first day of hospitalization onward to ensure that the posttraumatic course remains complication-free.

The use of **antibiotics** is of doubtful value. The lung wound is very resistant to infection. The best prophylaxis of pleural empyema is optimal drainage of the pleural cavity. Since all that a prophylactic application of antibiotics does is to promote the development of resistant organisms, we have not used prophylactic antibiotic medication since 1972. Changes in the course of recovery and more frequent occurrences of pneumonia or lung abscesses were not observed.

Indications for Thoracotomy

The experience of the last 10 years, both during the Vietnam War and also in peacetime due to the increased number of penetrating thoracic injuries, permits us today to precisely delineate the operative indications:

1. **Injuries to the heart and great vessels:** when there is cardiac tamponade (Fig. 32), massive blood loss, or when the direction of the gunshot tract indicates involvement of the heart or large vessels. As a stopgap or diagnostic measure, if there is suspicion of cardiac tamponade, pericardiocentesis can be done; if there is a hemopericardium, however, operation must follow immediately.

2. **Massive and persistent blood loss through the chest drains,** especially if the circulation cannot be maintained by volume replacement. The amount of blood initially drained by the insertion of a chest tube does not always reveal the true picture.

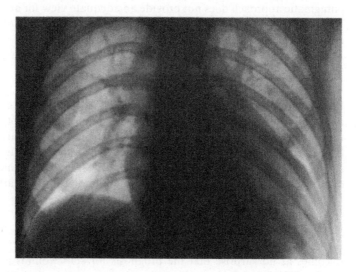

Fig. 32. Hemopericardium with cardiac tamponade occasioned by gunshot through the left ventricle by a Flobert gun

3. **Bronchial or tracheal injuries**

4. **Massive bleeding into the bronchial tree**

5. **Injuries to the esophagus,** confirmed by esophagography. Every penetrating thoracic injury involving the posterior mediastinum requires esophagography.

A massive hemothorax, which cannot be evacuated by thoracic drainage because blood coagulation has set in, provides an indication for **early removal of hematoma** from a few days to 2 weeks after the injury.

Thoracoabdominal Injuries

Penetrating injuries of the thorax with abdominal involvement produce a considerably higher mortality, most especially when it is the colon that shares the injury [157]. In the abdomen, it is by far the liver that is injured most frequently (in the large series of patients studied by Borja [157] it was 61%).
Penetrating thoracic injuries with suspicion or confirmation of abdominal involvement **offer in every instance an indication for a laparotomy.** Evidence of a projectile in the abdomen, injuries in the area of the lower thorax with the wound going in the direction of the abdomen, symptoms and findings of an acute abdomen, unexplained blood loss, and evidence of a perforating diaphragmatic injury provided by a thoracotomy point toward abdominal involvement.
The operative approach of choice is the **midline laparotomy** even when, in taking care of intrathoracic injuries, a thoracotomy was performed. Because of the possibility of colon injury and the greater morbidity of a thoracoabdominal incision with the danger of osteomyelitis or chondritis of the rib cage, separate approaches are recommended. A thoracoabdominal approach is indicated only if an injury in the upper belly (e. g., a severe liver injury) cannot be treated in any other way. A transdiaphragmatic approach does not provide an adequate view for abdominal inspection. The chest injury is treated with suction drainage as long as there is no operative indication for a thoracotomy.

Projectiles in the Thoracic Area

If projectiles from retained missiles lie intrathoracically, they generally need not be removed as long as the injury caused by the projectile does not require a thoracotomy. For the most part, they do not cause any trouble. If they are lodged subdermally or in the musculature, they can be removed at some later date. There is no urgent reason here for immediate intervention. A special case with unique problems, however, is represented by projectiles or bullet fragments in the heart (see Chap. 17).

III. Prognosis

It comes as no surprise that the prognosis for stab wounds is better than that of gunshot injuries and that, of the latter, those caused by projectiles of lower velocity have a more favorable prognosis. Comparisons of the lethality in individual studies are pointless: the causes of injury vary greatly; often patients who are dead on arrival at the hospital are not included, and although shorter transportation times between injury and reception at the clinic now give some patients a better chance of survival, their severe injuries tend to prejudice the statistics. Under civilian circumstances, the data on lethality show 2% for pure stab wounds [179] and 10%–14% for gunshot wounds [155, 156].

Later prognosis for surviving patients is astonishingly good; permanent damage or incapacity to work caused by thoracic injuries are rare.

Review of Our Patients

We surveyed 91 cases of penetrating thoracic injuries, 48% of which were gunshot wounds. There were 15 heart injuries, 11 injuries of the large vessels, and 16 injuries to the diaphragm. Additional abdominal involvement affected 19 patients.

In 21 patients a thoracotomy was performed, in 13 a laparotomy, and in 8 other patients an opening of both body cavities was necessary.

Of these 91 patients, 5 died, resulting in a mortality of 5.5%. One patient died immediately upon arrival at the hospital, and two died of abdominal complications following thoracoabdominal gunshot wounds. Of the remaining two patients, one had suffered from preexistent cardiac failure and in the other there was shock-induced damage to lung and kidneys.

A **follow-up review** of 33 patients [182] revealed no significant pathologic finding. The pulmonary function tests were comparable to those of a healthy population. In the thoracic roentgenograms there were often discrete findings: a conglutinated phrenicocostal sinus or an atypical diaphragmatic appearance.

Chapter 8
Aspects of Intensive Care of Patients with Thoracic Injuries

I. Basic Considerations

Like every other kind of intensive care, the intensive therapy of patients with thoracic injuries, and particularly patients with multiple trauma, is **interdisciplinary.** It presupposes a treatment team in which surgeons, anesthesiologists, and internists work together. This circumstance should not obscure the fact that, in the final analysis, one single physician, trained in emergency surgery and at the same time well versed in the problems of intensive medicine, must retain supervision over **all** problems of the patient and establish priorities. An "organ specialist" may indeed be a valuable advisor, yet can never guarantee such patients the necessary, comprehensive therapy. The seriously injured patient needs **one** doctor who feels responsible to the patient for everything and in every respect. It goes without saying that modern intensive care is impossible without the collaboration of competent and well-trained nurses and attendants.

1. The intensive care of patients with thoracic injuries is not so much a matter of heroic decisions or managing acute, life-threatening situations nor of expensive electronic equipment, but rather — even more than usually assumed — it is **detail work.** The real key to success lies in the **attention paid to detail:** uninterrupted surveillance, changing the patients' position, suctioning the patient, breathing exercises, counteracting effusion formations and atelectasis, and optimal treatment of incidental attendant injuries even if they appear to be trivial.

2. A **constant reevaluation** of the patient is absolutely necessary. Experience teaches us that there are many injuries in the chest area or consequences of such injuries that are not diagnosed until later developments occur or are overlooked altogether [2]: cardiac contusions, ruptures of the diaphragm, aorta, or esophagus, or the development of ARDS.

3. Thoracic injuries, but also many procedures in intensive medicine, involve a **considerable risk of complications. Every therapy program must be sensitive to the possibility of complication.** The prophylaxis of possible complications is of crucial importance.

It is obvious that neither the fundamental techniques of intensive care nor a general overview of the variety of problems involved in intensive medical treatment of the severely injured can be dealt with within the scope of this book. For that I refer you to the appropriate comprehensive works of Lawin [199], Kucher and Steinbereithner [197], and Zschoche [206]; for techniques and problems of ventilation: Wolff [205] and Bendixen et al. [187].

Patients with thoracic injuries often present **special problems** in intensive care, several of which will be discussed briefly.

II. Monitoring and Evaluating the Patient with Thoracic Injuries in Intensive Care

With the severely injured, to a greater degree than in the rest of intensive care, the rule applies that: the intensive care nurse belongs **at the side of the patient,** at the sick bed, and not in front of a control center with monitors. On the other hand, "clinical evaluation" by itself is completely inadequate; without continual recourse to reliable instrumental data, the treatment of critical patients is doomed to failure. The monitoring of the **state of consciousness, blood pressure, central venous pressure,** and **urinary output** should be a matter of course.

1. ECG

During the first several days, every severe thoracic injury requires surveillance by ECG monitoring. The concern is not for diagnosis of ischemic changes but for **early recognition of disturbances in heart rhythm** (see Chap. 16).

2. Periodic Arterial Blood Gas Analysis

Even if there is no electronic measurement of blood pressure, the insertion of a **permanent intra-arterial catheter** for taking arterial blood samples is recommended. We prefer the cannulation of the femoral artery, using the Seldinger technique. Complications are extremely rare; however, as a rule, no patient with an intra-arterial catheter may be sent back to a regular ward. The normal arterial blood gas analysis, which must be possible any hour of the day or night, is supplemented in critical patients by daily determinations of PO_2 after 20 min of ventilation with pure oxygen (oxygenation test, see Chap. 4).

3. Pulmonary Artery Catheter

A floating catheter in the pulmonary artery (Swan-Ganz) provides three essential items of information:

1. By making possible the withdrawal of **mixed venous blood,** the intrapulmonary **right-to-left shunt fraction** ($\dot{Q}_S/\dot{Q}_T$) can be calculated.

2. **Measurement of pulmonary artery pressure:** increased pulmonary vascular resistance can be lowered by application of alpha blockers (phentolamine initially 5 mg IV, then 0.1 – 0.5 mg/min; maximum dosage 2 mg/min) [198].

3. The measurement of **pulmonary capillary pressure** (PCP) or of the **wedge pressure** makes it possible to evaluate the **left side of the heart** [203].

In spite of all this, the indication for insertion of a pulmonary artery catheter should be implemented within narrow limits: the duration of its use is limited because of the danger of infection, whereas the illness of these patients may stretch out for weeks.

4. Determining Cardiac Output

In the evaluation of severe pulmonary disturbances, especially in ARDS, the function of the heart is of decisive importance (see Chap. 4). Practical experience shows that cardiac output in such cases **cannot be assessed clinically.** An substantial intrapulmonary right-to-left shunt always results initially in a compensatory increase of cardiac output (see Fig. 33 for example). It is important to **deal early** with a **reduction** of cardiac output secondary to cardiac decompensation and, if necessary, to increase it with medication. In such cases, we prefer using dopamine (150 – 1000 μg/min) because of its favorable renal effect [192]. It must be remembered, however, that dopamine is often not potent enough and must be replaced by epinephrine or isoproterenol.

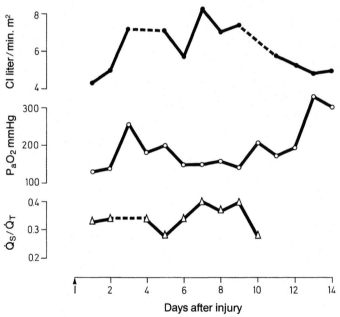

Fig. 33. ARDS: progress of cardiac index (CI), right-to-left shunt ($\dot{Q}_S/\dot{Q}_T$), and P_aO_2 in the oxygenation test ($F_IO_2 = 1.0$). In the period of greatest shunt fraction, the cardiac output increases compensatorily and attains a level of 16 liters/min (CI of 8 liters/min m²). The increased cardiac output may inversely have led to a larger shunt fraction. Not until the pulmonary situation had improved (reduction of shunt fraction, increase of P_aO_2) did the cardiac output decrease again (A. D., male, 29 years old)

5. Roentgenograms of the Thorax

In the acute phase, daily roentgenograms of the thorax make it possible to recognize a pneumothorax, atelectasis, effusion formation, pneumonic infiltrates, left-sided cardiac insufficiency, etc. The location of central venous catheters, pulmonary catheters, and endotracheal tubes is kept track of by radiologic means.

6. Laboratory Determinations

In addition to the usual laboratory investigations that are generally made, the daily determination of **serum protein** is important because of its significance in intravascular oncotic pressure (see Table 10). The determination of **specific cardiac enzymes** (particularly CPK isoenzymes and LDH isoenzymes) is important for the diagnosis of cardiac contusion.

III. Mechanical Ventilation

For the technique of **mechanical ventilation,** I refer you to the general works mentioned above. In general, volume-controlled ventilators are used, and a low rate as well as a positive end-expiratory pressure (PEEP usually of $+10$ cm H_2O) are selected. For long-term mechanical ventilation, we sedate and relax the patient, not the least of which is for psychological reasons.
I shall not discuss the **respiratory approach** (long-term intubation or tracheotomy) here. We use **nasal intubation without temporal limits** except for weekly changes of the tube. Tracheostomy for long-term ventilatory support is undertaken only when fractures of the facial bones require it, when intubation is very difficult for technical reasons, or when severe brain damage indicates that later the patient will not be able to maintain open airways during spontaneous breathing.
In the **transitional phase,** from controlled to spontaneous breathing, in addition to volume- or pressure-regulated instruments with trigger mechanisms, new procedures, such as **intermittent mandatory ventilation (IMV)** [191] and spontaneous breathing with **continuous positive airway pressure (CPAP)** [193], are used to good advantage.

IV. Principles for the Infusion of Fluids

When fluids are transfused in large quantities in lung injury (e. g., lung contusion) and with increased permeability of the lung capillaries (ARDS), more water gathers in the pulmonary interstitial tissue than in the rest of the body tissues [88, 97, 131]. Thus, free water should be infused in minimal quantities.

In patients without excessive loss of fluids, the prescribed **water balance** is +500 – +700 ml in the first days after trauma and is increased to a level of +700 – +1000 ml.

If larger quantities of fluids need to be infused (parenteral feeding, continuous infusion of medication by infusion pump), the desired water balance is achieved by means of diuretics (e. g., furosemide). Obviously, water balance should be regarded separately from volume infusion and volume loss.

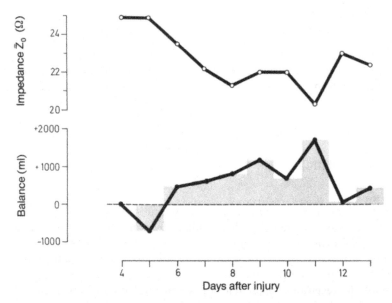

Fig. 34. Fluid content of the lung, determined relatively by measurement of the average impedance ($\bar{Z}_0$), is dependent upon the daily water balance. Increased water intake results in an accumulation of water in the lungs and consequently a drop in $\bar{Z}_0$. The process is still partially reversible by reducing the water balance (E. K., male, 75 years old)

This somewhat rigorous therapy of minimal free water infusion should only be carried out under appropriate **controls** to avoid renal failure. Of great significance is the **daily determination of urea and creatinine** in the serum. An increase of urea without a corresponding increase of creatinine is a reliable indication of exsiccosis and a warning that the balance should be raised. Other clues are provided by the **serum protein level, urine production,** and the **osmolality of the urine.** In this respect, determination of serum sodium is not as helpful because its level is affected by infusions and by the influence of diuretics.

By continuous **measurement of electrical impedance** of the thorax, relative changes in the fluid content of the lung can be assessed. It was thus possible to prove that the fluid content of the lung actually depends to a high degree upon the infusion of free water and that "errors in balance" caused by increased fluid infusion immediately lead to increased water retention in the lung (Fig. 34).

V. Subsequent Pulmonary Complications

Atelectasis

The intensive care of patients with thoracic injuries is an unremitting struggle against the formation of atelectasis (Fig. 35). The disturbed mechanics of respiration occasioned by chest fractures, pain, and formation of effusion and hematoma result in regional hypoventilation, on the one hand, and lead to difficulties in expectoration of secretions, on the other, with both resulting in the formation of atelectasis. Because of the supine position and the inability to actively cough, this also becomes a threat when a respirator is used, even with PEEP. Additionally, a high inhaled oxygen concentration causes the formation of atelectasis. In poorly aerated areas, oxygen is quickly absorbed and as a result resorption atelectasis occurs [190].
In this development, **prophylaxis** is of extreme importance, and **intensive breathing exercises** (see Chap. 9) play a major role. Adequate moistening of the inhaled air prevents the drying out of bronchial secretions.

1. In patients on a respirator, a **positive end-expiratory pressure** conteracts the formation of atelectasis by raising the functional residual capacity. Here, too, physiotherapeutic measures are unavoidable.

2. Changing the patient's **position from side to side** is especially important in prophylaxis. It is very tempting to be satisfied with minimal turning from the supine position, but this is inadequate. Even severe injuries to the thoracic wall with multiple rib fractures permit the patient to be placed on the injured side.

3. **Percussion and vibration** of the chest wall can serve to loosen the accumulation of secretions. Tracheobronchial suctioning then follows these physiotherapeutic procedures.

The **treatment of atelectasis** must be accomplished consistently and with a determination approaching stubbornness. In general, it is said one must treat the patient and not the X-ray picture. Nevertheless, in atelectasis formation it is necessary to "treat the X-ray picture," even if things are still going well with the patient. In other words, if the patient is feeling well and there is little change in the blood gas analysis, a roentgenogram indicating atelectasis formation may not be treated with indifference.
In atelectasis **therapy** (Table 14), **physiotherapeutic procedures** (laying the patient on his side, percussion, forced inspiration, expectoration) are put first. These will

Table 14. Therapy in atelectasis formation

---
1. Physiotherapeutic procedures (laying patient on his side, percussion, vibrating, IPPB, etc.)
   If unsuccessful:
2. Endotracheal suction (blind or with laryngoscope)
   If unsuccessful:
3. Bronchoscopic suction (possibly followed by intubation and brief ventilation with PEEP)

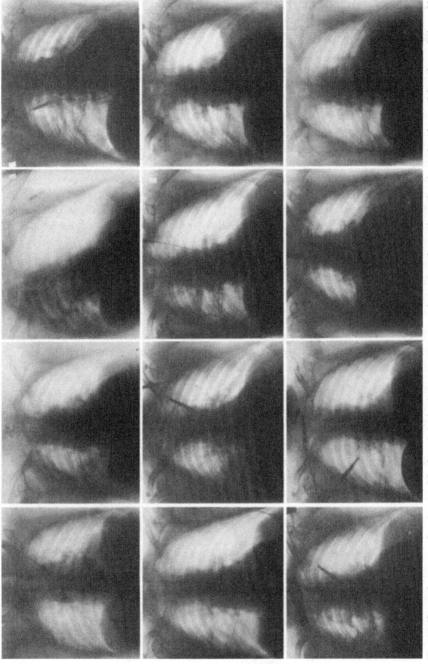

Fig. 35. Intensive care of patients with chest injuries is a constant struggle against formation of atelectasis; changeful atelectasis in a 65-year-old ventilated male patient with multiple rib fractures on the right, subdural hematoma, and cerebral contusion

suffice in almost all cases. These procedures are supplemented by **endotracheal suction** (blind or with the aid of a laryngoscope); not only is the removal of secretions by suction important in itself but in conscious patients also the stimulation of coughing.

Only in exceptional cases will it be necessary to resort to **bronchoscopic suction.** When the decision is made to take this step for the first time in a case of chest injury, bronchoscopy should also be used **diagnostically** for purposes of excluding the possibility of injuries to the bronchi.

However, we should not set our hopes too high for the treatment of atelectasis in chest trauma by means of bronchoscopic suction: the accompanying essential active inspiration of the patient will be impaired by any preceding anesthesia or sedation. In rib fractures, pain and mechanical factors restrict the expansion of the lungs so severely that removal of the secretions alone is not sufficient to clear up the atelectatic areas. In such cases, we usually follow bronchoscopy with a brief period of intubation with strong inflation of the lungs by means of an air bag or occasionally even by ventilation with PEEP for 24 h.

Example: An instructive example is shown in Fig. 36: a 20-year-old patient, after chest trauma, had a typical roentgenogram of **atelectasis in the left lower lobe** with displacement of the heart to the left (Fig. 36 a). After bronchoscopic suctioning, the findings remained unchanged. Ultimately, the result was **total atelectasis of the left lung** (Fig. 36 b). Renewed bronchoscopy with definitive opening of all bronchi out to the periphery brought about little improvement in the radiologic findings. Only then did it become obvious that the breathing mechanism of the patient, which had been disturbed by a sternal fracture, made adequate reexpansion of the atelectatic lung impossible. It was not until **positive pressure ventilation** had been applied with a respirator for 12 h after another bronchoscopy and manual inflation that conditions returned to normal (Fig. 36 c). The patient subsequently remained free of further pulmonary complications.

Tension Pneumothorax

All forms of respiratory support, especially in which positive end-expiratory pressure is applied, run the risk of producing tension pneumothorax [201, 202, 207]. This danger is especially great in patients with thoracic injuries because during ventilation even insignificant lesions of the lung can often lead to pneumothoraces. **In late stages of ARDS,** tension pneumothorax usually occurs; in these cases, high respiratory pressures are unavoidable, and due both to the loss of elasticity in the lung tissue and to infection, such lungs are especially fragile [200].

In the ventilation of a patient with multiple rib fractures there is, therefore, a firm rule: insert a **chest tube prophylactically** on the injured side. In contrast to the older rubber thoracic drains, the newer siliconized trocar catheters (Argyle) remain functional for a long time. A further rule for prophylaxis requires that **no** thoracic drains be **removed** while the patient is still being **ventilated.**

Naturally, chest tubes in patients receiving controlled ventilation are **not to be clamped off** during the change of suction bottles or during the time the patient is being moved. The use of a **Heimlich valve** (see Chap. 11) can serve as an alternative to simply leaving the drainage open. Experience teaches us that there is an almost irresistable temptation to provide the chest tubes with a clamp, even for patients on a respirator with massive air loss.

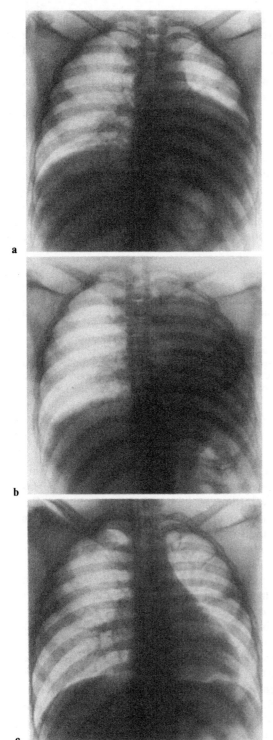

Fig. 36. a Atelectasis of the lower left lobe; b Later, total left lung atelectasis cannot be removed solely by bronchoscopic suction; c Reexpanded lung after bronchoscopic suction and mechanical ventilation with PEEP (see text)

A tension pneumothorax developing while a patient is on a respirator is a harmless complication if it is recognized immediately; otherwise, it is fatal. A sudden **rise in respiratory pressure** combined with a **rise in the central venous pressure** is an almost infallible indication. Generally, once alerted by it, one can readily confirm the suspicion and determine the side involved by the distended but hardly mobile half of the thorax, the hypersonorous sound in response to percussion, and the presence of diminished breath sounds. Taking thoracic roentgenograms merely means a loss of time.

Recognizing a tension pneumothorax can, however, also be a **very difficult clinical diagnosis.** This is the case if there are partially adherent areas of pleura and the tension pneumothorax is localized (Fig. 37) or when severely fibrosed lungs in a late stage of ARDS can no longer collapse (Fig. 38). Under these conditions, the breath sounds remain audible on the respirator. If the clinical diagnosis is impossible, thoracic roentgenograms are always resorted to immediately if there is a rise in respiratory pressure that cannot be explained.

Once a drop in blood pressure has occurred, only a few minutes are available for the immediate relief of pressure by insertion of a chest tube before cardiac arrest occurs. Relief of pressure by means of a large cannula can be momentarily helpful at best but is inadequate for a longer period of time on the respirator. Chest tubes must be available and ready for use in every intensive care unit.

Even a chest tube already in place does not exclude the possibility of a tension pneumothorax of the same side of the chest. It can be clogged; but more frequently,

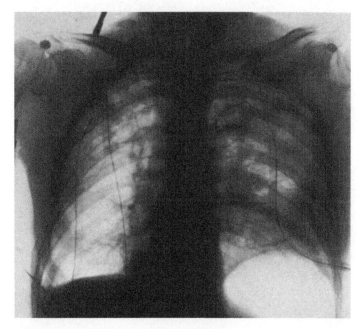

Fig. 37. In the presence of pleural adhesions, a localized left basal tension pneumothorax occurs with mechanical ventilation even with chest drainage. Mediastinal shift, falling blood pressure. Clinical diagnosis is hardly possible

however, there are local adhesions, and the tension pneumothorax is formed in another location. One should not hesitate to insert as many tubes as are necessary for complete evacuation of air (Fig. 39).

Pulmonary Infections

Twenty-five percent of all patients with thoracic injuries in our intensive care unit incur bronchial pneumonia. In virtually every case, these were **patients on the respirator.** If pulmonary infection is unavoidable despite all efforts to the contrary, it can normally be kept under control and only in exceptional cases results in death.
In the **prophylaxis** of bronchopulmonary infections, (1) **physiotherapy** also plays a decisive role. (2) Equally important is conscientious care of the trachea with **gentle** but effective **suctioning** of tracheobronchial secretions under the most sterile conditions possible. (3) An adequate but not excessive **moistening of the air passages** must be ensured.
The focus of prophylactic measures is centered in **nursing care.** Other beneficial definitive treatment is undertaken: drainage of hemothorax or pneumothorax for

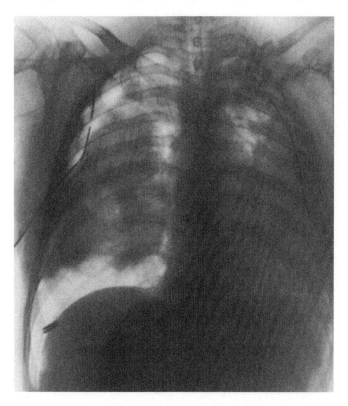

Fig. 38. Tension pneumothorax during mechanical ventilation in an advanced stage of ARDS: in spite of massive intrapleural positive pressure, the lung, filled with fluid and fibrosed, can no longer collapse. Breath sounds have changed very little

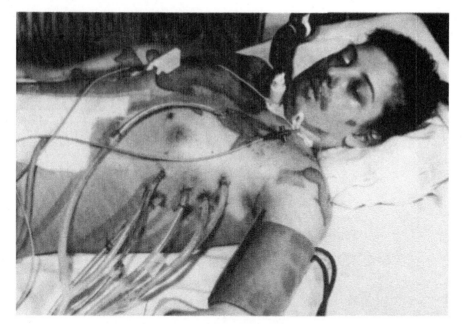

Fig. 39. An 18-year-old female patient with very severe thoracic trauma and ARDS. A recurrent tension pneumothorax required the insertion of a total of seven chest tubes on the left side

complete reexpansion of the lungs, treatment of atelectasis, operative treatment of diaphragmatic ruptures, bronchial ruptures, etc.

Prophylactic use of antibiotics is futile. Their use does not protect against pneumonia; all that happens is that an infection develops with a strain that is resistant to the particular antibiotic being used.

In 685 blunt thoracic injuries, half of which were treated prophylactically with antibiotics, Ashbaugh [186] determined that the frequency of pneumonia was twice as great in the group treated prophylactically. The mortality of this group was also almost twice as high (11%) as in patients receiving no prophylactic antibiotics (6%).

In every intubated or tracheotomized patient, pathogenic organisms are found in tracheal secretions 1–2 weeks after trauma [196]. This **colonization** is part of the normal course of events and does not as yet justify antibiotic therapy. Not until clinical and/or radiologic signs disclose pneumonia are antibiotics indicated. In this situation the nursing care is equally as important [194].

The antibiotic medication is then as germ-specific as possible. Bacteriologic examination of tracheal secretions at least once a week as well as surveillance of the actual organisms that occupy the intensive care unit usually permit a choice of the most specific antibiotic possible. A **strict "antibiotic regimen"** keeps critical antibiotics (e.g., aminoglycosides) in reserve according to precise guidelines as long as other medications are still effective. If chemotherapeutics or antibiotics are introduced, their application in the intensive care unit should be done intravenously at optimal dosages.

In my experience, **resistance seldom develops** under these circumstances. Rather, in individual patients there is an occasional **change of the causative organism.** In determining therapy, the **clinical course** is at least as important as the bacteriologic findings: with the appearance of new infiltrates or the increase of existing ones during antibiotic therapy, a change of the causative organism should already be suspected clinically and the medication altered.

Chapter 9
Physiotherapy of Patients with Thoracic Injuries

I. Basic Considerations

The significance of physiotherapeutic measures in the treatment of thoracic injuries cannot be overemphasized. Besides **coughing up secretions,** the **goal** of respiratory therapy consists in **maintaining the greatest possible functional residual capacity,** which aids in avoiding threatening complications, such as the formation of atelectasis and microatelectasis (with development of a right-to-left shunt) and infections. Undoubtedly, in many cases treatment with a respirator can also be avoided through intensive, optimal physiotherapy [213].

Physiotherapy for the severely injured should not be restricted to "normal" working hours on weekdays. As irreplaceable as trained, competent physiotherapists are for the care of these patients, it is only in exceptional cases that their services can be scheduled during evening hours. The nurse, especially the **nurse in the intensive care unit,** must then take over physiotherapeutic care and ensure the continuity of

Table 15. Physiotherapeutic measures for thoracic injuries

1. General:	Percussion, vibration	Indispensable
	Alternate positioning on side	Indispensable
	Deep breathing	
	Diaphragmatic breathing	When respiratory insufficiency threatens
2. Forced expiration:	Coughing/induced coughing	Indispensable
	Balloon inflation	
	Blowing against cotton wadding	Doubtful: only the prior unconsciously increased inspiration has favorable effect
	Breathing against resistance (water bottle)	
3. CO_2-induced increase in ventilation:	Enlargement of dead space (Giebel tube)	Possible increase in ventilation by increasing respiratory frequency is ineffective; only with frequency below 20
4. Intermittent positive pressure respiration (IPPB):	IPPB Monaghan Bird	Good and effective measure, possibly combined with inhalation of bronchial dilators
5. Maximal voluntary inspiration	Bartlett-Edwards incentive spirometer	Excellent, simple exercise

the treatment. Special emphasis should be placed on methods of treatment that the patient, after prior instruction by the physiotherapist, can carry on alone or with only minimal assistance.

Of the many methods that find general application, some are based on clear concepts of lung physiology, some have proved their value empirically, and again others have no basis whatsoever. The following presents a survey of the most important and helpful measures, together with references to advantages and disadvantages (Table 15). The choice of an optimal method does not by itself guarantee success; it requires devotion and the competence of the therapist and most especially frequent application.

Because there are various methods available, which also find a variety of acceptance among patients, **respiratory therapy** should be **custom-tailored** to suit the individual patient with thoracic injuries. This therapy should not be made the sole responsibility of the physiotherapist; greater commitment on the part of physicians and more supervision by medical doctors than is normally the case would be desirable.

II. General Measures

Every respiratory therapy applied in fractures of the chest causes **pain** that makes success doubtful. Preceding medication with potent analgesics is crucial. **Deep**

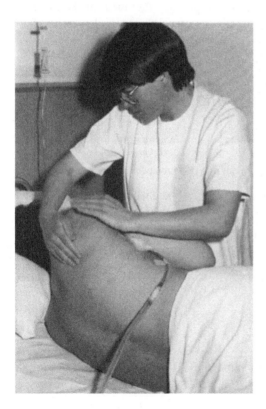

Fig. 40. Loosening up secretions by percussion and vibration of the patient in a lateral position

breathing exercises and **induced coughing** are better tolerated by the patient if the hands of the therapist keep the fracture sites immobile to lessen the pain. **Percussion** and **vibration** bring about the release of secretions, which are then coughed up or removed via endotracheal suctioning.

As with the patient on a respirator, it is also essential that the patient breathing spontaneously is **positioned on his side** (Fig. 40) for purposes of atelectasis prophylaxis and better aeration of otherwise basal parts of the lung. In accomplishing this, the position taken is not simply modified supine but an actual 90° lateral position.

Even in severe multiple rib fractures, no damage is done by appropriate percussion, vibration, and laying the patient on the side of his injured chest. The fear that a "lung injury" or "bleeding" will be brought on by such physiotherapeutic means is unfounded.

In patients with extensive rib fractures, even in certain cases of paradoxical respiration, an appropriate, well-directed **introduction to diaphragmatic breathing** can on occasion help to avoid respiratory insufficiency [213]. Diaphragmatic breathing even makes spontaneous breathing possible in an opened chest, as reports from China on lung operations with acupuncture indicate. The injured person is made aware of diaphragmatic breathing by feeling his abdomen with his hand.

III. Forced Expiration

Except for **spontaneous coughing** or **induced coughing** (e. g., by means of an endotracheal suction catheter), the value of exercises in this group is minimal. The goal of trying to attain maximal continuous inflation of as many alveoli as possible is not reached by these means. Rather, the increased expiration will result in alveolar collapse. A more desirable effect is achieved only in roundabout ways, namely, by unconsciously increasing inhalation before the exhalation exercise. What is involved is

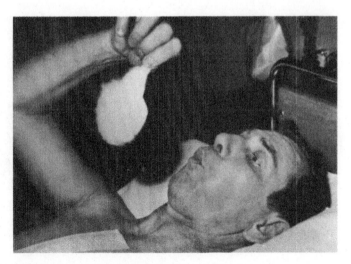

Fig. 41. Forced expiration by blowing at a wad of cotton-wool

a laborious, indirect, and often painful route with low efficiency to reach increased alveolar ventilation.

However, such exercises require only a few, simple aids (balloon blowing, blowing at a wad of cotton-wool [Fig. 41], exhaling over water bottles that serve as resistances). The prerequisites for their use are minimal; they can be implemented even if the patient exhibits limited willingness to cooperate and has a low level of intelligence.

IV. CO_2 -Induced Increase in Ventilation

By **enlarging the dead space,** partial rebreathing is achieved; the CO_2 retention stimulates the breathing center and results in increasing the ventilation minute volume. This is not alveolar hyperventilation since it does not result in a decrease in the arterial PCO_2.

The method involving enlargement of dead space introduced by Schwartz and Dale [218] in 1957 was improved upon for clinical usage in German-speaking countries by Giebel, who made it possible to adjust dead space enlargement to individual needs [214, 215]: every unit of the **Giebel tube** enlarges the dead space by 100 ml: the demands made of the patient can be increased (Fig. 42).

The favorable effect of such an enlargement of dead space for atelectasis prophylaxis in the postoperative period has been repeatedly described [212, 214, 215, 218]. The increase in ventilation minute volume, which is always attained, is ideally achieved by raising the tidal volume. This is the only desirable effect, whereas increasing the respiratory frequency is senseless and only an encumbrance.

Therein lies the difficulty of applying this method to patients with a traumatized thorax. Many of these patients develop considerable **tachypnea,** which only in-

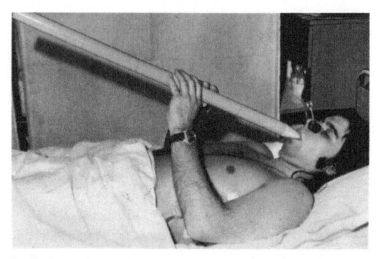

Fig. 42. Every unit of the Giebel tube enlarges the dead space by 100 ml

creases with use of the Giebel tube. With a respiratory frequency rate of more than 20/min, respiratory therapy by enlarging dead space is not indicated. With a normal rate before the exercise, careful monitoring of the respiratory frequency and pulse is essential. The enlargement of dead space should be adjusted in such a way that the respiratory frequency remains below 20/min. Therapy to enlarge dead space is contraindicated in paradoxical respiration.

V. Intermittent Positive Pressure Breathing (IPPB)

Ventilation of the lungs with a **small pressure-controlled respirator** connected to a mouthpiece (IPPB by Monaghan, Bird) has the desired effect of forcing inspiration and can open alveoli and keep them open (Fig. 43). The principle, introduced in 1958 by Rudy [217] and Noehren [216], is universally recognized and constitutes one of the most important exercises in our plan of treatment. It can be combined with the inhalation of bronchodilators.
Despite the convincing theoretical basis, however, there is one "fly in the ointment" in the practical application of such equipment: the tidal volume is not a constant volume as such, but is limited by the (adjustable) respiratory pressure. Every **resistance by the patient** to the air stream, whether it is deliberate or caused by the pain of a rib fracture, results in an increase of the respiratory pressure and diminishes the inspiratory volume. A decrease in the functional residual capacity (e. g., in atelectasis formation) necessitates a diminished volume to attain the preselected pressure; with diminished tidal volume, the proportion of ventilated dead space increases.

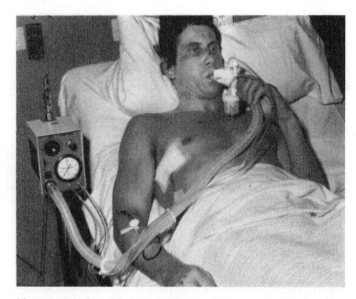

Fig. 43. Intermittent positive pressure breathing as respiratory therapy using a Monaghan IPPB respirator

In controlled studies of postoperative atelectasis prophylaxis, not all results were reported as favorable (e. g., 210). One possible reason may lie in the fact that an application repeated four times daily during a 10 – 15 min period is not sufficient for attaining the therapy goal; the patient should be able to reach for the equipment himself during the course of a 24-h period and engage in the exercises, again always under the supervision and control of the therapist or intensive care nurse.

Active cooperation of the patient is a necessity. What is more, proper equipment and appropriately trained personnel may not be available everywhere.

VI. Maximal Voluntary Inspiration

A **deep, sustained inspiration** undoubtedly achieves the goal of opening the greatest possible number of alveoli and maintaining the highest possible residual capacity. This can be achieved voluntarily with proper guidance and occurs, for example, during **yawning.** Such breathing exercises have proved their worth in atelectasis prophylaxis [219]. Ward [221] was able to prove that **holding** the breath at the maximum point of inspiration is of substantial significance for alveolar distention.

Use of the **Bartlett-Edwards "incentive spirometer"** is a great help [208, 209]. The ideal requirements for opening up the alveoli, namely, **the highest possible intra-alveolar pressure over the longest possible period of time at the highest possible inhalation volume,** are met by this device [209].

With this equipment the patient himself inhales a volume of air, fixed beforehand and adjusted to his capabilities. If this tidal volume, which is set as high as possible,

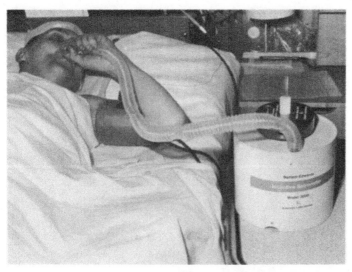

Fig. 44. Application of the Bartlett-Edwards "incentive spirometer" (see text). This 58-year-old male patient with severe multiple rib fractures successfully did the exercise 1442 times during the first 3 days after his accident

is attained, a red light goes on. If the inhalation continues beyond the preselected volume, the light continues to glow until no air is being inhaled anymore. Every one of such inhalations is registered on a counter (Fig. 44).

The patient's cooperation is essential. After instruction has been given in the use of the device, breathing exercises are possible at any time, even without the therapist being present. The accompanying circumstances (red light, counter) should offer the patient a certain amount of sporting incentive.

The effectiveness of this method was analyzed by Van De Water et al. [220] in a controlled study with impedance measurements. They obtained somewhat better results than with intermittent positive pressure breathing, at costs of less than one-tenth that of IPPB therapy.

Since 1972 therapy with the incentive spirometer has been part of our standard procedure for respiratory therapy of patients with thoracic injuries. Most of the conscious patients like to work with the equipment; only a few are unwilling to cooperate. Analysis of 116 patients revealed that during the treatment period the exercise was carried out on an average of 130 times a day.

The results of working with this equipment have impressively confirmed how severely the vital capacity is reduced in rib fractures. The volume of inhalation achieved by exercise is very small during the first few days and for the most part in multiple rib fractures only amounts to around 500 ml.

Part II

Diagnosis, Clinical Significance, and Treatment of Specific Injuries

Chapter 10
Rib and Sternum Fractures

I. General Considerations

Clinical Significance

There are three reasons why fractures of the thoracic wall can be dangerous injuries:

1. **Simultaneous internal injuries of the thorax.** Even individual rib fractures that might otherwise be insignificant can, under these circumstances, cause a threat to life. Of special importance and especially frequent are **cardiac contusions** occurring in connection with sternal fractures and the **pneumo- and hemothorax** occurring in rib fractures (Table 16).

2. **Pain.** As with every other fracture, movement causes pain in chest fractures. The patient attempts to avoid pain by breathing gently, with the most superficial respiratory motions possible. The normal expansion of the affected parts of the lung does not take place, which is conducive to the formation of minor or massive atelectasis. In addition, impairment of expectoration due to pain is also important because it in turn leads to the accumulation of secretions. In conjunction, they enhance the development of pneumonia.

Table 16. Most frequent intrathoracic companion injuries in 306 patients with multiple rib fractures

Location of the fractures	Ventral	Lateral	Dorsal	Fragmented fracture	Fracture both sides	Total
	29	86	69	39	83	306
Hemothorax	20[a] (69%)[b]	51 (59%)	37 (54%)	34 (87%)	79 (95%)	221 =72%
Pneumothorax	3 (10%)	19 (22%)	16 (23%)	7 (18%)	28 (34%)	73 =24%
Lung contusion	11 (38%)	12 (14%)	13 (19%)	25 (64%)	37 (45%)	98 =45%
Heart contusion	15 (52%)	4 (5%)	10 (14%)	7 (18%)	43 (52%)	79 =26%

[a] Number of cases.
[b] Percentage of patients with fractures in each area.

3. **Mechanical impairment of breathing.** Multiple rib fractures and an unstable thoracic wall have the same effect as pain inhibition, but also cause an increase in the work of breathing and can lead to respiratory insufficiency due to the mechanical impairment of breathing.

A favorable diagnosis immediately after trauma does not exclude the possibility of vital endangerment several days later. A pneumo- or hemothorax can also develop slowly. Pain and instability of the thoracic wall do not reveal their full effect until several days after the accident when secretions have continually accumulated and the increase in the work of breathing may have resulted in exhaustion. I have found the **critical time to be 2 – 4 days** after the accident.

In measurements of **vital capacity** and **maximal breathing capacity** in multiple rib fractures, one is always surprised how low these values can be in some cases, even in the presence of normal arterial blood gases.

Example: In a 59-year-old patient with multiple fractures of ribs III – XI on the left side, the forced vital capacity on the day of the accident, after administration of analgesics, was 13% of normal. In a 19-year-old patient with multiple fractures of ribs III – XII on the left side, it was 19% of the desired value (normal values according to Anderhub [33]). Neither patient required ventilatory support.

An even more significant fact for clinical practice is that these values **continue to decline** until the 2nd day after the accident. In approximately half of the patients there is a marked drop in forced vital capacity in the period 24 – 48 h after the injury (Fig. 45). In this group of patients, the forced vital capacity was initially less severely restricted than in the total group, and after the low point on the 2nd and 3rd day after the accident, recovery proceeded at a substantially more rapid rate.

These reflections precede a systematic discussion of multiple rib and sternal fractures because they reveal the **kinds of problems** involved in injuries to the bony thoracic wall and also indicate where **therapy** must begin: in the **treatment of companion injuries,** in **counteracting pain,** and in **active respiratory therapy.**

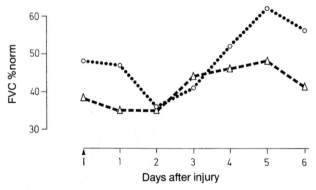

Fig. 45. Mean values of forced vital capacity (FVC) of patients with multiple rib fractures during the course of the 1st week after the accident (n = 23; see also Fig. 14). In patients with a decline between the 1st and 2nd day (n = 10), mean impairment after the accident is less; the FVC on the 2nd day after the accident corresponds to that of the other patients, but the recovery is more rapid (·····) (see text)

Historical Note

Already in the earliest epochs of the history of mankind, injuries of the chest probably often presented grave and unsolvable problems concerning their treatment. Therefore we are not surprised to find that in the oldest historical medical document, the Edwin Smith Papyrus, which was written 3500 years ago and whose contents are supposedly 5000 years old, the prognosis of an open rib fracture is evaluated very negatively:
> If you are examining a man with a rib fracture because of which a wound has erupted and you find that his ribs are displaced under your fingers, you should say of him, "here is a person who has a rib fracture that has caused the eruption of a wound. This is a disease for which nothing can be done" [239].

The fact that even very severe multiple rib fractures were not necessarily fatal in ancient times is proved by the preserved skeleton of a Roman soldier of the fourth century B.C. with healed fractures on both sides of the chest totaling 16 fracture sites [246].

Mechanism of Injury

The upper **four sets of ribs** are well protected by the shoulder girdle. It takes a powerful blow to fracture ribs in this area. Fractures in the posterior part of the upper ribs can result from the mechanical forces of deceleration (e. g., when in riding in an automobile the outstretched arms attempt to brace a person against a collision) [266].

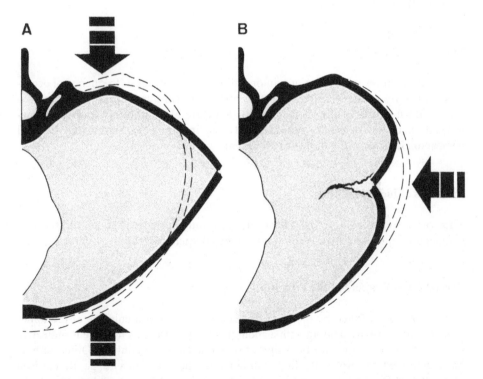

Fig. 46 A, B. Rib fracture resulting from indirect (**A**) and direct (**B**) violence. Lung injuries are more common as the result of the latter

The **lower ribs** are seldom injured and then only by a direct blow because they are more capable of giving way to the effects of force.

By far the greatest number of rib fractures involve the **middle ribs, V – IX.** After direct violence, lung injuries occur more frequently as the result of bone fragments penetrating the interior of the thorax than in fractures brought on by indirect violence (Fig. 46).

In 90% of the cases, **fractures of the sternum** occur as the result of direct violence [264] (determining the type of accident mechanism has no practical significance).

Spontaneous fractures of the ribs are common, especially among elderly patients with chronic lung ailments when, as the result of a sudden muscle pull, e. g., when coughing, a fracture occurs. Even isolated fractures of the first rib can originate in this manner. In such cases, however, one must always consider the possibility of a **pathologic fracture** involving a metastasis.

Because of the elasticity of the thorax, rib fractures among **children** are seldom observed. The higher the age, the less the amount of force required to cause a fracture. Among our patients, 32% of all patients with rib fractures were over 60 years old. The number of rib fractures is not a criterion for the severity of a thoracic injury, unless the age of the patient is taken into consideration.

II. Specific Types of Fractures

Sternal Fractures

While rib fractures take first place among all thoracic injuries in frequency of occurrence, fractures of the sternum are rather infrequent (in our hospital, 5% of the patients with fractures of the thoracic wall). They are almost always **transverse fractures.** Dislocation is usually minimal and only in rare cases significant. Internal **companion injuries** of the thorax are frequent.

Fractures of Individual Ribs

They can be regarded as trivial. However, this is only the case when no intrathoracic companion injuries exist and secretions can be adequately cleared.

Special Case: Fracture of the First Rib

The first rib is protected by the clavicle, scapula, and the musculature of the upper thorax. Unless we are dealing with a spontaneous fracture, this fracture is indicative of a powerful blow and can be a sign of severe intrathoracic injury. Other authors have described an especially high mortality in these patients (e. g., Richardson [265]: 36% of 55 patients), something that we cannot confirm on such a scale, however. Frequently, there is a combination involving a fracture of the clavicle. In every fracture of the first rib, injuries to the subclavian artery and vein or to the innominate artery must be considered a possibility. Furthermore, lesions of the brachial plexus or Horner's syndrome occasionally accompany fractures of the first rib. After the fracture has healed, callous formations can cause a vascular or a neural thoracic outlet syndrome [247, 259, 261, 265] (see p. 245).

A careful examination to determine dysfunction and injuries of these structures is therefore indicated for every patient with a fracture of the first rib. Of all the possible internal thoracic injuries, it will be necessary to exclude cardiac contusion, bronchial rupture, and rupture of the aorta.

Special Case: Basal Rib Fractures

Inasmuch as the movable lower ribs are fractured only by the effect of direct violence, it is understandable that rupture of the liver or spleen often occurs.

Multiple Rib Fractures

Three or more rib fractures, even when there is no instability of the thoracic wall, regularly lead to the previously described problems of guarded breathing and impaired expectoration due to pain. Functional consequences of fractures in the pos-

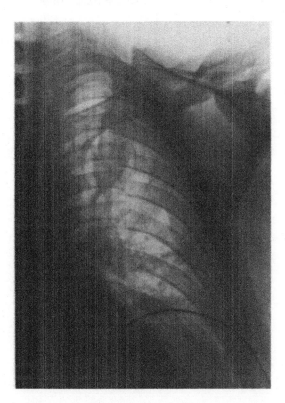

Fig. 47. Because of the strong protective musculature, dorsal multiple rib fractures are tolerated more easily than lateral or anterior fractures. This 50-year-old male patient with multiple fractures of ribs I–XI on the left side suffered no respiratory insufficiency

terior rib section are clearly less severe because the strong musculature in this area provides better support (Fig. 47). Bilateral multiple rib fractures occur with astonishing frequency, among our patients in 29% of the cases.

Flail Chest

Synonyms: stove-in chest, crushed chest, volet mobile.

A freely moving fragment of the chest wall caused by double fractures of three or more adjacent ribs or by multiple rib fractures in combination with a fracture of the sternum generally leads to **paradoxical respiration.** Severe multiple fractures without comminution can also affect the stability of the chest mechanism so severely that paradoxical respiration results. Although a flail chest can be caused by several different atypical fracture locations, a distinction is usually made between **two principal forms** (Fig. 48):

1. **Anterior type of flail chest** caused by multiple parasternal rib fractures in the chondral area, possibly combined with a fracture of the sternum.

2. **Lateral type.**

Distinguishing between these two forms is important because of the possible companion injuries and the therapy to be applied.

Pathophysiology of Paradoxical Respiration

In spontaneous breathing, because of innervation of the respiratory musculature at inspiration, there is an enlargement of thoracic space, which causes a negative pres-

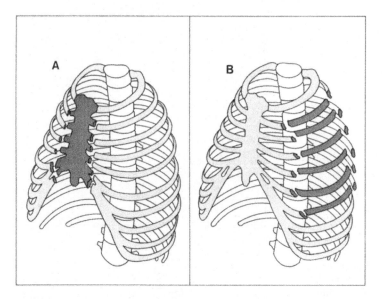

Fig. 48 A, B. The two principal forms of flail chest. **A** Anterior type; **B** Lateral type

Specific Types of Fractures

sure in the pleural area of −10 mmHg, and even much more with forced inspiration. This negative pressure pulls any freely moving fragments of chest wall toward the interior of the thorax during inspiration. Expiration lowers the intrapleural negative pressure and forced expiration even converts it to positive pressure: the free fragment returns to its original position or may be forced further outward. The free portion of thoracic wall, therefore, behaves **contrary** to normal respiratory movement: it moves **paradoxically** (Fig. 49).

The extent of paradoxical respiration is therefore determined by the **depth of inspiration and expiration.** For this reason, in normal breathing it is often impossible to detect paradoxical respiration despite the presence of a free fragment. By calling upon the patient to inhale and exhale deeply, paradoxical respiration is demonstrated.

Textbooks contain the theory of **"Pendelluft,"** said to be an explanation of respiratory difficulties in paradoxical respiration. It was Brauer who in 1909 postulated this concept suggested by paradoxical respiration following thoracoplastic operations [226]. It states that during inspiration, air rich in CO_2 is inhaled via the injured side of the thorax into the noninvolved lung and that during expiration, this same air, rich in CO_2, flows back to the injured side. This back-and-forth movement of "used" air is said to be the cause of respiratory insufficiency in such patients. This theory was so plausible that it gained popular acceptance, but it has never been supported by proof.

The mere reflection upon the fact that during inspiration there must be a negative pressure in the pleural space to produce paradoxical respiration and that therefore during also this phase of breathing air **must** flow into the affected lung should create doubts about the validity of this theory. Maloney et al. [256] in their experimental

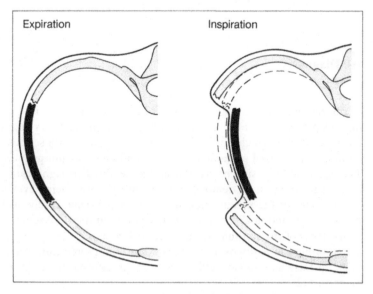

Fig. 49. Behavior of a free thoracic wall fragment during paradoxical respiration caused by double fracture of the ribs

investigation of this question have demonstrated that "Pendelluft" does not occur in a closed thorax. Admittedly, measurements on dogs with their easily shifted mediastinum are not readily transferable to human beings: yet the findings of Duff et al. [238] in experiments with human beings demonstrated that the ventilation minute volume of both lungs is identical during paradoxical respiration. This, as well as the observation that paradoxical respiration in cases of parasternal rib fractures causes the same respiratory difficulties on both sides, allows the conclusion to be drawn that there is **no validity** in the concept of "Pendelluft" in the respiratory insufficiency that develops in paradoxical respiration.

Inspiration and expiration are dependent to a large extent upon **differences of pressure** in the pleural space. The fragment, which is moving paradoxically, impedes by its inward movement the buildup of an adequate negative pressure in the pleural space and **thereby** hampers respiration.

Even with very slight paradoxical respiration the necessary **work of breathing is increased** [238]. By **increasing the work of breathing,** the patient can achieve adequate respiration. This explains why a patient can under certain circumstances compensate for his paradoxical respiration for several days but on becoming fatigued suddenly develops respiratory insufficiency.

In this precarious state of equilibrium, the **retention of secretions** becomes a significant additional complicating factor. In a freely mobile thoracic wall, it is not only difficult to attain a negative intrapleural pressure but also a positive pressure through coughing, thus reducing the thrust of the cough.

Through the completely different mechanism of an intrapulmonary right-to-left shunt, a severe **lung contusion** under the paradoxically moving fragment of thoracic wall can likewise result in hypoxia. It is essential for therapy to keep these two constituent parts of respiratory failure separate (see Chap. 4). Trinkle [274] has also made a strong point of this.

III. Diagnosis

In **rib fractures,** the patient complains of **localized pain** that is aggravated by coughing, deep breathing, and change of body position. There is **guarded breathing** on the affected side, which can lead to a diminishing of breath sounds even without hemothorax. **Localized palpable tenderness** and **compression pain** are always present. The classic clinical sign of **crepitation** has retained its significance in this instance because it can often be demonstrated by auscultation, being evoked by the respiratory motions of the patient. **Subcutaneous emphysema,** rarely evident in single rib fractures, is found in 27% of the patients with multiple rib fractures.

In **fractures of the sternum, local compression pain** is very prominent. Occasionally a **step formation** is discovered by palpation and **crepitation** heard with the stethoscope. A **false motion** can seldom be detected. Sternal fractures are often belatedly diagnosed [266].

The presence of **paradoxical respiration** is determined by careful observation. During respiration at rest, it occasionally does not show up until later when the muscu-

Diagnosis

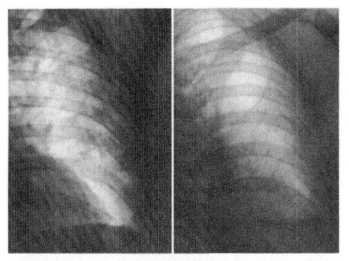

Fig. 50. Rib fractures can often not be detected radiologically or do not show up until later roentgenograms of the thorax are taken

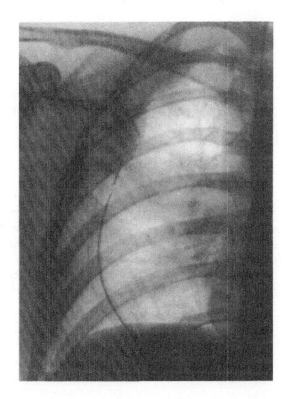

Fig. 51. Extrapleural hematoma in rib fractures

lature becomes fatigued and breathing becomes labored because of higher energy requirements, whereby the negative pressure in the pleural space rises. It is for this reason that during the first examination the patient is asked to inhale and exhale maximally.

Rib fractures must be **diagnosed clinically!** Many rib fractures are not visible on **roentgenograms** (see p. 18). This does not only just apply to fractures in the cartilaginous part of the ribs, which cannot be shown radiologically anyway. Many fractures are visible, however, in a later roentgenogram (Fig. 50). If the parietal pleura has not been torn, a **subpleural hematoma** occasionally shows up on the roentgenogram (Fig. 51).

It is not decisive that the roentgenogram reveal all the sites of rib fractures, but it should provide information about conditions in the **interior of the thorax.** Because of concomitant injuries, radiologic follow-up should be made, the first no later than 24 h after the accident.

Radiologic evidence of a **sternal fracture** can only be brought out by a good **lateral** picture, and in extraordinary situations only by the use of tomograms.

Severe multiple rib fractures or the presence of paradoxical respiration always require clarification of the respiratory situation through **arterial blood gas analysis,** which is also significant for the evaluation of subsequent developments.

IV. General Considerations for Therapy in Rib and Sternal Fractures

Assistance at the Scene of the Accident

For patients with respiratory insufficiency and severe paradoxical respiration, temporary splinting can provide decisive help: manual pressure on the paradoxically moving thoracic wall or better still, **placing the patient on the side** of the thoracic wall instability, also serve to provide relief.

Hospitalization?

Only patients with **single rib fractures** without pneumothorax and at most a low-grade hemothorax can be considered for treatment as an outpatient. Even in these cases a roentgenogram should always be taken the following day. The decision to hospitalize the patient should, of course, take into account the age of the patient, the pain involved, and the general condition.

In my view, **sternal fractures,** because of the great frequency of serious attendant injuries, are always an indication for hospitalization, at least for a brief period.

Attendant Injuries

It is taken for granted that attendant injuries are given appropriate treatment and that a pneumothorax or significant hemothorax are drained.

Fig. 52. Rib fractures are known for their good healing tendencies, even when there are dislocations (*A*). Even when no osseous healing with bridging callous occurs (*B*), the healing by scar tissue is so pronounced that for the most part there are no functional disturbances or complaints

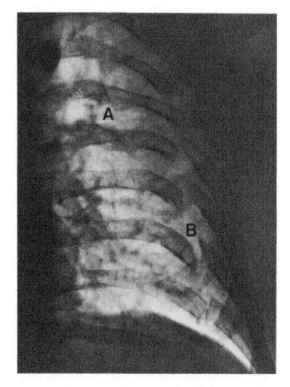

Chest Strapping?

Rib fractures, known for their good healing tendencies (Fig. 52), do not require immobilization to bring about consolidation. At most, the function of a fixed bandage (adhesive plaster strapping, rib girdle) is to **reduce pain** and possibly to render **assistance in coughing.** For anatomic reasons, such immobilizing bandages are inefficient in fractures of the upper ribs.
These methods of fixation, however, have decided **disadvantages:** they definitely reduce ventilation of the half of the thorax in question and in so doing promote the formation of atelectasis and respiratory insufficiency. Drewes [237] has documented this restriction of respiratory function by compression bandages with spirographic examinations. It is precisely the desired maximal inflation of the lung for purposes of opening the greatest possible number of alveoli that is considerably restricted. The rib girdle is especially dangerous in this instance because it also impedes ventilation in the healthy half of the thorax.
From what has been said we can adduce the indication for these remedies: patients with simple rib fractures and in generally good condition will profit from it. If their pain is almost eliminated, they will discontinue wearing the irksome bandage of their own accord.
However, the worse the condition of the patient and the more extended and threatening his rib fractures are with regard to ventilation, **the more dangerous the therapy**

with an immobilizing bandage will be. In severe multiple rib fractures, in pronounced paradoxical respiration, and in manifestations of respiratory failure from some other source, it is **contraindicated.** The fact that the patient perceives it as being comfortable is no proof of its effectiveness. The diminution of pain is a costly bargain when paid for by the danger of subsequent pneumonic complications or an increase in respiratory insufficiency.

Example: A 65-year-old female patient with multiple left-sided fractures of ribs III – VI. On the 5th day after the accident, a rib girdle was applied. Arterial blood gas analysis with spontaneous respiration on 6 liters of O_2:

	PCO_2	PO_2	SO_2
11:00 A.M., without rib girdle	35 mmHg	126 mmHg	99%
5:00 P.M., with rib girdle	44 mmHg	53 mmHg	87%
8:30 P.M., without rib girdle	38 mmHg	76 mmHg	94%

Tracheostomy?

The advantage of reducing the dead space by means of a tracheostomy is slight when compared with the potential of other measures. If a tracheostomy is not required for other reasons (e. g., severe injuries and fractures of the face and pharynx areas), I no longer see the indication for a primary tracheostomy. In conscious patients, there are other, less mutilating ways available for removing secretions. In unconscious patients and in respiratory emergencies, one would resort first to intubation anyway.

Decisive: Physiotherapy

The goal of every kind of therapy in fractures of the thoracic wall is good ventilation of the underlying lung sections and the avoidance of an accumulation of secretions. Physiotherapeutic measures (see Chap. 9) are without doubt of decisive importance. By energetic breathing exercises, complications (atelectasis, pneumonia) can largely be avoided. It also helps to obviate the need for mechanical ventilation.

Drug Therapy

The use of **mucolytic agents** is probably accorded too much significance in treating patients who are otherwise healthy. In exceptional cases, their use can be justified. What is important is the **moistening of air passages** by vaporizers or nebulizers. Atropine is contraindicated and merely leads to annoying dehydration of all the mucosa and to inability to expectorate tenacious secretions. In asthmatic situations, **spasmolytic therapy** is decisive.

Therapy of Sternal Fractures

It is predominantly **conservative.** Only in very severe dislocations is an operative reduction advised. Even so, in no way is it a question of an emergency operation; the other problems of the patient can be dealt with first. If it is an open reduction, fixation is done with wire sutures or heavy synthetic nonabsorbable suture material. A closed reduction (according to Scudder [cited in 245] by hyperextension with deep inspiration) in a severe dislocation of the fragments is hardly successful, if at all. The attempt is not worth it.

V. Pain Control

One of the most important pillars of every kind of therapy in fractures of the thorax is the control of pain.

Analgesics

Oral analgesics, particularly those not containing morphine, are only adequate in the therapy of individual fractures and can be prescribed on the basis of "need".
For severe fractures, that is, multiple rib fractures and fractures with paradoxical respiration, parenteral application of a potent analgesic, a **morphine derivative,** is necessary. The fear of a respiratory depressing effect of morphine derivatives is generally unfounded; as could be demonstrated by tests of lung function, the respiratory improvement achieved by the effects of analgesics is much greater. The dosage must naturally be chosen in such a way that there is no excessive sedation of the patient.
I usually prefer the morphine derivative nicomorphinum HCl because of its potent analgesic and its limited breath-depressing effect, applied every 4 h subcutaneously. Controlling pain by means of analgesics often encounters a difficulty that is seldom thought of: before long it is discontinued by the nurses on the basis of the fact that "the patient doesn't have any more pain." This is based on a faulty consideration: the goal of therapy is not freedom from pain but breathing as deeply as possible with strong inspiration. The patient will instinctively attempt by very superficial breathing to achieve a minimum of pain or freedom from pain altogether, and most of them do. But by means of analgesics he must be relieved also of those pains that occur when he breathes deeply. Only then are such deep inspirations possible at all.

Intercostal Nerve Block

Intercostal nerve block immediately achieves a diminution of pain or painlessness without respiratory depression. There is a disadvantage in the fact that the analgesia lasts only for 6 – 12 h, even when long-lasting local anesthetics are used, which renders this method laborious and unpleasant for the patient. Nevertheless, in certain situations, it represents an important therapeutic alternative.

Technique

Although intercostal nerve block can be given along the entire course of the nerve proximal to the site of the fracture, there are several preferable points of injection.

1. The dorsal **costal angle,** immediately lateral to the erector musculature of the spine, where the rib lies near the surface (Fig. 53).

2. The **posterior axillary line.** Nerve block further ventrally no longer encompasses the lateral cutaneous branch of the intercostal nerves.

The patient is placed in a lateral position for the posterior intercostal block or in an oblique position for a block in the posterior axillary line. After applying a skin prep, the injection cannula is inserted perpendicularly to the lower part of the rib and the needle advanced 3 mm below the edge of the rib. At this point, after aspiration to avoid an intravascular injection, 3 – 5 ml of local anesthetic is injected. We use bupivacaine 0.5% because of its long-lasting qualities (Fig. 54).

Inasmuch as the areas of innervation of the intercostal nerves are not sharply delineated, the infiltration should be extended 1 or 2 spaces above and below the fractured rib.

Epidural Anesthesia

Thoracic epidural anesthesia has been used in isolated cases of multiple rib fractures for the alleviation of pain [244]. Recently, Dittmann [235] adopted this method with good success. Undoubtedly this is a potent and very welcome alternative for neutralizing pain since the local anesthetic can be injected on a prn basis through the catheter, which has been left in place. The effect upon vital capacity is impressive, and it can be assumed that in certain instances with a cooperative patient the need for mechanical ventilation can be avoided.

The method requires absolute familiarity with the technique of epidural anesthesia. Because of the danger of positioning the anesthesia too high or the occurrence of a

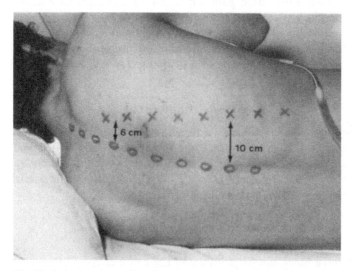

Fig. 53. Injection sites at the costal angle for intercostal nerve block

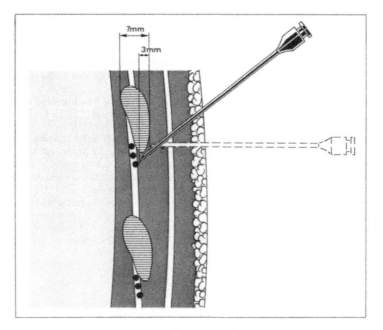

Fig. 54. Technique of intercostal nerve block

drop in blood pressure, these patients should be placed in an intensive care unit. In multiple trauma cases, it conceals whatever symptoms there are involving abdominal problems. No definite assertions can as yet be made regarding the danger of infection and of epidural scarring with subsequent attendant pain.

By and large, this method offers a valuable enrichment of therapeutic alternatives when in the hands of a trained professional. Unfortunately, this method is not generally well-known and in my opinion is utilized all too infrequently. It is decisive that epidural anesthesia is applied early, shortly after the patient is admitted, without waiting for severe respiratory insufficiency to develop.

VI. Therapy of Flail Chest

Up to the middle of the 1950s, treatment of an unstable thoracic wall consisted of various attempts to provide **external support** (strips of adhesive tape, sandbags, fitted plaster casts according to Tiegel [273]), of all possible sorts of **skeletal traction** of the free fragment (towel clamps, flexible wires inserted behind the sternum or implanted in the rib, Kirschner wires, extensions of adhesive tape, even wires implanted subcutaneously), or of the attempt at **operative fixation** (wire sutures of the ribs, pericostal sutures, internal fixation with Kirschner wires).

A new era began in 1956 when Avery et al. [224] reported for the first time on the application of **long-term ventilation,** maintained until there was adequate stabilization of the thoracic wall. Already in 1952 Jensen [249] had recommended the use of a respirator for treatment of patients with paradoxical respiration. Under the slogan "internal pneumatic stabilization," this concept soon gained popular acceptance also in Europe and is regarded today as the standard therapy for flail chest.

After initial uncritical enthusiasm, people became aware of the fact that long-term ventilation incorporated the possibility of a whole series of **complications.** The latter could indeed be markedly reduced by improved techniques and better training of physicians and nurses manning the intensive care stations. Nevertheless, certain complications, especially infection, have not been eliminated. In addition, the treatment is lengthy, expensive, and requires a large staff.

It is not surprising, therefore, that more and more reports are again being made of attempts at **operative stabilization of the thoracic wall.** The impetus was provided especially by the works of Dor [236], Eschapasse and Gaillard [240], and Couraud [232] in France. They used internal fixation with **Kirschner wires** of the ribs as the only method (Dor) or, depending upon the location of the fractured part, as an alternative they used **skeletal traction** of the sternum (Eschapasse and Gaillard, Couraud). A report was also made by Moore [258] on further experiences with internal fixation with Kirschner wires. Other authors employed **steel bars** (Brunner and colleagues [227], Regensburger [263]), **metal implants on the outside of the rib** to which the rib was fastened with wire (Carlisle [229], Paris [260]), **agraffes** (Judet [251], Stoianov [271]), **intramedullary plates** (Paris [260], Schüpbach [268]), or **small fragment plates** (Aigner [222], Sinigaglia [269]).

However, a purely conservative procedure that avoids mechanical ventilation is increasingly finding its advocates [213, 274]. In 1975 Trinkle [274] even accused long-term ventilation of being a "triumph of technique over judgment."

Now What?

There is so much in question today that time should be taken for reflection:

1. Respiratory insufficiency in flail chest is not always only a mechanical problem. Lung contusions or other lung damage with an intrapulmonary right-to-left shunt, as in ARDS, may also be present.

2. To what extent alleviation of pain is possible and how cooperative the patient is are questions of decisive importance. In a patient with craniocerebral injuries, for whom hypoxia is not acceptable under any circumstances, the approach is altogether different from that for a patient with only thoracic injuries.

One thing is clear: **paradoxical respiration by itself is not an indication for long-term mechanical ventilation.** This is indicated only when there is simultaneous respiratory failure. If the hypoxia is occasioned by a substantial intrapulmonary right-to-left shunt, mechanical ventilation is resorted to early on, and if improvement is shown after a short time, spontaneous breathing is again attempted. If the respiratory insufficiency has a mechanical cause, the attempt is made to circumvent long-term mechanical ventilation by means of intensive respiratory therapy and even to temporarily accept a moderate hypoxia (PaO_2 with oxygen supplied nasally as low as 60 mmHg) provided there are no cerebral injuries. Thus, 25% of our patients with paradoxical respiration were treated successfully without mechanical ventilation. In cases of paradoxical respiration, the respirator is probably sometimes employed prematurely.

Such a statement, however, applies more often to the **indications for performing rib fixations.** After reviewing a number of postoperative roentgenograms, I am convinced that many internal fixations of a rib were carried out and are being carried out in cases of multiple rib fractures that with adequate treatment should have run their course without any problems whatsoever and without the necessity of mechanical ventilation.

No one questions the fact that internal fixation of a rib, as an alternative to long-term mechanical ventilation, offers many advantages; nevertheless, the **indication** for its meaningful use is **limited** by a whole series of restrictions (see below) so that **only a few** cases can really benefit from it.

In these rare cases, it seems to me to be thoroughly commendable. Especially favorable is the **fixation of the anterior type of flail chest in parasternal multiple rib fractures** by the use of a flat metal bar inserted retrosternally. This operation is simple, requires no exposure of the rib fractures, and results in good stabilization. I am skeptical about **internal fixation with Kirschner wires** since it requires a thoracotomy, results in only limited stability, and runs the risk of migration of the wire. **Implantation of plates** come into consideration when the fractures are located laterally. In my opinion, they cannot be used in the chondral rib section since the screws are difficult to anchor in the cartilage, and furthermore, postoperative chondritis constitutes a burdensome complication.

The use of **external sternal traction** makes the care and necessary changing of body positions of the patient infinitely more difficult and, in my judgment, they are not to be recommended, especially for a patient with multiple trauma.

I should like to issue a warning against an argument used to publicize internal rib fixation: the fact that it is impossible to carry out long-term ventilatory support in a particular hospital is not to be interpreted as an indication for operation. Today, all patients can be transferred to a nearby medical center that has the necessary facilities.

The **basic therapy** for respiratory insufficiency resulting from an unstable thoracic wall is still **mechanical ventilation.** In certain clearly defined cases, it can be replaced advantageously by operative stabilization of the thoracic wall.

Long-term Mechanical Ventilation

For the technique of mechanical ventilation, I refer you to the special literature and to the references in Chap. 8. A **chest tube** is always inserted into the affected half of the thorax.

Within a short time, ventilation results in a **repositioning** of thoracic wall fragments that have become displaced toward the interior of the thorax (Fig. 55). Stability of the thoracic wall sufficient for spontaneous breathing is generally attained after 2 or 3 (up to 4) weeks. The first attempts at spontaneous breathing are usually made after 14 days. If paradoxical respiration is still very pronounced, controlled ventilation is continued for another week and then, applying intermittent mandatory ventilation (IMV), the transition to spontaneous breathing is initiated.

In the future, more and more novel forms of ventilation and other variations will be used. Interesting is the report of Cullen et al. [233] who, by combining IMV with positive end-expiratory pressure (PEEP), were able to achieve a significant reduction in the duration of mechanical ventilation.

Indication for Operative Measures

The **indication** for operative stabilization of the thoracic wall appears to me upon critical observation to be given **only when the following special conditions exist:**

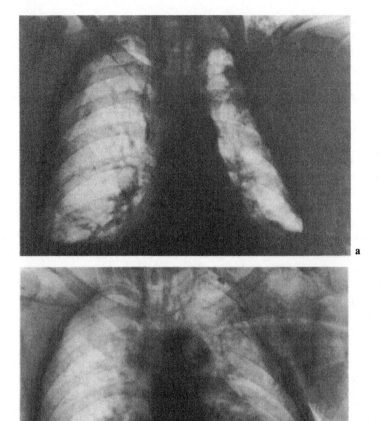

Fig. 55 a, b. The impressed thoracic wall with multiple fragmented rib fractures (**a**) is repositioned by controlled positive pressure breathing (**b**)

1. If without these measures mechanical ventilation would be unavoidable (unilateral multiple rib fractures without paradoxical respiration therefore do not represent an indication for an operation).

2. If there is no other indication for mechanical ventilation except the instability of the thoracic wall (e. g., ARDS, cerebral respiratory insufficiency, concomitant injuries in the thoracic area).

3. If the patient is conscious.

4. If a convincing method of operative repair is available for the type of fracture in question, one that really results in stabilization.

Therapy of Flail Chest

5. If stabilization can be undertaken within days after trauma and before a pulmonary infection has occurred through treatment with a respirator [234, 236, 240, 269].

6. If there are no other contraindications.

Stabilization of the Anterior Type of Flail Chest in Multiple Parasternal Rib Fractures

For this stabilization I use a slender, pointed steel bar as used by Sulamaa [272] in funnel chest operations. It is inserted retrosternally. In contrast to other authors who have described similar operating procedures [223, 227, 252, 263], I put this bar in diagonally and bend it at each end so that it is well-supported by the ribs beyond the fracture sites. The length of the rod, which is approximately 1 cm wide and 2 mm thick, is determined by the size of the patient and the location of the rib fractures (Fig. 56).

Operative Technique (Fig. 57)

1. Preoperative: marking the extent of the freely moving thoracic wall and the location of the rib fractures. Identifying the supporting ribs on the right and, one to two ribs more cephalad, on the left half of the thorax. The bar should cross the sternum

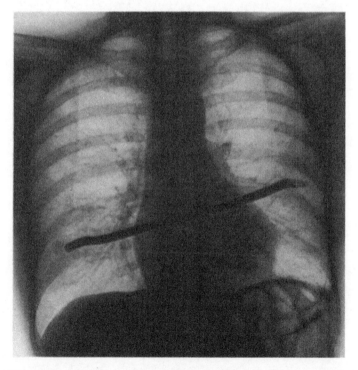

Fig. 56. Stabilization of bilateral parasternal multiple rib fractures accompanied by paradoxical respiration by means of a metal bar inserted retrosternally into a 51-year-old female patient resulted in spontaneous breathing without paradoxical movements immediately after the operation

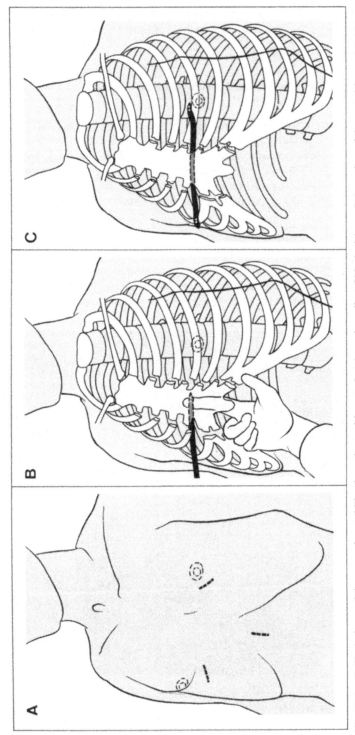

Fig. 57 A–C. Technique of the operative stabilization of unstable anterior thoracic wall. **A** Skin incisions; **B** Insertion of the metal bar guided by a finger in the retrosternal space; **C** Final position of the stabilizing bar, which runs behind the sternum and on both ends rests on the front of a rib laterally to the line of fracture (see text)

as close to the middle of the flail chest as possible but also low enough so that the place where it crosses can be reached with the finger under the sternum from the xyphoid process.

2. Exposing the "supporting ribs" laterally to the fracture zone by means of two small incisions.

3. Small longitudinal cut below the xyphoid process and blunt dissection with the index finger into the retrosternal space but always in contact with the posterior side of the sternum.

4. After bending the steel bar properly, it is pushed into the intercostal musculature and without injuring the pleura is brought under the sternum. The finger, which has been inserted through the incision and underneath the xyphoid process, takes over the guidance of the bar blindly and does it in such a way that it appears again in front of the left side below the rib intended to be used as a support base. Final bending of the surfaces of the bar to conform to the anchor ribs and fixing them by sutures of nonabsorbent material, one through and one around the rib.

Table 17. Therapy in multiple rib fractures (not taking companion injuries into consideration)

Stable thoracic wall	Unstable thoracic wall Paradoxical respiration
1. Controlling pain	– Analgesics (morphine derivatives) every 4 h even if there are "no pains" (see text) – If necessary, intercostal nerve block – If necessary, epidural anesthesia
2. Intensive breathing exercises	
	Only in cases of respiratory insufficiency: – **Mechanical ventilation;** prophylactic insertion of a chest tube – In exceptional cases, operative stabilization of the thoracic wall

Internal Fixation of Ribs with Kirschner Wires and Plates

This procedure is considered only in fragmented fractures of the posterior or lateral thoracic wall in which no fractures course through the chondral rib section.

Dor [236], Eschapasse and Gaillard [240, 241], Couraud [233], and Moore [258] make use of **intramedullary positioned Kirschner wires.** This method requires a thoracotomy.

Sinigaglia [269] and Aigner [222] recommend **internal fixation** of the ribs with **small fragment plates.** The incision is made individually according to the location of the rib fractures. A thoracotomy is unnecessary. The intraoperative fixation of the plate on the ribs with two forceps may facilitate the drilling of the holes and mounting of the screws [269]. It is not necessary to provide all fractured ribs with a plate to achieve adequate stability; this can largely be restricted to ribs IV–VIII.

Chapter 11
Pneumothorax and Hemothorax

Example: In a 17-year-old girl who was being ventilated during general anesthesia, a **bilateral tension pneumothorax** developed (Fig. 58). The diagnosis was based on the radiologic findings. Without a relief puncture or thoracic drainage, she was transported 15 km to the university hospital for treatment. It was a miracle that she survived.

Cases of pneumothorax and hemothorax can be provided with extremely effective therapy for the most part with **simple methods**. It must, however, be given **early**. Furthermore, the drainage of air and blood must be **efficient**.

I. Pneumothorax

Injuries of the lung, the bronchi, and the trachea (in communication with the pleural cavity) as well as exposure of the pleural area to the outside, even temporarily, lead to pneumothorax. There is often a concomitant hemothorax.
Recently, **iatrogenic** causes have become more frequent: as a complication occasioned by puncture of the subclavian vein [278] but also by mechanical ventilation [201, 202, 207], by external cardiac massage, by thoracentesis, by improper removal of a chest tube, and even by acupuncture.

Pathophysiology

A low-grade, closed pneumothorax is generally tolerated quite well without significant dyspnea. Even in the complete collapse of a lung, the respiratory functions of the other side are adequate insofar as there is no immediate endangerment to life. Usually at that point, however, there is already a pronounced dyspnea and the patient's physical stamina is restricted.
Apart from the reduced ventilation, a functional, intrapulmonary right-to-left shunt appears in the collapsed lung, which likewise contributes to the hypoxia. The latter remains, however, marginal since with the collapse of the lung the vascular resistance on the affected side increases and the supply of blood is thereby significantly reduced [266].

Diagnosis

In the **clinical examination,** the leading findings are hyperresonance, diminished breath sounds, and a reduced mobility of the affected half of the thorax while breathing.

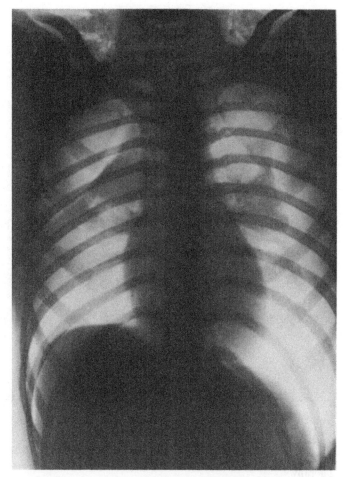

Fig. 58. Bilateral tension pneumothorax as a complication of mechanical ventilation during general anesthesia (see text)

In the **roentgenogram,** particularly in the upper third of the thorax, the outline of the lung in the pleural space is visible or a completely collapsed lung is seen in the vicinity of the hilum. Along the border of the thoracic wall, there is an air-filled space without lung structure.

A pneumothorax of less than 10% sometimes does not show up on the roentgenogram. This is especially true of a roentgenogram of a patient in a recumbent position. Identification is much easier in the upright position, especially during expiration [266]. The difficulties of diagnosing pneumothorax when there is subcutaneous emphysema were already pointed out in Chap. 3. The characteristic picture of subcutaneous accumulation of air can simulate elements of the lung (see Fig. 7).

If the pneumothorax is combined with a hemothorax, a characteristic **fluid level** will show up in the roentgenogram of a patient in an upright position (Fig. 59).

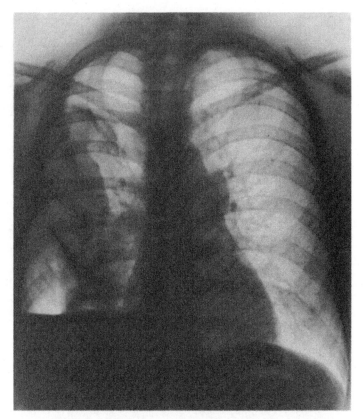

Fig. 59. Pneumo- and hemothorax with characteristic fluid level (roentgenogram taken in upright position)

Therapy

Only a **minimal pneumothorax** may be treated **expectantly**. If there is no further air leak, it can be absorbed within several days. Watchful waiting, however, is permitted only

1. In single rib fractures

2. When there is a possibility of close supervision and repeated radiologic monitoring of the thorax and

3. If there is no need for anesthesia or mechanical ventilation.

Even then there is danger of significant deterioration brought on by a sudden increase in intrapulmonary pressure (e. g., by coughing). In most cases, therefore, especially in a recent trauma, it is best to insert a chest tube. The more seriously a patient is injured, not only in the thoracic area, the less often should watchful waiting be considered.

Inserting a **chest tube** is the **therapy of choice** in cases of pneumothorax. The total evacuation of air can hardly be accomplished by thoracentesis alone, at least not permanently. Furthermore, there is danger of renewed injury from the needle as the lung reexpands.

Chest drainage with continuous suction almost always produces a reexpansion of the lung. If this is not the case, either the chest tube is located improperly, the lung injury is very extensive, or there is a rupture of a bronchus or the trachea. There are still other advantages of drainage over puncture:

1. It permits an assessment of air loss and indicates when the leak in the lung is closed. A simple grip (Fig. 60) provides general information.

2. The immediate reexpansion of the lung and the reliable drainage of air enable the surgeon to confidently address other problems of the patient without having to worry about the development of a tension pneumothorax.

3. The expansion of the lung results in a tamponade of the leak and, by formation of adhesions and coalescence with the parietal pleura, results in rapid healing of the lung lesion.

4. Continuous suction drainage is more comfortable for the patient than repeated thoracentesis.

If there is **nothing more** than a pneumothorax, a **chest tube** (Charrière 20) is placed in the midclavicular line through the second or third intercostal space. If there is a pneumothorax in combination with a **hemothorax,** the tube is inserted laterally, as in the case of a hemothorax alone.

A suction of 25 cm H_2O is applied. If the position of the intrathoracic tube is proper, the inside of the tube will be covered with moisture by the warm air being evacuated. The reexpansion of the lung almost always causes a temporary, but quite intense, pleural pain; therefore, a preceding administration of an analgesic is recommended.

A **follow-up roentgenogram** provides information about the position of the tube. If, with the drainage located properly, the lung is only partially expanded several hours after insertion of the chest suction, drainage of the residual pneumothorax can perhaps be achieved by changing the position of the patient. If this is impossible or ineffective, a second tube is introduced into the remaining accumulation of air.

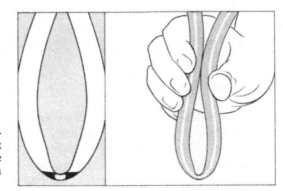

Fig. 60. Simple grip for general estimate of the loss of air during chest suction: by buckling the drainage tube, the passage of air bubbles can be observed as the fluid collects

If steady passage of air through the tube does not produce reexpansion of the lung, the suction can be increased. If this is unsuccessful or if there are other moments of doubt about a bronchial rupture, a **bronchoscopic examination** is indicated, provided an immediate thoracotomy is not necessary to manage an increasing deterioration of the patient's condition.

The rule is: **the condition of an incompletely expanded lung despite pleural drainage may not be left as it is.**

Acute Unilateral Lung Edema After Reexpansion of the Lung

The occurrence of acute lung edema upon reexpansion of the lung following drainage of massive **pleural effusion** has been known for a long time. As far back as 1875 Foucart reported on this, and Ortner (1899), Riesmann (1902), and Hartley (1906) shared similar observations [280, 298].

In 1959 Carlson et al. [280] published for the first time a report on these complications after expansion of a lung that had collapsed due to **pneumothorax.** To date, a total of 18 cases of such acute unilateral lung edema have been reported [e. g., 287, 295, 298]. Common to all these cases is a long-standing condition of lung collapse (between 3 and 82 days). The only exception has to do with one of the cases of Humphreys and Berne [287] in which a pneumothorax had existed for only 1 h. A quick expansion of the collapsed lung by suction drainage appeared to strengthen the inclination toward edema.

These observations were confirmed in animal experiments by Miller et al. [290]. In rhesus monkeys with a pneumothorax lasting 3 days, the evacuation of air with suction of 10 cm H_2O resulted in unilateral lung edema, whereas edema did not occur with underwater-seal drainage. In a pneumothorax lasting only a short time (1 h), this complication was not observed even when suction was applied.

It must be assumed that in a prolonged collapse of the lung a disturbance of the permeability of the collapsed wall, most likely caused by hypoxia, occurs and that the surfactant content of the alveoli is also lost [290]. A strongly negative intrapleural pressure during drainage raises the pulmonary capillary pressure and the blood flow in the affected lung and also promotes the development of interstitial lung edema.

The complication is certainly more frequent than one would expect on the basis of the few published cases; nevertheless, there is little danger of this in traumatic pneumothorax since the reexpansion of the lung usually occurs immediately. Almost all reported cases pertain to **spontaneous pneumothorax.**

If such an acute, threatening lung edema occurs, the therapy consists of brief ventilation with positive end-expiratory pressure (PEEP).

II. Tension Pneumothorax

The normal, closed pneumothorax is not immediately life-threatening if there are no other significant injuries. By way of contrast, there is a most **acute threat to life** in tension pneumothorax. Every traumatic pneumothorax can develop into a tension pneumothorax; however, this complication is rare with spontaneous breathing. Very frequently, in a more dangerous form by far, a tension pneumothorax occurs

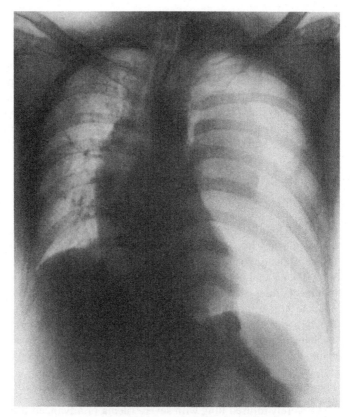

Fig. 61. Tension pneumothorax on the left side after closed thoracic trauma during internal fixation of a femur (see text)

during mechanical ventilation, whether in ventilation as a first-aid measure, during anesthesia, or during long-term ventilation.

Especially during manual ventilation, because of increasing cyanosis, the insidious impression arises that the patient is being poorly ventilated. As a result, the ventilation is delivered with greater pressure and more volume, a procedure that serves to strengthen the pneumothorax all the more.

Example: In a 39-year-old patient with paravertebral fractures of ribs II – IV on the left side, difficulties of ventilation developed during anesthesia for internal fixation of the femur. The patient became increasingly hypoxic and cyanotic. Because of the fracture of the femur, fat embolism was assumed to be the cause of the sudden deterioration, and on the basis of this diagnosis the patient was directed to the university hospital for long-term mechanical ventilation. The roentgenogram showed the massive tension pneumothorax on the left (Fig. 61).

Pathophysiology

Through **a valve effect,** often with only minor lung or bronchial lesions, air accumulates with increasing positive pressure in one of the pleural spaces. The mediastinum is shifted to the opposite side. The other lung is increasingly compromised.

Experimental animal research conducted by Rutherford et al. [294] has shown that the most significant change is **progressive hypoxia** and not, as one might assume, a decrease of cardiac output caused by impaired venous return resulting from the displacement of the mediastinum. These experiments were conducted under conditions of spontaneous breathing, however. With artificial respiration, the aspects of the case take on a much more perilous form. In a short time, intrapleural positive pressures develop (40 mmHg and higher), which greatly exceed the central venous pressure. When that happens, the **impairment of venous return** to the heart by positive pressure and dislocation of the mediastinum is of greater significance than hypoxia.

Diagnosis

Clinical diagnosis is usually easy: hyperresonance, reduced breath sounds, elevation of the affected side of the chest with weak respiratory motion. The trachea is displaced to the opposite side. Often the influx of air is obstructed.

With such a characteristic picture, therapy ought to begin **without delay or taking roentgenograms.** If the blood pressure has already dropped because of a tension pneumothorax, there are often only a few minutes remaining before cardiac arrest.

In Chap. 8 we have already referred to tension pneumothorax as a **complication of mechanical ventilation.** An **increase in ventilation pressure when tidal volume remains the same** combined with an **increase of central venous pressure** points to tension pneumothorax.

There are two situations that make clinical diagnosis difficult, if not impossible:

1. A severely injured lung with **severe edema** or advanced **fibrosis** can no longer collapse (Fig. 62). Despite tension pneumothorax, the breath sounds are still quite audible.

2. If there are pleural adhesions, a **local tension pneumothorax** can develop, which is almost impossible to diagnose clinically (Fig. 63).

The **thoracic roentgenogram** usually reveals the collapse of the entire lung, a mediastinal shift to the opposite side, and a depression of the diaphragm with flattening of the domes (Fig. 61). It is difficult to interpret the radiologic findings when a localized tension pneumothorax is involved (Fig. 63) or when subcutaneous emphysema — a frequent combination with tension pneumothorax — simulates lung parenchyma in the pleural space (Fig. 7). The **shift of the mediastinum** is of important diagnostic significance in these cases.

Therapy

Treatment consists of the immediate relief of pressure. If there is a **chest tube drain** available, it is inserted. In so doing, definitive therapy is initiated and what is more, large amounts of air can quickly escape. If a chest tube is not immediately available, a relief puncture is made with as thick a cannula as possible in the third intercostal space in the midclavicular line.

The **primary goal of treatment** consists only in the **relief of pressure,** thereby transferring the tension pneumothorax into a normal pneumothorax. During manual or mechanical ventilation the lung is expanded anyway by the intrapulmonary positive pressure. Chest tubes or cannulas are initially **left open to the outside** until the drainage system with suction is installed. Tiegel's puncture cannula, with the famous fingerstall, is no longer appropriate in clinical situations.

Relief puncture with a cannula is **never** definitive therapy. It is to be replaced immediately by a chest tube.

If the conjectured clinical diagnosis turns out to be wrong and if a chest tube was inserted without the presence of a tension pneumothorax, this seldom has negative consequences, and cannot be compared to the catastrophic consequences of an overlooked or belatedly treated tension pneumothorax.

III. Open Pneumothorax

This situation describes a pneumothorax that communicates with the **outside** atmosphere and not simply a pneumothorax caused by penetrating injuries. Most of the stabbing injuries and many gunshot wounds actually result in a pneumothorax, but not in an open pneumothorax.

Wartime surgeons have long been aware of the danger of this situation, even though it was not until World War I that it was generally recognized that the immediate threat to life could be overcome by closure of the thoracic wound, i. e., conversion into a closed pneumothorax [291].

In the Battle of Mantinea (362 B. C.) a spearhead penetrated the chest of Epaminondas, the Theban general. Since he was apparently aware of the danger of an open pneumothorax, he did not remove the spear until after the victory of his own troops was assured and then died as a consequence of his injury.

In 1267 Theodoric, the Bishop of Cervia, contrary to accepted academic opinions, recommended the closure of open chest wounds so that "the natural heat cannot escape and cold air cannot enter the chest" [266]. This advice went unheeded. In the sixteenth century Ambroise Paré was still recommending that larger chest wounds be left open [494].

Hewson reported in 1767 on an observation that in gunshot wounds in the thoracic area the patient was able to breathe better after the wound had been covered. He concluded from this that the air entering the thorax prevented an aeration of the lung through the trachea [284]. A similar observation was made by Larrey, Napoleon's field surgeon, as he covered the chest wound of a dying soldier to spare the other wounded from the sight. To his astonishment the patient's breathing improved and he survived [266].

Pathophysiology

In a free pleural space, the broad exposure of the chest cavity to the outside results in total collapse of the lung with atmospheric pressure in the pleural space. The mediastinum is not stable, like the chest, but is mobile. At inspiration it is drawn toward the healthy side by the negative pressure in the intact pleural space. During expiration the movement is just the opposite. This mediastinal movement is called **mediastinal flutter.** Basically **paradoxical respiration** in the uninvolved thoracic side occurs with the mediastinum as the mobile part.

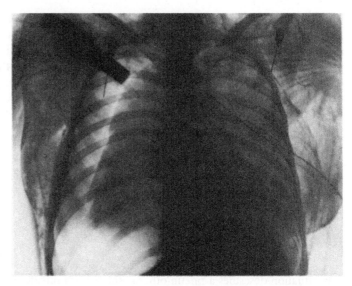

Fig. 62. Tension pneumothorax under mechanical ventilation for ARDS: in spite of massive intrapleural positive pressure, the lung, which is filled with fluid, can no longer collapse completely

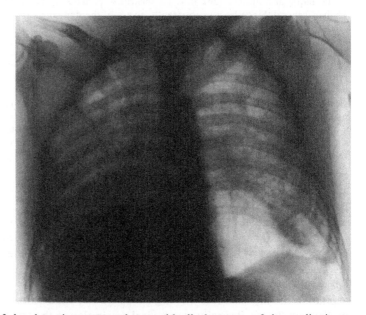

Fig. 63. Localized left basal tension pneumothorax with displacement of the mediastinum (patient on a respirator)

A hampering of the heart function and venous return to the heart were held responsible for the deleterious progression in this situation. In fact, the shift of the mediastinum is not nearly as pronounced as it is in a tension pneumothorax. On the other hand, however, because of the loss of function of the one lung and the very massive paradoxical respiration of the other side, a very **severe hypoxia** develops.

Carey and Hughes [279] have investigated this mediastinal flutter in dogs and monkeys and have proved that it causes no restriction of cardiac output nor of the venous filling of the right side of the heart. As expected, however, the open pneumothorax resulted in lethal hypoxia. If the defect in the thoracic wall is sufficiently large to produce unrestricted communication between the pleural cavity and the outside without a valve effect, the **size** of the thoracic opening toward the outside has no effect on the amount of functional impairment.

Diagnosis

A penetrating thoracic wound with a sucking sound of incoming and outgoing air ("sucking wound") adds to the clinical and radiologic evidence of pneumothorax.

Therapy

Every open pneumothorax represents an acute threat to life and demands immediate treatment. Under **clinical conditions,** there are two possibilities today for gaining control of the situation:

1. **Immediate airtight closure of the thoracic wound,** e. g., with gauze, attached to the thoracic wall with a covering foil or with adhesive tape: the open pneumothorax is converted into a closed pneumothorax. However, one has to keep in mind the danger of the possible development of a tension pneumothorax.

2. **Immediate intubation and mechanical ventilation.** In severe injuries this is the **method of choice.** This treatment not only eliminates mediastinal flutter immediately, it also makes possible the reexpansion of the lung. Most of the time, there is an operative indication anyway and because of it the necessity for general anesthesia. The wound can be examined very calmly, the chest drained, and the thoracic wall closed.

During **first aid,** whether on the street or during armed conflict in wartime in the field, only the first of these measures is possible, i. e., the closure of the thoracic wound. For very large defects, Müller has suggested a procedure for emergency situations: with the hand, a compress, or forceps the lung is forced into the wound and held there, thus sealing the defect of the thoracic wall.

IV. Hemothorax

Rib fractures and **other injuries of the thoracic wall accompanied by laceration of the parietal pleura** and **lesions of the lung** or of the **intrathoracic vessels** usually result in hemothorax. Often forgotten is the fact that **vertebral fractures** of the thoracic spinal column, particularly at the level of T-4 – T-6 [295], can lead to a hemothorax. This often does not take place until several days after the injury [293].

In addition to local problems (compression of the lung, displacement of the mediastinum) there is also the **loss of blood.** In hemorrhaging into the free pleural space, there is no tamponading effect. One must keep in mind that the pleural space can take up to 6 liters of blood.

Diagnosis

A massive hemothorax causes a **diminution of breath sounds;** percussion produces a **muffled sound.** A minor hemothorax can hardly be detected clinically, however.

In the **roentgenogram,** an accumulation of less than 200 ml of blood is usually not visible, especially if taken with the patient in a recumbent position. Such amounts

Table 18. Differential diagnosis of hemothorax

Immediately after trauma:	Rupture of diaphragm
	Atelectasis
	Preexisting pleural effusion
Several days after trauma:	Chylothorax
	Cholothorax
	Pleural empyema

of blood are clinically insignificant. In more severe hemorrhage, an increasing opacity is found; in a recumbent patient, there is never the classic picture with the line of effusion sloping up toward the thoracic wall but a more or less pronounced **clouding of the affected half of the thorax** up to complete **opacity** (Fig. 1). A severe hemothorax causes displacement of mediastinal structures to the opposite side.

In the **diagnosis** of hemothorax (Table 18), formation of atelectasis and rupture of the diaphragm should be **differentiated** since they also cause shadowing of the thorax in a roentgenogram of recent chest trauma (see Chap. 3).

Therapy

Resuscitative treatment through volume replacement and **local treatment** of the hemothorax go hand in hand, in which the restoration of a normal blood volume has priority. A **minimal** hemothorax with accumulation of blood in the phrenicocostal sinus does not require therapy but does make continuing supervision obligatory.

Thoracentesis, repeated if necessary, is considered only in cases of **slight hemothorax.** In most instances, and always in a hemothorax of larger proportions, a **chest tube** is inserted as a first step.

Goal of Treatment

1. Emptying the pleural space as completely as possible of the accumulated blood. This is done most easily shortly after trauma before coagulation or even fibrosis has set in.

2. Reexpansion of the lung compressed by the effusion of blood.

3. In moderate hemorrhages from the surface of the lung and thoracic wall, the goal is to achieve a tamponading effect by bringing the lung into contact with the parietal pleura.

4. Evaluating the amount of blood loss.

A **large** chest tube (at least Charrière 28) is inserted in the midaxillary line directed posteriorly. A suction of 25 cm H_2O is attached to the drainage. In a very massive hemothorax, the insertion of two tubes can be advantageous [150].
If a state of shock caused by intrathoracic bleeding cannot be controlled in spite of volume transfusion, if an injury of the large blood vessels or of the heart is suspected, and if massive bleeding persists, a **thoracotomy is indicated** (see Chap. 5).
With the insertion of the chest tube, large amounts of blood are often evacuated. The corresponding loss of blood has, of course, already taken place, not merely at the moment of drainage. In most cases, the bleeding will slowly come to a halt after the evacuation of the primary hemothorax.
The fear that evacuation of the hemothorax will promote further bleeding is, by and large, unfounded. From World War I up to the beginning of the 1960s, this fear was the reason why very cautious aspiration of the hemothorax and drainage of a maximum of 1 liter of blood was recommended [292].

V. Clotted Hemothorax, Fibrothorax

Moderate amounts of blood remaining in the thorax are **absorbed** astonishingly well in the course of a few months (Fig. 64).
On the other hand, the pathologic picture of a **clotted hemothorax with coagulated blood** and the resultant **fibrothorax** is generally well-known. If blood has coagulated, it can no longer be removed via chest drainage.
Immediate effective thoracic drainage is the best prophylaxis against fibrothorax. If performed consistently, fibrothorax will become a rarity [275, 281, 297]. Among 358 consecutive patients in our clinic with traumatic hemothorax, there was never an indication for late thoracotomy to remove a hematoma or for decortication.

Instillation of Fibrinolytic Enzymes

In a moderate hemothorax that can no longer be drained, it is worthwhile to make an attempt with fibrinolytic enzymes, especially if a chest tube has already been installed. Tillet and Sherry [298] recommended this therapy in 1949.

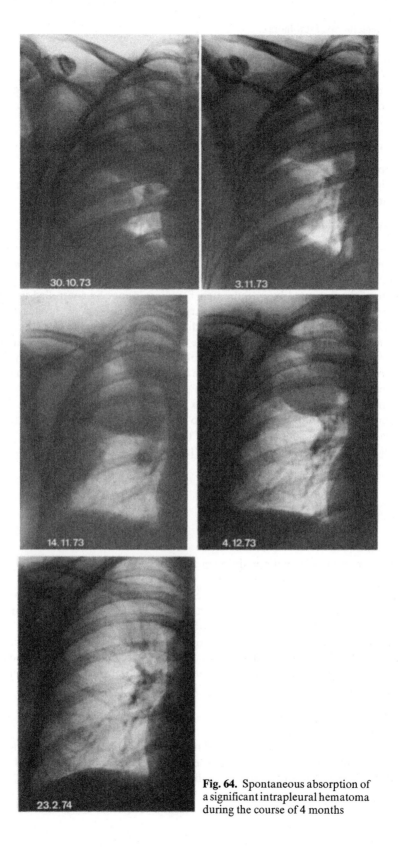

Fig. 64. Spontaneous absorption of a significant intrapleural hematoma during the course of 4 months

The expectations from this conceptually ideal therapy are not to be placed too high, however. We instill these enzymes on a trial basis, at the most twice, and often achieve an improvement. In my view, however, there is no justification in applying this therapy more frequently or even over a period of weeks. It is not in any way pleasant for the patient and often results in generalized symptoms.

The contents of an ampule of the combination preparation of **streptokinase** (100 000 units) and **streptodornase** (25 000 units) are dissolved in 120 ml of physiologic saline solution and instilled via the chest tube already in place. To avoid instilling air at the same time, the chest tube is clamped at the point of emergence from the skin, the drain is filled while being held in an upright position, and not until then is the syringe connected to the tube and the solution instilled. The chest tube is clamped for a period of 8 h, after which drainage is resumed with a suction of 25 cm H_2O.

The instillation of these fibrinolytic enzymes can cause febrile reactions and vomiting, something to which the patient's and nurses' attention should be called. If the general condition of the patient worsens significantly or dyspnea develops, the drainage tube is opened beforehand.

Operative Removal of Hematoma, Decortication

When a massive hemothorax can no longer be drained, the indication is given for operative removal of the hematoma or for decortication. This is usually the case when half or more of one side of the thorax is shaded.

It is important to make such a decision **early,** within 1 week, or at most 2 weeks, after trauma. Within this period, the coagulated blood can be evacuated without technical difficulties by means of a **small thoracotomy.** An actual **decortication** is **not necessary** as yet [275, 285]. Later on, a decortication will actually have to be performed. Although a distinct layer of organized hematoma can usually be found, there are always adhesions, and the danger of lung injury and of significant postoperative bleeding is not a trivial matter. Restraint in the indication for delayed decortication is certainly justified.

Technique

In the early evacuation of hemothorax a **small anterolateral thoracotomy** in the fifth intercostal space is sufficient. The coagulated blood is loosened and removed from the surface of the lung by hand or, if already in the process of being organized, by means of stick swabs. Extended thoracic drainage is recommended.

VI. Thoracentesis

In acute thoracic injuries, thoracentesis is seldom resorted to. Usually a chest tube is preferred. It is indicated primarily when effusions occur **later** or when there are **effusions after removal of the chest tube;** it can also serve as a diagnostic tool.

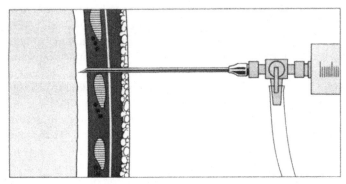

Fig. 65. Technique of thoracentesis (see text)

Contrary to common practice, which calls for thoracentesis with the patient in a sitting position, I recommend in all cases that it be performed with the patient in **a recumbent** position.

1. The sitting position is uncomfortable for the patient and painful if there are multiple rib fractures. Weakness and collapse are frequently the results.

2. In a sitting position, the puncture must be made low enough to evacuate the effusion. Injuries to the diaphragm, liver, spleen, or stomach can result. In the recumbent position, good evacuation at the level of the fifth intercostal space is possible if puncture is made in the posterior axillary line.

3. In a recumbent patient, there is no danger of an arterial air embolism caused by puncture of a lung vein.

Thoracentesis is made in the posterior axillary line at the level of the nipple in the fifth or sixth intercostal space. After local anesthesia, which includes the periosteum at the upper edge of the rib in question, a large needle is inserted toward the target rib and cautiously pushed about 7 mm further above the upper edge of this rib (Fig. 65).

A three-way stopcock between syringe and needle allows the effusion to be aspirated and the syringe to be emptied without admitting air into the pleural cavity.

VII. Intercostal Tube Drainage

We are indebted to Bülau for this simple and effective principle of closed chest drainage with long-term suction, which today bears his name. He used it for the first time in 1875 to treat pleural empyema [277]. Beyond its original indication, it subsequently attained far-reaching significance for the drainage of air, blood, and effusion from the pleural area.

The extended debate on the question of whether, because of the danger of infection, repeated thoracenteses are preferable to thoracic chest tube drainage, can now be laid to rest. Reports from the Korean War [176, 178] still blamed chest tube drainage for the great frequency of empyema and puncture was virtually the exclusive procedure. In the Vietnam War, with extensive use of chest tubes, the frequency of infection was much lower than in the Korean War [174]. The experiences of the 6-Day War in 1967 and the Yom Kippur War in 1973 have confirmed this [177].

Also under civilian circumstances, there have been reports on the use of chest tube drainage in penetrating injuries with very low infection rates [275, 285].

This is also in accord with my experiences in dealing mainly with closed thoracic injuries: pleural empyema has become a great rarity. The fear of an infection due to thoracic drainage is false. On the contrary, **early, complete evacuation of blood and air** is the **best prophylaxis against empyema** (Table 19).

Table 19. Drainage is the best prophylaxis against pleural empyema

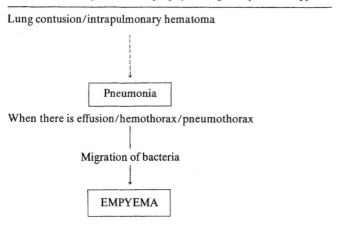

Technique of Intercostal Tube Drainage

Material

For a long time we have been using **siliconized thoracic trocar catheters made of plastic,** which are slipped over metal rods and inserted (Argyle trocar catheter) (Fig. 66). Compared to trocar methods formerly in use, these chest tubes have several significant **advantages:** they are made of material of good compatibility, which is flexible yet firm and does not collapse. Because of the silicone cover, clogged drains have become very rare. Insertion is quick. The metal rod aids in placing the drains with extreme accuracy.

The caliber is larger than in the earlier trocar method, making drainage more effective. The metal rod inside the drain usually prevents air from entering the thoracic space as it is inserted.

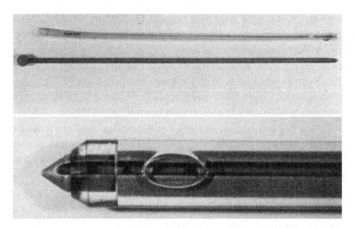

Fig. 66. Thoracic trocar catheter (Argyle): the flexible plastic drain is slipped over a metal rod and then inserted

Location and Position of the Drainage (Fig. 67)

In Pneumothorax

A. The drain enters the thorax from in **front,** at the **midclavicular line in the second intercostal space,** and is guided upward against the top of the pleura. The distance to the edge of the sternum should be at least the width of two and one-half fingers to avoid the danger of injuring the internal thoracic artery.

In Hemothorax or Pneumohemothorax

B. **Classic position:** the drain enters the thorax at the **midaxillary line, not below the level of the nipple.** The tube is directed posteriorly and superiorly.

C. **Suitable variation:** point of entry same as in B. The drain is guided posteriorly and inferiorly into the phrenicocostal sinus, offering ideal drainage for the lowest sections of the thorax (Fig. 68). In this drainage position, supplemental drainage openings have to be made in the tube since the openings at the tip become clogged very quickly in the narrow sinus by the tissues that are sucked in.

The rule is that **no chest tube should enter the thorax below the level of the nipple** to avoid injuries to the diaphragm and intra-abdominal organs. In blunt thoracic trauma, the diaphragm is often elevated due to restricted breathing, which in the presence of a hemothorax is frequently not visible on a roentgenogram.

Inserting the Tube

A **subcutaneous tract** about 5 cm in length is planned for the course of the tube. **Local anesthesia** should include the area of the skin incision, the subcutaneous tract,

Intercostal Tube Drainage

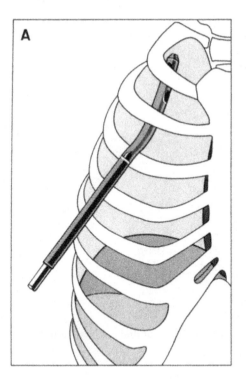

Fig. 67 A – C. Ideal position of a chest tube in pneumothorax (**A**) and in hemothorax: classic position (**B**) and variation for the selective drainage of the lowest sections of the thorax (**C**)

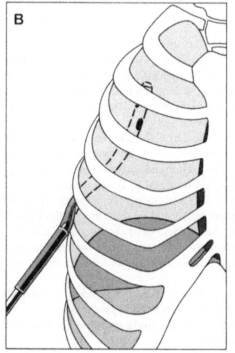
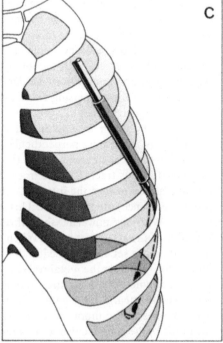

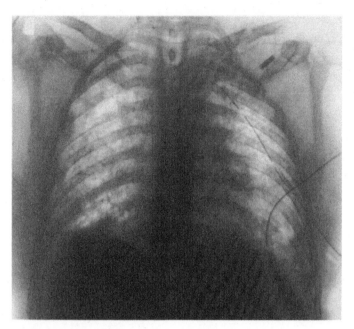

Fig. 68. Ideal position for thoracic drainage in a hemothorax: a drain is inserted in a basal direction and placed into the posterior phrenicocostal sinus

and the rib at the anticipated spot of entry into the thorax, along with the periosteum and pleura at the upper edge of this rib.

In making additional drainage openings in the thoracic tube, care should be taken to cut the last opening on the radiopaque contrast thread.

The **skin incision** should be made conveniently large. The left hand takes hold of the chest tube together with the guide rod with a **specific grip** (Fig. 69) to prevent the guide rod upon entry from suddenly being shoved uncontrollably into the interior because of the decreasing resistance. I have known of cases of severe lung and even aortic injuries when this precaution was not observed.

Guide rod and drain are now inserted according to a **specific sequence.** The direction of thrust is initially perpendicular to the interior of the thorax to get through the skin to the subcutaneous tissues (Fig. 70A). Then the thrust is tangential to form the subcutaneous tract (B). The trocar is again returned to the perpendicular position and aimed toward the interior of the thorax with its tip palpating the rib at the point of entrance into the thorax. This serves as orientation as to the depth of the rib location. With one powerful, short thrust, the thoracic cavity is entered at the superior edge of the selected rib (C). When the point of the trocar has entered the chest, the guide rod is set in the direction that the drain is to follow and the plastic catheter pushed forward over the metal rod (D).

In the spontaneously breathing patient, the tube is clamped. The length of insertion is checked by means of the guide rod, and the drain is fixed in place.

The tube lies in the thorax when in withdrawing the guide rod blood follows or if the inside of the tube is covered with moisture.

Intercostal Tube Drainage

The fear of injuring the lung in the process of inserting the chest tube is largely unfounded since it has been pushed aside, away from the thoracic wall, by the effusion of blood or by air.

The same principles also apply to the former technique of **inserting a rubber drain** through the **metal sleeve of a trocar.** If even this equipment is unavailable, a drain will have to be used that is introduced into the thoracic area with a **medium-sized clamp.**

Difficulties in Inserting a Chest Tube

In **rib fractures,** the insertion of a tube is always **painful.** Local anesthesia offers no protection against movement of ribs at the point of fracture. The thrust to achieve entrance into the chest cavity, which must overcome considerable resistance, should be short and forceful.

In comminuted rib fractures, there is a danger when the tube is inserted that a **mobile fragment of thoracic wall** might be displaced into the thorax (Fig. 71). In such cases, the point of entrance is to be selected in the **stable** section of the thorax even though an atypical drainage results.

Applying Suction to the Drainage

By installing **permanent suction,** better evacuation of fluids and air and more rapid reexpansion of the lung is achieved. Normally it totals 25 cm H_2O, but after a pneu-

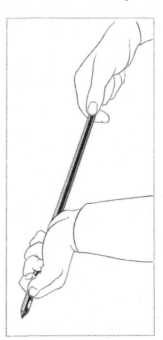

Fig. 69. Grip used to avoid penetrating too far into the thorax with the puncture rod in the process of inserting the tube

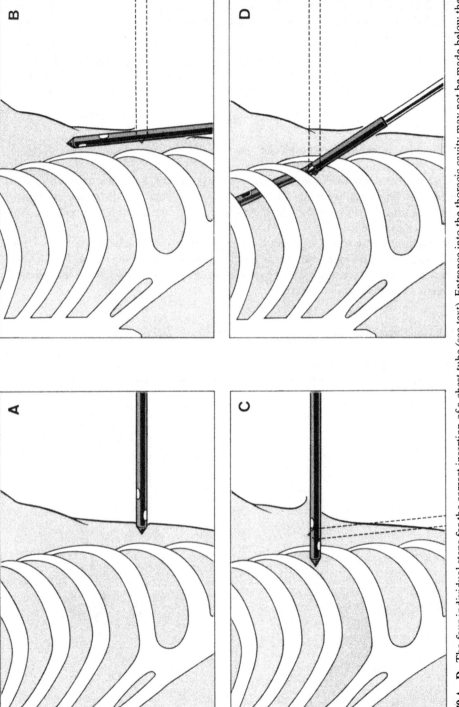

Fig. 70 A–D. The four individual steps for the correct insertion of a chest tube (see text). Entrance into the thoracic cavity may not be made below the level of the nipple

Fig. 71. The free fragment of chest wall in a multiple double rib fracture was shifted into the chest cavity when a chest tube was inserted

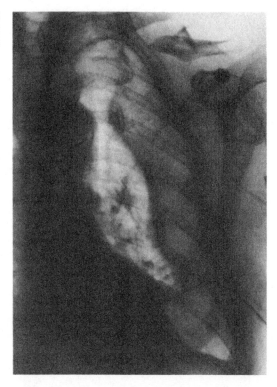

monectomy it is at most 5 cm H_2O. With a large air leak on a respirator, there are situations in which there is an advantage to dispensing with suction. If a pneumothorax cannot be expanded under normal suction, it may occasionally be worthwhile to raise it to 45, 60, or maximally to 100 cm H_2O.

The **connecting piece** between the thoracic drain and chest tube should not have any narrow places. Experience shows that they easily become clogged (Fig. 72).

A large **bottle** serves to collect blood and effusions. The **water column,** next in sequence, regulates the level of negative pressure. A small intermediary receptacle prevents water from entering the suction pump or the vacuum system on the wall

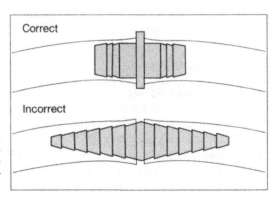

Fig. 72. The connecting piece between the chest tube and the drainage system should not have any narrow places

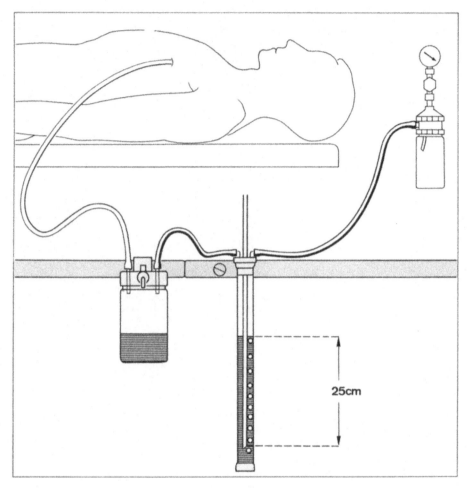

Fig. 73. Drainage system of a thoracic suction drain (see text)

(Fig. 73). Under suction, air bubbles rise in the water column. If this does not happen, there is a mistake somewhere: either the system is not airtight and is sucking air, the suction applied by the suction equipment is insufficient, or (very rarely) the loss of air from the lung is greater than the suction capacity of the system being used.

Heimlich Valve (Fig. 74).

In 1965 Heimlich [286] reported on a valve that permits the exit of fluids and air and positively precludes the entrance of air into the thoracic cavity. It involves a further development of the well-known rubber fingerstall of Ehrman and Tiegel. A sleeve is attached to the thoracic drain, inside which there is a flattened length of rubber tubing, which during inspiration prevents air from entering the chest tube while air and fluid can drain when the pressure is higher than the atmospheric pressure. In addition, a suctioning apparatus can be connected to this system.

The Heimlich valve was widely used during the Vietnam War [300]. The use of this valve proved its value in transporting patients with chest tubes, e.g., into the operating room and to radiologic and other special examinations [289]. It prevents tension pneumothoraces and enables a patient with a chest tube to be moved independently of the suction.

Complications and Problems with Thoracic Suction Drainage

1. **The tube is not placed into the chest:** the inexperienced person occasionally slides the tube off a rib and then inserts it into the subcutaneous tissue. One is often misled by the extent of the fat and muscle layer of the thoracic wall.

2. **Inserting the tube too caudally** results in injuries to the diaphragm and intra-abdominal organs (Fig. 75). The principle that chest tubes should never be installed below the level of the nipple was imposed because of such experiences.

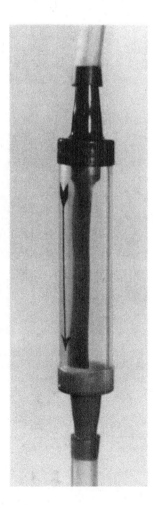

Fig. 74. The Heimlich valve permits the drainage of air and blood but prevents the entrance of air into the chest tube

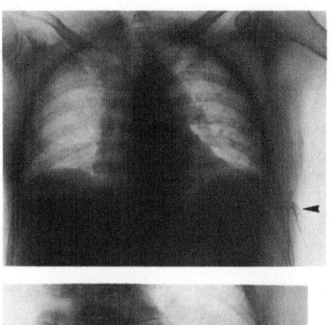

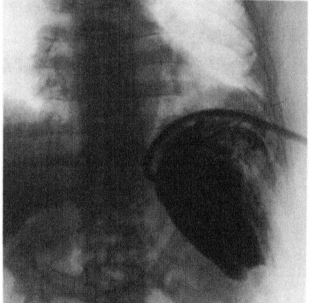

Fig. 75. a Chest tube introduced intra-abdominally injuring the spleen because of disregard of the rule that a chest tube must never be introduced below the level of the nipple. **b** Locating the drain using contrast medium

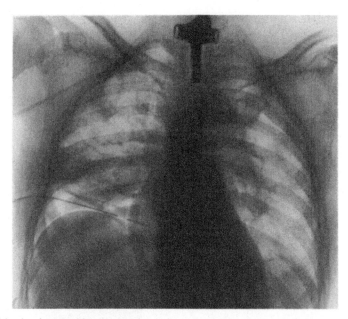

Fig. 76. By contact with the heart, this chest tube led to frequent supraventricular extrasystoles; the rhythm disturbances disappeared when the drain was withdrawn

3. **Lung injuries occurring during installation:** superficial lung injuries have no clinical significance. If there is suspicion of intrapulmonary positioning of the tube, however, it is examined by means of a lateral roentgenogram and, if necessary, the tube is removed and replaced with another. Only after the tube has been removed can the lung injury heal. A tube situated in the lung often erodes larger vessels.

4. **Damage by tubes situated in the pleural space:** by contact with the heart, rhythm disturbances can appear (Fig. 76). The erosion of larger vessels, e. g., in the top of the pleura, is a rarity.

5. **Clogged tubes:** because of the use of siliconized materials, this occurs less frequently than formerly. Often the patient is lying on the chest tube, the drain is under the mattress, or is pinched off somewhere else. The connecting tube should not be too long.

Removal of the Chest Tube

When no further blood or effusion is produced and if the lung wound is airtight, the tube can be removed. One must take into consideration the fact that irritation caused by the tube itself can produce an effusion of 100 ml/day. Effusions of this amount are no reason for not removing the tube.
Before removal of the tube, **a test for air leak is made by means of a gravity siphon system (Perthes' system)** (Fig. 77): using two bottles arranged one above the other,

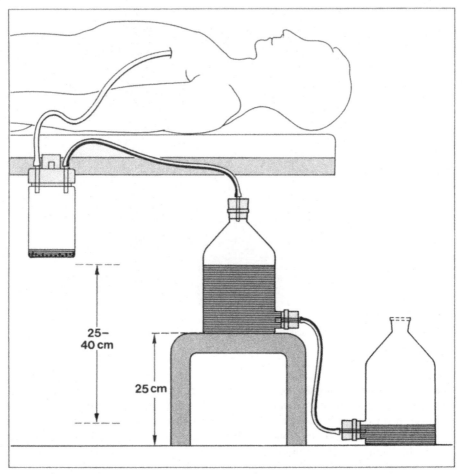

Fig. 77. Testing for air leak after pneumothorax with the Perthes version of a gravity siphon (see text)

suction continues to be maintained in the pleural space by means of gravitation in a closed system. If air is being drained, the level of the water in the upper bottle drops. If the level remains constant over a period of 12 h, the lung (provided the tube is open) is airtight and the chest tube can be removed.

If there are doubts about the airtightness of the system itself or of the chest drain, the chest tube should be temporarily clamped at its exit from the chest. If the water level in the Perthes' system decreases farther, the system itself is not airtight.

If a test for airtightness by means of the Perthes' system is impossible, the chest tube is clamped, and 24 h later a follow-up roentgenogram is taken with the tube still in place.

Removal of the chest tube is made under suction. While the subcutaneous skin tract is held under compression, a prepared rectangular plaster with a small swab will close the entrance spot the moment the tube is removed with a quick jerk.

Chapter 12
Traumatic Emphysema

I. Subcutaneous Emphysema

An accumulation of air in the subcutaneous tissue is not infrequent in both closed and open thoracic injuries. Upon admission to the hospital, 27% of the patients with multiple rib fractures are found to have subcutaneous emphysema.

1. If a **pneumothorax** occurs and the parietal pleura is simultaneously injured, air enters the subcutaneous tissue of the thoracic wall (Fig. 78). A **tension pneumothorax** in multiple rib fractures nearly always goes hand in hand with acute emphysema. Also, after insertion of a chest tube in cases of pneumothorax, air often escapes into the subcutaneous drainage tract.

2. In injuries to the lung or pleura, subcutaneous emphysema can also form without the presence of a pneumothorax when the pleural membranes have **adhered.**
However, there are cases of subcutaneous accumulations of air in which there are definitely no pleural adhesions present and in which no pneumothorax can be verified. If none of the causes listed below are suspected, it must be assumed that there is indeed a minor pneumothorax that is not visible on the roentgenogram.

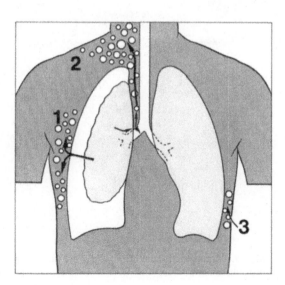

Fig.78. The three possible causes of subcutaneous emphysema (see text)

3. Upon escaping from **mediastinal emphysema,** air spreads out in the throat area and forces its way into the soft tissue of the head and thorax.

4. Air can enter the thorax from an **external wound;** subcutaneous emphysema of this genesis does not expand very much.

In subcutaneous tissue, with its very minimal resistance, air spreads out very rapidly. The swelling of the tissue is most impressive where it is least compact: in the face, especially in the area around the eyelids, and in the scrotum (Fig. 79). The scrotum can become as large as a soccer ball. We have observed the diffusion of air throughout the entire body down to the tips of the toes.

Disquieting for relatives is the swelling of the face, which makes it impossible for them to recognize the patient. The injured person, however, feels well, the only difficulty being that in advanced subcutaneous emphysema the eyes can no longer be opened.

Treatment with a respirator, especially in ventilation with high inspiratory pressures and positive end-expiratory pressure, leads to especially pervasive emphysema, which expands very rapidly.

Findings on palpation are completely characteristic and unmistakable: crepitation under the skin, which has been described as sounding like "crunching snow."

Just as characteristic is the **roentgenogram.** The subcutaneous accumulation of air shows up as an irregularly flecked picture with radiolucency. If the emphysema is more diffuse, the spread of air along the muscle fibers of the major pectoral muscle

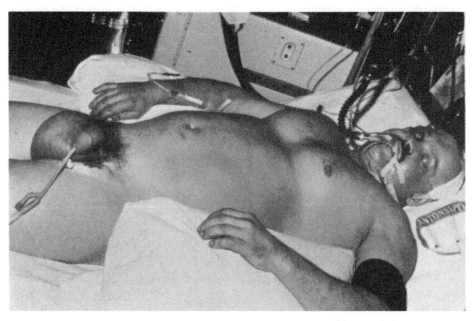

Fig. 79. Characteristic picture of patient with subcutaneous emphysema, with swelling in the face, thorax, and scrotum

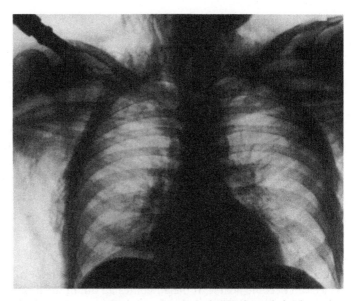

Fig. 80. Roentgenogram of subcutaneous emphysema: fan-shaped diffusion of air along the fibers of the major pectoral muscle, accumulation of air along the thoracic wall and in the throat area

shows up in the shape of a fan (Fig. 80). A massive subcutaneous emphysema makes it impossible to evaluate the underlying lung in a roentgenogram.

The **differential diagnosis** of gas-forming infections never presents difficulties if attention is paid to the history and the general condition of the patient.

Therapy

Despite its impressive appearance, the treatment of subcutaneous emphysema itself is mostly **unnecessary.** Obviously, the underlying cause should be eliminated as far as possible and a pneumothorax drained. In this connection, it is helpful to observe from what point of origin the emphysema has derived its further diffusion. If it has been determined that it was in the throat at first, a question will be raised as to the cause of **mediastinal emphysema.** At the thoracic wall the first localization of emphysema points toward the **place where rib fractures have occurred.** Usually, a diffuse subcutaneous emphysema is also absorbed spontaneously within a few days. It is interesting to note that **subcutaneous infections** practically **never** develop.

Occasionally on the respirator, however, subcutaneous emphysema can increase irresistibly despite a correctly placed chest tube. In such a situation, it is advisable to install a similar tube in the subcutaneous tissue at the site where the air is presumed to be escaping, usually in the area of the chest tube, and also to promote drainage by means of a thoracic suction system.

II. Mediastinal Emphysema

Severe injuries can be the underlying cause of the invasion of air into the interstitial connective tissue of the mediastinum: rupture of the trachea, rupture of a bronchus, tension pneumothorax, or rupture of the esophagus.
These lesions have to be excluded. In more than one-half of all cases, however, mediastinal emphysema does not form because of these life-threatening injuries but because of **alveolar ruptures involved in lung contusions or in mechanical ventilation.** The air coming from the alveoli follows the vascular structure of the lung and hilus and from there it reaches the mediastinum.
In the accumulation of mediastinal air, however, the delicate mediastinal pleura can be torn. Then a **secondary pneumothorax** develops.

Diagnosis

Often the patients complain about a **feeling of pressure** or of **retrosternal pains.** The voice can become **hoarse.** If the air comes up out of the mediastinum above the sternal notch and spreads out in the **cervical area,** the characteristic crepitation will be detected there. In very pronounced cases, the **cardiac dullness disappears.** Of much greater significance, however, is the **characteristic sound on heart auscultation** as described by Hamman [301]: air in the mediastinal tissue in front of the heart brings about a loud crunching, clicking sound that is synchronous with the heartbeat. This unmistakable auscultatory finding often makes it possible to establish a diagnosis of a mediastinal emphysema before this can be verified by a roentgenogram or palpated in the vicinity of the neck. On occasion, however, it is falsely interpreted as pericarditis or pneumohemopericardium [304].
Larger accumulations of air in the mediastinum are visible in the **roentgenogram.** The most important indication is a **double line on the left contour of the heart** caused by displacement of the mediastinal pleura (Fig. 81). The **deep cervical emphysema** can be verified by specific anteroposterior roentgenograms of the upper mediastinum or of the throat before it can be palpated [351].
Substantial mediastinal emphysema always demands **investigation for** a possible **tracheal or bronchial rupture** by means of bronchoscopy or for a possible **esophageal rupture** by means of esophagography with contrast medium. The very rare esophageal injury often results in only a slow development of mediastinal emphysema.
In rare instances, the accumulation of air in the mediastinum with increasing pressure impairs **venous return** to the heart. Such patients exhibit a picture of venous congestion with distended neck veins. Tachycardia, dyspnea, and finally collapse of cardiac output can be the result [306]. In 1927 Jehn and Nissen [302] described the similarity of this condition to cardiac tamponade. Since then, a term used for it is "extrapericardial cardiac tamponade."

Therapy

The **cause** of mediastinal emphysema must be treated: a tension pneumothorax needs to be drained, immediately upon recognition; a significant tracheal, bronchi-

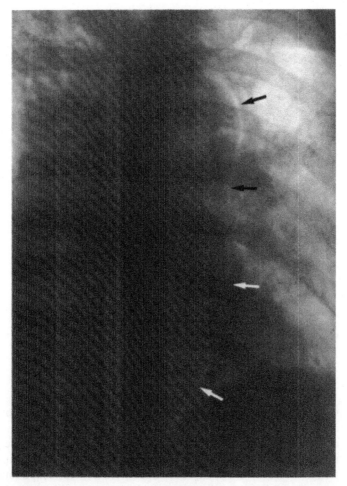

Fig. 81. Mediastinal emphysema: typical double line on the left heart contour silhouetted by the mediastinal pleura

al, or esophageal injury must be treated surgically. If these life-threatening causes of mediastinal emphysema can be excluded, therapy is generally expectant. However, when a picture of **threatening pressure increase with venous congestion** develops a **cervical mediastinotomy** [305] can be necessary. Admittedly, this is seldom the case.

 Laennec relates the episode of how he punctured by candlelight the suprasternal area of a 4-year-old child with mediastinal emphysema under tension. The candle was blown out by the air streaming out under pressure. The child, previously at the point of death, recovered.

Technique of Cervical Mediastinotomy (Fig. 82)

A transverse incision of the skin is made between the origins of the sternocleidomastoid muscle, the width of one finger above the suprasternal notch. After divid-

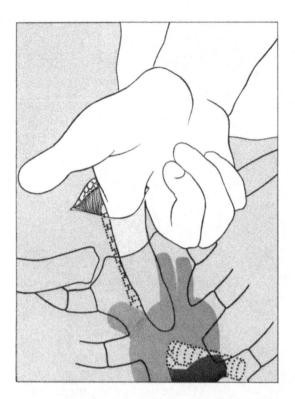

Fig. 82. Cervical mediastinotomy (see text)

ing the subcutaneous tissue and the platysma, the sternothyroid muscles are spread apart with scissors and the front wall of the trachea exposed. With the finger, blunt dissection is carried out along and in contact with the trachea. In this way, one is able to reach as far as beneath the aortic arch without bleeding or injury to important structures. During the entire operation, air will escape under pressure from the tissues. In the prepared tract, a thick, noncollapsible drain is introduced (a thick thoracic drain with additional drainage openings is well suited for this). The edges of the incision are then brought into apposition.

Chapter 13

Lung Injuries from Blunt Trauma

I. General Considerations

Three mechanisms cause damage to the lung parenchyma in a closed chest injury:

1. **Rib fractures** can result in lacerations or contusions of the lung components lying beneath them.

2. A **compression** of the thorax causes lung contusions or ruptures of the lung.

3. In closed injury, contusions can occur as a **"contrecoup" lesion** far from the point of impact.

The extent of an injury to the thoracic wall gives no indication as to the severity of the pulmonary injury. On the contrary, in rib fractures the pulmonary damage is often localized; in compression of the elastic thorax in a young person diffuse damages to the parenchyma occasionally ensue.

The healing tendency of lung tissue is astonishingly good so that lung parenchyma injuries are generally tolerated quite well.

At times, classification into precise forms of injury is questionable since transitions and combinations of various lesions occur; nevertheless, for practical purposes, individual injury types can be differentiated (Table 20). One of them is especially significant. It is the severer of the two forms of lung contusion, namely, **contusion with respiratory insufficiency.** The critical nature of this injury is often hidden initially, thereby delaying early therapy.

Of decisive importance for **diagnosis and evaluation** of closed lung parenchymal injuries are:

1. **Repeated** roentgenograms of the thorax

2. **Repeated** blood gas analyses

A single finding tells very little. Lung hematoma or lung contusions may not become visible on roentgenograms until hours after the accident and continue to increase for days; pseudocysts may not show up for 1 or 2 weeks after trauma.

 Contusion injuries of the lung were already described in 1761 by Morgagni [331] who reported on autopsy findings in two cases. In one of them there were no external signs of injury nor any rib fractures in evidence.

Table 20. Clinical significance and therapy of various forms of lung parenchymal injuries

		Clinical significance	Therapy
	Lung laceration/ lung rupture	Mostly harmless (exception: central lung rupture) Significant: hemo- and pneumothorax	Conservative Thoracic drainage in pneumothorax and hemothorax Operation only in exceptional cases because of bleeding or massive air loss
	Intrapulmonary hematoma	Harmless	None
	Traumatic lung pseudocysts	Harmless	Mostly none
	Simple lung contusion	Mostly harmless Can develop into lung contusion with respiratory insufficiency	Breathing exercises Careful monitoring of progress
	Lung contusion with respiratory insufficiency	Progressive respiratory insufficiency: hypoxia, right-to-left shunt, interstitial edema, considerable mortality	Intubation and positive end-expiratory pressure ventilation (PEEP) Maintenance of a normal oncotic pressure (fluid infusion limited, human albumin 20%) Steroids
	Blast injury	Severest injury Progressive respiratory insufficiency Danger of arterial air embolism Hemothorax, pneumothorax, abdominal injuries (colon!)	As in lung contusions with respiratory insufficiency

II. Lung Laceration, Lung Rupture

Lacerations of lung tissue produce **bleeding** and **local escape of air.** Because of the low pressures in the pulmonary circulation, bleeding is usually minor, and hemostasis is spontaneous if no large vessels are injured.

If the visceral pleura is torn, a **pneumothorax** occurs, possibly combined with a hemothorax. If the visceral pleura is intact, a **central lung rupture** has occurred. In extreme cases, there are total ruptures of entire lobes of the lung, which can result in massive hemorrhage.

Diagnosis

The **clinical picture** is dominated by either pneumothorax or hemothorax. Hemoptysis can be present and in central parenchymal ruptures is often the only clue to an injury. The **roentgenogram** reveals a poorly delineated, localized opacity. At times, this condition cannot be distinguished from a lung contusion. In less severe, superficial lung lacerations that lead to pneumothorax, there is often no change in the parenchyma on the roentgenogram.

Therapy

A pneumothorax or hemothorax is drained. In almost all cases air leakage soon ceases and bleeding comes to a halt.

An **operation is indicated** only when there is persistent, severe bleeding or it is impossible to attain complete reexpansion of the lung by means of suction drainage (see Chap. 5). If, in exceptional cases, an operation must be resorted to, the use of a double-lumen endotracheal tube is recommended when there is significant hemoptysis because of the danger of aspiration into the undamaged lung.

In severe bleeding from the injured lung, the hilus is temporarily clamped intraoperatively with a soft vascular clamp. The injury can then be explored calmly and hemostasis as well as the suturing of the larger bronchi carried out. Not every wound encountered during a thoracotomy has to be sutured. Small air leaks always stop under suction drainage. In view of the good healing tendencies of injured lung tissue, there has to be major destruction before a resection is indicated.

Attention must be called to the fact that in blunt thoracic injuries pneumonectomy has a poor prognosis. In such severe injuries, there are almost always foci of contusion in the other lung. Moreover, since the latter must accept the entire cardiac output and as a consequence is unavoidably flooded with blood, the danger of edema formation with very severe respiratory failure is quite great (Fig. 83).

Example: A 21-year-old military driver ended up lying under an overturned jeep. Upon admission to the hospital, he was in a very severe state of shock. In the presence of large fields of opacity in the right lung (Fig. 83a), massive bleeding from the chest tube required an emergency thoracotomy. Because of massive lacerations of the entire right lung, there was no other alternative except a pneumonectomy. Three hours after the operative intervention, the roentgenogram already revealed very severe lung edema on the left side (Fig. 83b), which could not be controlled. The patient died 3 days after the accident.

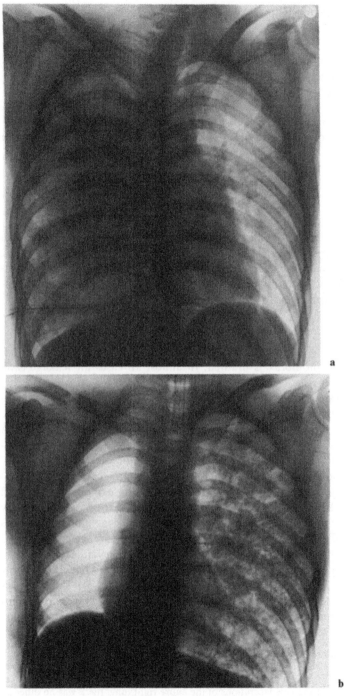

Fig. 83. a Very severe lacerations of the right lung with massive bleeding required a pneumonectomy in this 21-year-old male patient. **b** Lethal edema in the remaining lung 3 h after the conclusion of the operation (see text)

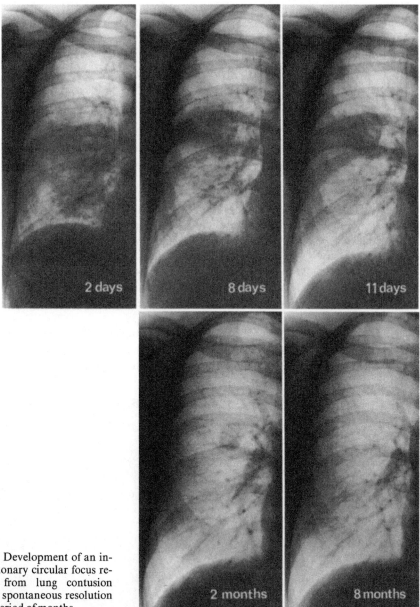

Fig. 84. Development of an intrapulmonary circular focus resulting from lung contusion and the spontaneous resolution over a period of months

III. Intrapulmonary Hematoma

This injury is a special, usually very minor form of central lung rupture. The roentgenogram initially reveals a localized, faint opacity, which within a few days typically develops into a distinct **circular focus** characteristic of intrapulmonary hematoma [317]. The spherical form is caused by the elasticity of the lung tissue [330].

Therapy is always conservative and on a wait-and-see basis. Hematomas regress spontaneously. The time necessary for resolution depends upon the size of the hematoma and usually takes from 2 weeks to 3 months, seldom any longer (Fig. 84).
This radiologic finding is of practical significance for the **differential diagnosis of tumor** [342]. Thought must be given to the possibility of carcinoma if there is still no decrease in the size of the focus within 2 months after trauma.

IV. Traumatic Lung Pseudocysts (Pneumatoceles)

The development of air-filled cavities (Fig. 85) occurs less frequently than intrapulmonary hematoma. These cavities are not lung cysts since the essential wall components of a cyst, especially the epithelium, are lacking. To be precise, they should be designated **pseudocysts.** The term **"pneumatoceles"** has also come into use. Frequently, there are transitional forms between a hematoma and a pseudocyst.
Their origin can be thought of in two ways: as a result of rupture of lung parenchyma or a bronchiole, there is a localized accumulation of air, or (extremely rare in the case of posttraumatic pseudocysts) they are the sequelae of prior inflammatory processes.
Such pseudocysts can already become visible on a **roentgenogram** immediately after trauma, but as a rule they are not recognized until 1 or 2 weeks after the accident when the hematoma in the surrounding lung tissue has been reabsorbed.

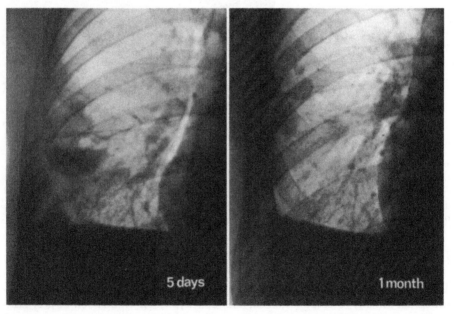

Fig. 85. Posttraumatic lung pseudocyst, partially filled with fluid (air-fluid level). Spontaneous regression

The **course** of developments is usually favorable. Since the wall of the cavity contains no epithelium, the air can be reabsorbed, with spontaneous regression of the pseudocyst within a period of 2 weeks to 5 months [329].

Therapy

Therapy is hardly ever necessary. Only if a connection to the bronchial system remains open can the pseudocyst continue to exist or even enlarge itself. In such cases, there is also the danger of infection. Then the installation of a Monaldi drain followed by suction treatment is indicated. Thin (e. g., Charrière 12) trocar catheters (Argyle) are suited to this purpose and are introduced under control with an image intensifier. The suction selected should be high enough to produce collapse of the cavity.

V. Lung Contusion

The clinical significance of this very common injury in blunt chest trauma has in recent times frequently been the occasion for confusion. It so happens that a lung contusion can appear in two clinical forms, which are different with regard to their morbidity and prognosis: **simple lung contusion** and **lung contusion with** a (precisely defined) **respiratory insufficiency.**
It seems essential to me to keep these two forms clearly separate and distinct.
The degree of opacity or the distribution of the foci of contusion on the **roentgenogram** provide no points of reference as to the form of lung contusion present. **Blood gas analysis** during respiration on room air and, in cases of doubt, with pure oxygen (oxygenation test), is the **only** way the two forms can be distinguished. Since the simple form can convert into the second, the blood gas analysis must be made **repeatedly** in the early stages of treatment.

1. Simple Lung Contusion

One finds individual blood-filled foci or extended hemorrhagic areas of the lung mostly localized at the point of impact and occasionally also as a "contrecoup" lesion.
The clinical picture is often influenced by other thoracic injuries (e. g., rib fractures). This lung complication is usually tolerated rather well, and there is hardly any dyspnea. Hemoptysis can be present.
The findings on the **roentgenogram** (Fig. 86) are extraordinarily diverse: they range from faintly delineated smaller shadows to expansive "infiltrates" to opacity of the entire lobe of the lung. The radiologic changes often develop because of bleeding into a bronchus and of subsequent aspiration in uninjured areas of the lungs.
The arterial PO_2 in the **blood gas analysis** is normal or only slightly decreased. With respiration or ventilation on pure oxygen, the P_aO_2 clearly remains above

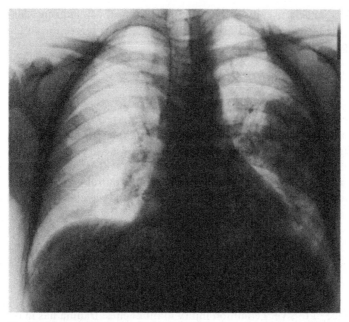

Fig. 86. Lung contusion on the left side without respiratory insufficiency

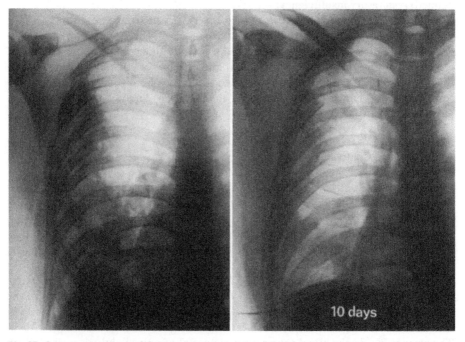

Fig. 87. Lung contusions and minor hemothorax in a patient with multiple rib fractures. Almost complete regression within 10 days

300 mmHg, and the calculated alveolar-arterial oxygen gradient is not elevated or only slightly (below 350 mmHg); there is therefore no significant intrapulmonary right-to-left shunt.

If this simple lung contusion does not evolve into the second form with respiratory insufficiency, spontaneous absorption of the intraparenchymal hemorrhages will take place in a few days to a few weeks (Fig. 87).

Therapy

Treatment is expectant. The progress is monitored by means of repeated blood gas analyses. Intensive respiratory therapy is essential (see Chap. 9).

2. Lung Contusion with Respiratory Insufficiency

Pathophysiology

Within contused areas of the lung, not only hemorrhaging into the tissue but also an **interstitial,** and partly also alveolar, **edema** occurs caused by changes in the permeability of the capillary wall. Microatelectasis occurs. The surfactant content decreases. Apparently undamaged areas of the lungs also suffer the same changes [322, 324, 332, 340].

These changes lead to a **reduction of the functional residual capacity,** to the development of a massive **intrapulmonary right-to-left shunt,** and through it to **arterial hypoxia.** Morphologically as well as functionally, therefore, the same changes occur with progressive respiratory insufficiency as in adult respiratory distress syndrome (ARDS) (see Chap. 4).

In spite of all the known factors, it is often impossible in any given incident to elucidate why local lung parenchyma, damaged by contusion, leads to respiratory insufficiency of such magnitude. Certainly, the **force of the impact,** and above all, its velocity, plays an important role [310, 340]. Valenta [340], in his experimental research using falling weights as heavy as 22.5 kg, was able to produce lung contusions but no respiratory insufficiency. It was not until he raised the impact velocity by propelling a cylinder weighing 180 g with a speed of 37 m/s or 50 m/s against the chest that lung contusions with respiratory insufficiency were produced.

As in ARDS, there are iatrogenic factors that play an essential role in the development of respiratory insufficiency in lung contusion. Undisputed, indeed of great clinical significance is the fact that **infusion of crystalloids in large amounts** can trigger the onset of or significantly worsen the pathologic aspect of the illness [34, 55, 78, 80, 81, 322, 326, 339, 340].

Diagnosis

The **patient's history** will always disclose signs of **severe trauma.** Added to the findings of simple lung contusion are the clinical signs of respiratory insufficiency.

The **thoracic roentgenogram** does not differ between the beginning stages of the illness and that of simple lung contusion and reveals nothing about the degree of functional impairment! Later, also those parts of the lung that were initially normal exhibit a growing cloudiness.

Of significance for diagnosis is the **arterial blood gas analysis,** which shows a pronounced hypoxia. The P_aCO_2 is either normal or lowered, although it may be increased when alveolar hypoventilation is present. The intrapulmonary right-to-left shunt quotient ($\dot{Q}_S/\dot{Q}_T$) is significantly raised and attains 20% or more. As an expression of the increased right-to-left shunt, the P_aO_2 under pure oxygen respiration or ventilation is lower than the values normally attained (in practice, below 300 mmHg), and the alveolar-arterial oxygen gradient is significantly raised (over 350 mmHg). As a compensatory mechanism, cardiac output increases; the arteriovenous oxygen difference (AVD) is lowered.

Immediately after the accident, these findings are characteristically not present, or if so, only to a minor extent, and do not develop until hours or days later.

Prophylaxis

Precisely because iatrogenic factors are of essential significance in the development of this form of respiratory insufficiency, it is conceivable that this severe form of lung contusion can be avoided in many cases:

1. **Active chest physiotherapy.** Avoidance of atelectasis and microatelectasis by physiotherapeutic measures (see Chap. 9). Important for good ventilation in addition to this is control of pain and forced removal of secretions.

2. It was demonstrated experimentally [332, 339, 340] and clinically [335, 345] that **mechanical ventilation,** most effectively with **positive end-expiratory pressure (PEEP),** can prevent the development of pathologic alterations in many cases.

In view of the frequency of lung contusions, it is impossible to ventilate every patient prophylactically, especially since this severe form of lung contusion is rare and other prophylactic measures are quite effective. There are certain indications for **prophylactic mechanical ventilation:**

1. The more severe the other injuries of a multiply injured patient are, the more preferable is the application of prophylactic mechanical ventilation.

2. A patient who has been intubated anyway for an operation will be ventilated advantageously with PEEP for 1 or 2 days.

3. When there is a significant decline of cardiac output as the result of cardiac insufficiency (e. g., contusion of the heart), the patient with severe lung contusion should be ventilated.

4. Paradoxical respiration would not be an indication for mechanical ventilation if there is no respiratory insufficiency. However, if there are lung contusions at the same time, then paradoxical respiration makes it impossible for the lung in this area to expand, and early prophylactic ventilation should be considered. Taken with a grain of salt, the same is true for severe multiple rib fractures.

In general, it is true that it is easier to prevent ARDS in severe lung contusions by means of early ventilation than to treat this pathologic condition later.

Therapy

As for the pathophysiologic disturbances, there are also parallels to ARDS with respect to treatment. Also in this situation, in consideration of the severity of the pathologic picture and the poor prognosis of spontaneous recovery, **aggressive therapy** is advised:

1. Immediate **ventilation with positive end-expiratory pressure (PEEP)**.

2. Immediate short-term application of **steroids** in high dosages (1 g methylprednisolone IV repeated after 6 h). The effectiveness of steroids in this situation is still not well documented; some reports [313, 320], as well as my own experiences, are favorable.

The **operative therapy,** the removal of damaged lung parts by lobectomy or pneumonectomy, is extremely questionable because the functional disturbances are not localized. Even though reports have been made on individually favorable cases [150], this was before the time of early application of PEEP. Experimentally, early pneumonectomy of the damaged lung produced only negative results [340].

VI. Blast Injuries

A **pressure wave generated by explosions and detonations** causes very severe damage to the lung by virtue of its force and high impact velocity. This organ is particularly vulnerable because certain physical phenomena occurring on the border between fluid (body tissues) and air (alveoli) damage the borderline structures: "spalling effect," "implosion effect," and "inertia effect" [309, 336, 341]. This also explains the involvement of other air-filled organs of the body, especially the intestines. Parenchymatous organs are damaged far less.

The damages caused by pressure waves are all the greater when they are conveyed by a fluid medium. Water is less compressible than air and transmits the pressure wave with less damping.

Such damages from explosion were already known in World War I [327]. The mechanism of damage was not well understood for a long time, however. It was thought that the suction following the pressure wave was responsible for it. Other theories made the transmission of pressure over airways into the lungs responsible, or the toxic effects of carbon monoxide or phosgene.

Zuckerman [344] was the first to prove that the pressure wave, exerting influence upon the body from the outside, is responsible for the pulmonary and abdominal damages.

The injuries to the lung correspond to a **combination of very severe ruptures and contusions** that affect great portions of the lung. Pneumothorax and hemothorax are often present. Very frequently the end result is progressive respiratory insufficiency with formation of edema.

A special danger is the development of **arterial air embolism.** The laceration of lung tissue under pressure can allow air to enter the pulmonary veins, which have also been opened up. Air emboli in the brain and coronary arteries can cause immediate death in connection with this injury.

Diagnosis

Dyspnea, hemoptysis, and the clinical signs of pneumo- and hemothorax or lung edema dominate the picture. In the severe cases, the result is a rapidly increasing respiratory insufficiency.

As a rule, patients have experienced the pressure wave as a blow. Occasionally, there is no evidence on the body of an external impact. Temporary symptoms of paralysis are frequently described.

On the **roentgenogram,** in addition to a pneumothorax, hemothorax, or mediastinal emphysema, infiltrates are found in both lungs. Most often the picture of an increasing interstitial and alveolar lung edema soon appears.

The **abdomen** always deserves attention. The most frequent injuries are hemorrhages and ruptures of the colon, less often of the small intestine. The spleen, liver, and kidneys are rarely injured. Explosions in the air and under water can produce lung damage and abdominal injuries; in the transmission of pressure waves through air, however, lung problems are the most common; in their transmission through water, intestinal lesions are more frequent.

Therapy

Pneumo- and hemothoraces are drained, volume replacement is undertaken, and abdominal injuries are treated. If there is **respiratory insufficiency,** the therapeutic guidelines suggested for lung contusions and respiratory insufficiency apply. Patients with blast injuries would therefore be ventilated early to good advantage.

Attention was called, however, to the fact that in mechanical ventilation during the first 24 h there is danger of **arterial air embolism** [308]. This possibility should not to be taken lightly inasmuch as it has also been reported that patients with blast injuries to the lung "do not tolerate anesthesia for an operation very well" [328], in which air emboli could play a role during mechanical ventilation.

In consideration of these potential special complications involving mechanical ventilation, a decision will have to be made in each individual case and presumably this risk taken to come up with whatever chance there is for survival.

Chapter 14
Tracheal and Bronchial Injuries

I. Injuries to Trachea and Bronchi Caused by Blunt Trauma

Closed injuries to the large air passages are rare among clinical patients and are observed only occasionally even in the large emergency wards. Their recognition and early treatment is either life-preserving or protects the patient from total atelectasis of a lung when a bronchus is torn off or from the severe infectious complications of a bronchial stenosis.

In 1848 Webb [370] issued the first report about a bronchial rupture, and as the consequence of a traffic accident at that (even in those days!): in India a pedestrian was run over by a horse-drawn wagon. Further reports followed in 1850 by Jackson [346], in 1863 by Biermer (this patient survived for 22 days with his left main bronchus completely severed) [346], and in 1873 by Seuvre [363]. In 1913 Hotz attempted to suture a ruptured lower lobe bronchus, but the 2-year-old child died on the 2nd postoperative day from atelectasis. In 1927 Krinitzki [356] reported on the first patient to survive a bronchial rupture (without therapy): in the autopsy of a woman who had suffered severe thoracic trauma 21 years ago as a 10-year-old girl, he accidentally found a complete severence of the right main bronchus with retraction of the bronchial stump.
It is not generally known that the first successful pneumonectomy by Nissen (1931) was performed on a girl because of infectious complications following rupture of a main bronchus [305]. In 1949 Griffith [353] was successful for the first time in resecting a posttraumatic bronchial stenosis with reanastomosis of the bronchus 7 months after injury.

Location and Mechanism of Injury

By far the most frequently affected are the **main bronchi** and mostly in the vicinity of the carina [354]. Both main bronchi are injured equally often [355]. The typical bronchial tear runs transversely and is usually complete.
Ruptures of the **thoracic trachea,** which are extremely rare, consist mainly of longitudinal lacerations of the pars membranacea [352, 359]. More frequently there are tears, and occasionally complete avulsions, of the **cervical trachea,** no doubt due to its superficial location.
In 1912 Schönberg assumed that the **principal mechanism of injury** was thoracic compression in the sagittal direction striking the air-filled lung with a closed glottis during inspiration: the resulting intraluminal positive pressure caused the bronchial rupture by bursting it at a typical site [362]. Subsequently, this theory was accepted by many authors and supported experimentally by Lloyd [252] and Peter [373].

Actually, it is mostly a powerful **thoracic compression** from in front that causes bronchial rupture: previously this occurred by being run over but nowadays most likely occurs by the steering wheel impacting on the driver of an automobile. The validity of this injury mechanism is supported by the observation that at the site of bronchical damage there is usually no significant injury to the surrounding tissue [355] and also by the rarity of the simultaneous occurrence of a bronchial rupture and a peripheral lung laceration: air escaping the lung into the pleural cavity protects the large air passages from the formation of a high intraluminal pressure.

Schönberg had already pointed out that obviously the elasticity of the thorax in a youthful person plays an important role in the rupture of a bronchus. Indeed, 65% of bronchial injuries occur in the age group below 30 years [355]. However, the possibility of a direct effect of shearing forces on the tracheobronchial tree is still discussed by some authors [373].

Diagnosis

Clinical signs and symptoms of tracheal and bronchial ruptures **vary** widely and are nonspecific. The pathologic picture may be immediately threatening or it may gradually worsen.

There are three situations that **always** require clarification in regard to possible bronchial rupture (Fig. 88):

1. A pneumothorax in which there is no expansion of the lung when suction drainage is applied

2. Significant mediastinal emphysema

3. Appearance of atelectasis that cannot be counteracted by the usual conservative treatment.

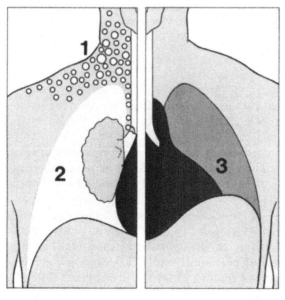

Fig. 88. The three significant suspicious facts pointing toward bronchial injury. *1* Mediastinal emphysema; *2* Pneumothorax: no complete expansion of the lung despite good drainage; *3* Formation of atelectasis

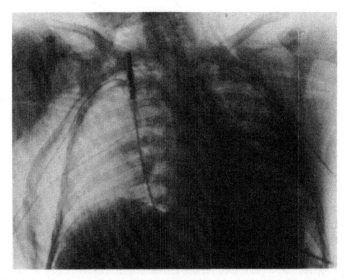

Fig. 89. Despite abundant thoracic drainage, a tension pneumothorax cannot be eliminated: rupture of the bronchus of the upper lobe on the right side and injuries to the lung parenchyma (see text)

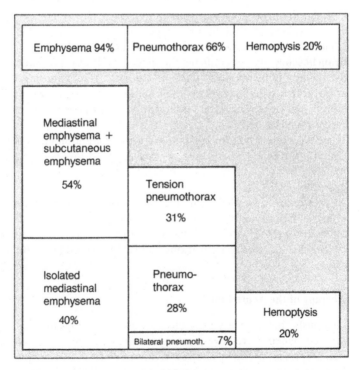

Fig. 90. Findings among 309 bronchial ruptures recorded in the world literature (Krauss and Zimmermann [355])

Example: A 28-year-old truck driver was wedged in between his truck and trailer. There was pronounced dyspnea, with multiple rib fractures and bilateral hemothoraces. With mechanical ventilation, extensive subcutaneous emphysema developed. In spite of pleural drainage with massive venting of air, a tension pneumothorax on the right side could not be eliminated (Fig. 89). A thoracotomy revealed a laceration of the right upper lobe and a large tear in the upper lobe bronchus. In addition, the upper lobe artery was injured. After lobectomy, he progressed with no complications to complete recovery.

Krauss and Zimmermann [355] analyzed 316 cases of **bronchial ruptures** from the world literature (Fig. 90): in 31% there was a tension pneumothorax, in 28% a simple, and in 7% a bilateral pneumothorax. Subcutaneous emphysema was found in 54% and isolated mediastinal emphysema among 40% of the patients. In only 20% of the cases was there hemoptysis. Nowadays, as a result of increased use of intubation in a severely injured person, bloody sputum in the suctioned secretions would be found more frequently. According to Burke [348], who also surveyed the literature, the only thing all patients had in common was that they had suffered **severe thoracic trauma.** Among patients over 30 years of age, rib fractures were always found, usually involving ribs I – III.

Eijgelaar and Van der Heide called attention to "deep cervical emphysema" as an early sign of a tracheal or bronchial rupture. Radiologically, it shows up before mediastinal emphysema is visible or a subcutaneous emphysema in the cervical area can be palpated [351].

According to an observation by Wolff [372], a higher CO_2 concentration in the air lost via the thoracic drainage than in the exhaled air points to the fact that there is no tracheal or bronchial rupture but that the leak is in the lung parenchyma.

One must keep in mind that the issue is not the making of the diagnosis on the basis of clinical signs. The issue is the **indication for bronchoscopy.**

Bronchoscopy always confirms the diagnosis. It also provides the basis for deciding the therapy to be adopted. The indication for this examination should be as liberal as possible because even a negative finding is valuable since with it the question of a bronchial rupture is settled once and for all. I have never regretted making use of early bronchoscopy.

There is no indication for bronchography or for a tomogram in cases of acute injury. Only in rare cases, when there is massive blood loss or adequate ventilation is impossible, will an immediate operation have to be resorted to without preceding endoscopy.

Attention must be called to the fact that in the past the diagnosis of a bronchial injury in the majority of cases was made **too late** (only in 15% [347] to 25% [355] was the injury recognized within the 1st week after the accident) and then, unfortunately, often not until later complications had set in (according to Burke [348] in 68% of all cases).

Therapy of the Acute Injury

Obviously, before everything else, a tension pneumothorax or a pneumothorax is drained; when there is respiratory insufficiency or significant hemoptysis, intubation is applied; a state of shock is treated.

Lesions in the trachea and bronchus that are **insignificant** and have **few symptoms** can be treated **conservatively; significant lacerations** and **bronchial avulsions** are

operated on as soon as the general situation has been clarified. Delay does not improve the situation; the operation becomes technically more difficult and infectious complications of the affected lung are more frequent.

Tracheal and bronchial lesions make great demands on the **anesthesiologist.** Based on the bronchoscopic findings, the intubation technique will have to be adapted to the individual case. In bronchial injuries, a double-lumen tube is usually indicated.

Access to the affected **main bronchus** is gained by means of an anterolateral thoracotomy in the fifth intercostal space. The bronchial suture or — in a total avulsion — the reunion is always possible and is made with chromic catgut (by using nonresorbable suture material there is danger of formation of granulation tissue in the interior of the bronchus). After additional coverage of the suture site with a pleural or pericardial flap, a leakage test is made with normal saline solution.

If a **lobar bronchus** is affected, a suture repair is worthwhile only if there are no severe injuries to the lung or vessels; otherwise, a lobectomy is indicated.

A follow-up bronchoscopy 2 months after suturing of the bronchus is recommended for early diagnosis of possible stenosis at the suture site.

Injuries to the **thoracic trachea** are taken care of in the upper intrathoracic section of the trachea with a median sternotomy, and in lesions immediately above the bifurcation with a high right-sided anterolateral thoracotomy.

Also in the case of total avulsion of the **cervical trachea,** a primary end-to-end anastomosis is probably always possible; the more frequent longitudinal tears can be taken care of by direct suturing. In these cases, it is advantageous to keep the intubation time as brief as possible. The simultaneous tracheostomy, which was formerly recommended, is indicated nowadays only in exceptional cases (e. g., in severe simultaneous injuries to the larynx). The most frequent complication of suturing cervical trachea injuries is recurrent laryngeal nerve paresis [365], especially when the rear wall of the trachea is exposed.

II. Old Bronchial Ruptures

Clinical Picture

Bronchial ruptures of larger dimensions that were either overlooked or for other reasons not treated operatively, will, in the course of time, lead via granulation and scar tissue formation to **bronchial stenosis.** The clinical picture is then very characteristic:

1. Through accumulation of secretions, a **partial** closure of the bronchus results in **inflammatory phenomena:** pneumonias, abscess formation, bronchiectases.

2. The **total** avulsion of the bronchus leads, through complete interruption of ventilation, to total **atelectasis.** The latter can be tolerated quite well for some time. Interestingly, no infection develops in these atelectatic lungs.

Therapy

The completely different disease patterns of bronchial stenosis and total bronchial interruption require distinctive therapeutic approaches.

1. **Bronchial stenosis:** only if no significant signs of infections have appeared, as a rule only up to 3 weeks after the accident, can the **bronchial suturing** — or the **bronchial resection** with end-to-end anastomosis — be attempted after removal of the intraluminal granulations. If signs of chronic infection are already present, the only thing left is a **lobectomy** or **pneumonectomy**.

Attempts at **dilating** a traumatic bronchial stenosis **bronchoscopically** are useless since this kind of intervention only leads to new and more extensive scar formation.

2. In **atelectasis occurring after old bronchial ruptures,** the treatment of choice is **resection** of the closed bronchial section with **end-to-end anastomosis.** There seem to be no time limits for this intervention, and it is astonishing that the atelectatic lung can still be reexpanded after years have passed.

Samson [360] reported on a successful operation of this kind 15 years after trauma on a boy who, at the age of 1 year, had suffered an accident. Vossschulte and Bikfalvi [369] operated with success 14 years after the injury, and Mahafey [357] 11 years after the injury.

Naturally, of interest here is the question as to the **function** of such a lung, which has been atelectatic for years. In some of the cases, there are corresponding investigations [355, 357, 360, 367, 369, 371]. Common to all is the fact that while the atelectatic lung could be reexpanded, the absorption of oxygen, postoperatively, by this lung was consistently poor. The lung remained undersupplied with blood and there was a significant right-to-left shunt. However, the function of such lungs, in subsequent development over a period of years, constantly improves and can become normalized after several years [355].

III. Penetrating Injuries to Trachea and Bronchi

Of particular clinical significance here are wounds with injury to the **cervical trachea.** The sound of incoming and outgoing air during respiration provides a basis for making the diagnosis. Dyspnea, hemoptysis, and subcutaneous emphysema are additional frequently found symptoms.

If oral intubation is impossible, as an emergency measure the tube can be inserted into the trachea through the site of the injury. By itself the prognosis of tracheal suture repair is good, and the fate of such an injured person depends more upon the **other damages occurring in the throat area.** Injuries to the larynx require treatment by a specialist in otorhinolaryngology. In these cases, a tracheotomy is often resorted to.

After suture repair of the cervical trachea, the patient is extubated as early as possible.

Example: After a motorcycle accident, a 20-year-old girl was brought to the emergency room unconscious, with fixed and dilated pupils and without pulse. A wound on the left side of the throat had stopped bleeding until circulation was restored through resuscitation and massive transfusion. Then the bleeding could be controlled by digital compression. An immediate operation revealed that half of the cervical trachea was sharply severed, the common carotid artery was totally severed, and there was a tear in the internal jugular vein and fractures of the vertebrae with avulsion of nerve roots. Application of an internal shunt in the carotid artery, suturing of the trachea with chromic catgut, suturing of the internal jugular vein, and venous interposition for reconstruction of the common carotid artery were performed. Extubation occurred 2 h postoperatively. No postoperative problems developed, and with the exception of paresis of the left arm, there was complete recovery.

Penetrating wounds with injuries to the **thoracic trachea** or a **bronchus** are usually fatal because of injury to other structures in the vicinity (aorta, other large intrathoracic vessels, heart) [350]. This was seen also among surgical patients in wartime; despite the great frequency of thoracic injuries, lesions of the large intrathoracic air passages were seldom observed [354].

 However, the first successful surgical repair of a bronchial injury was made by Sanger during World War II on two patients with gunshot wounds [361].

Because of concomitant bleeding, the operation on open lesions of the large intrathoracic air passages is usually more urgent than in closed injuries. There is hardly time for a bronchoscopic examination.

Chapter 15
Injuries to the Esophagus

I. Rupture of the Esophagus, Penetrating and Iatrogenic Esophageal Injuries

Causes, Location (Table 21)

1. **Blunt trauma:** esophageal ruptures caused by blunt trauma are **rarities.** Only a very few surgeons will encounter this injury in the course of their lifetime. Besides, since the symptoms in the initial state are not evident, such injuries are often not recognized at all or not until very late [393].
It is assumed that the esophagus is ruptured by inner pressure when air and the contents of the stomach are pressed into the gullet by compression of the lower section of the thorax and the epigastrium [386]. The site of the rupture in the majority of cases is located near the cardia, in the same area as the more frequent "spontaneous" rupture during sudden vomiting with a distended stomach.

2. **Penetrating injuries:** perforations of the esophagus by shot or stab injuries can appear over its entire length; they are most numerous in the area of the cervical gullet. They also rarely occur among clinical patients. The deep, protected location of the

Table 21. Etiology of mechanical esophageal injuries

External violence
  Blunt trauma
  Penetrating wounds of the throat and thorax

Iatrogenic injuries
  Endoscopy
    Esophagoscopy, biopsy
    Gastroscopy
  Dilatations of the esophagus
    Bougienage
    Stark's dilatator
  Introduction of tubes
    Nasogastric tube
    Sengstaken-Blakemore tube
  Intraoperative injuries

Foreign bodies
  Sharp, especially during extraction
  Large, embedded (pressure necrosis)

thoracic esophagus hardly permits an injury in this area without a simultaneous involvement of the heart, aorta, or other large vessels.

Thus, in the review of wartime surgery, esophageal lesions are seldom mentioned; their frequency is around 0.5% of all open thoracic injuries given hospital treatment [178, 380, 390].

3. **Iatrogenic esophageal injuries:** by far the most frequently occurring are iatrogenic esophageal injuries. In first place is perforation during esophagoscopy. Although most of the reports of this complication go back to the days of the rigid metal esophagoscope, esophageal perforations are known to have occurred with the flexible endoscope [376].

The perforation always occurs at points of constriction of the gullet: either at one of the three physiologic narrowings or above an inflammatory or tumor-related stenosis.

Beyond this, injuries to the esophagus occur in connection with dilatation of stenoses (bougienage) or as intraoperative complications during preparation of the gullet (e. g., for a truncal vagotomy) or in operations on neighboring organs.

4. **Foreign bodies:** angular or pointed foreign bodies can perforate the esophagus wall at the physiologic narrowings. Frequently, the injury does not occur until the attempt at endoscopic removal is made. Large foreign bodies that have lodged during passage can cause pressure areas and necrosis of the esophageal wall with subsequent perforation.

Spontaneous Course of These Perforations

In the further course of development, the **localization of the injury** plays a significant role:

1. Injuries to the **cervical** part of the gullet result in a locally limited inflammation of the surrounding area, including possible formation of an abscess. In smaller lesions, this inflammation can heal without negative consequences, but in exceptional cases, it spreads downward and results in mediastinitis.

2. Injuries to the **thoracic** esophagus follow an entirely different course. Saliva, permeated with anaerobes, and the contents of the stomach enter the slack mediastinal tissue. The intrapleural negative pressure during inspiration, the peristalsis of the esophagus, and an air insufflation during endoscopy promote the escape of this highly infectious material. **Mediastinal emphysema** results usually followed by extended **mediastinitis** soon afterward.

In a simultaneous injury to the pleura or in spreading of the infection into the pleural cavity, a **pyopneumothorax** is formed. Only in rare instances does the infection remain localized while forming a **mediastinal abscess.** During the ensuing course, most of these patients succumb to sepsis after a few days in a toxic condition.

3. In a perforation of the short **intra-abdominal esophagus,** an acute **peritonitis of the upper abdomen** develops, sometimes also a **subphrenic abscess.**

Diagnosis

Only if an esophageal injury is considered, despite its rarity, will it be possible to make the diagnosis early enough. The **patient's history** is helpful; above all, with prior history of instrumental interventions the possibility of an esophageal lesion must be kept in mind.

Acute injuries to the cervical esophagus are characterized by pain, dysphagia, and hoarseness. Subcutaneous emphysema in the cervical area points toward the diagnosis and requires investigation.

In open wounds in the cervical area in which an esophageal lesion is suspected, Sheely [389] recommended placing a stomach tube into the cervical esophagus, compressing the distal cervical esophagus by hand from the outside, and gently supplying air to the tube: air exiting the wound is diagnostic. By expanding the esophageal wound by means of air, it can also be located more readily during the operative exploration.

The leading symptom in **acute injuries to the thoracic section of the esophagus** is **mediastinal emphysema.** This is not always the case, however, and it can develop very slowly. With further expansion of air, subcutaneous emphysema in the cervical area can be palpated. Severe pains are always present. In distal lesions, the latter will be felt in the area of the epigastrium.

A perforation into the pleural cavity results in **pneumothorax with pleural effusion.** The thoracic drainage sometimes transmits food particles and later pus.

In a later stage, symptoms of inflammation dominate the picture: fever, leukocytosis, and toxic condition. Venous congestion can also occur.

Roentgenograms make it possible to identify the mediastinal emphysema and the cervical emphysema. On occasion, only a widened mediastinum is found.

Of crucial significance diagnostically is a **radiologic examination** of the esophagus, using a water-soluble contrast medium [meglucamine diatrizoate (Gastrografin)]. It is the method of choice for clarification when an esophageal lesion is suspected; since it is a simple examination without complications, its indication cannot be too liberal.

Attention must be called, however, to the fact that esophagography is often falsely negative. (Foster [381] reported 15% false-negative results of radiologic examinations using contrast media and Berry [377] 25%; [388, 389, 391].)

If there is clinical suspicion, a negative esophagography must be repeated. In a cervical esophageal injury, the reliability of this method is even worse: Sheely [389] found it to be positive in only 47%. Despite a negative esophagography, operative exploration of a wound in the cervical area should not be superficial.

Esophagography is also indicated even if the diagnosis has been made clinically; the knowledge of the localization of the injury is decisive for the planning of therapy and especially for the operative approach. An **esophagoscopy** is not indicated; in this situation, I regard it as a dangerous method of examination.

Therapy

For the treatment of a penetrating cervical wound with injury to the esophagus, instructions are found already in the oldest historical medical document, in the Edwin Smith Papyrus [239]:
"Instructions for wounds of his throat:... and when he drinks water, it will choose to come out of the opening of his wound; it burns very much, and as a result he develops fever. You should grasp this wound with a clamp and you should say of him: this is a man who has a wound in his throat that has perforated all the way to his gullet; this is a disease with which I shall do battle."

An **early operation** brings good results. If an acute esophageal injury has been diagnosed, surgery is always indicated. Only minor lesions of the cervical esophagus are regarded as exceptions to this, but more recently early operation has been preferred over the wait-and-see of conservative measures.

The **operative approach** depends upon the location of the injury:

1. In **cervical injuries,** it is made by an incision along the anterior border of the sternocleidomastoid muscle and extended down to the suprasternal notch. In general, the left approach is preferred because of the slight curve of the cervical esophagus to the left. After cutting through the platysma and the superficial cervical fascia, access to the esophagus is by blunt dissection between the sternohyoid and sternothyroid muscles on the one side and the laterally situated sternocleidomastoid muscle on the other. As a rule, the median thyroidal vein must be severed, and in exceptional cases also the inferior thyroidal artery. Precaution is called for because of the recurrent laryngeal nerve, which passes between the esophagus and trachea.

2. In injuries to the **upper part of the thoracic esophagus,** the approach is made by a right-sided posterolateral thoracotomy.

3. In injuries to the **lower part of the thoracic esophagus,** a left-sided posterolateral thoracotomy is performed. This is also the approach for a lesion in the upper part of the esophagus if a perforation into the left pleural cavity has already occurred.

4. Injuries to the **abdominal esophagus** are dealt with by an upper midline laparotomy.

The **injury** is repaired by two rows of **sutures:** the inner suture with chromic catgut, the outer suture of the musculature with silk. It is covered by surrounding tissue, e. g., with a pleural flap or with a piece of omentum pulled up through the diaphragm [388], and in lesions of the cardia area by means of a fundoplication. If intraoperative detection of the lesion is difficult, the **instillation of methylene blue** into the esophagus can be helpful.

The area of operation is extensively **drained,** by approach through thoracotomy via pleural drainage.

In severe injuries requiring extensive suturing, and also in the patient with multiple injuries who must be ventilated for a long time for other reasons, the primary performance of a **gastrostomy** is recommended.

Postoperative evacuation of the stomach is accomplished by means of a nasogastric tube or gastrostomy. **Parenteral nutrition** has improved the prognosis markedly [387]. **Antibiotic therapy** is introduced to good advantage preoperatively.

The **poor general condition** of a patient, indeed even a moribund patient, is no contraindication or reason for postponement of an operation. On the contrary, in this situation, only an operation can provide improvement (Loop: "The patient is too ill not to operate" [385]).

In **delayed cases,** the repair will on occasion have to be dispensed with if there is no prospect that the sutures will hold in the damaged tissue. In that case, the esophagus can be excluded by performing a cervical esophagostomy and a gastrostomy with ligature of the distal esophageal section [392]. Also, drainage alone or an esophageal resection with a cervical stoma can be considered in exceptional cases (e. g., in a carcinoma).

The compilation of 1232 cases with esophageal injuries by Bittner [378] reveals that the suture closure is superior to all other forms of treatment: the mortality with this procedure was 13.4% compared to 20.8% for resectional treatment, 25.5% for drainage alone, and 28.6% for conservative treatment.

The **prognosis,** however, is largely dependent upon the timely moment of the operative intervention (mortality in repair within 24 h after injury is 7.7%, in delayed closures, 19.3%). It is especially poor in blunt esophageal injuries because here the lesion is often not recognized at all [393].

II. Traumatic Esophagotracheal Fistula

As a consequence of **blunt thoracic trauma,** the esophagotracheal fistula occurs more frequently than the esophageal lesion by itself. However, it is also recognized as a **complication of long-term ventilation** if the tube cuff causes pressure necrosis to the tracheal wall and the esophagus, especially if there is a nasogastric tube in the esophagus at the same time.

Characteristically, the traumatic esophagotracheal fistula appears 3 – 7 days after the accident; only in rare instances is it already formed immediately after trauma [352, 375].

We are indebted to the works of Kronberger [384] for first providing convincing information about its formation: vehement compression of the thorax, by raising pressure in the trachea with the glottis closed, not only causes rupture of the trachea; before the rupture occurs, it can also be squeezed against the spinal column, and the esophagus lying in between can thereby be crushed. In that case, there is no primary esophageal rupture. Not until there is necrosis formation on the front wall of the esophagus is there development of a fistula. Inflammatory reactions have, in the meantime, led to adhesions and formation of scar tissue so that in the vicinity of the fistula no significant infections can spread any further.

The **prognosis** of a traumatic esophagotracheal fistula is distinctively better than that of an isolated esophageal injury; even without treatment there is less mortality.

Diagnosis

The leading symptom is the strong **cough stimulus** that occurs whenever food is ingested ("swallow cough"). Here, differential diagnosis for disturbances in swallow-

ing must be made. This can be done with insertion of a nasogastric tube into the proximal esophagus with instillation of methylene blue.
The diagnosis will be confirmed conclusively by esophagography with water-soluble contrast media [meglucamine diatrizoate (Gastrografin)], bronchoscopy, or esophagoscopy.

Therapy

Through repeated aspiration, esophagotracheal fistulas will lead to pulmonary infections. Only exceptional cases heal spontaneously.
Operation is successful in a high percentage of cases [374, 382]. Since the fistula is often situated just above the carina, the best approach is a right-sided thoracotomy. The trachea is closed with a single row of sutures, the esophagus with a double row, and some tissue interposed, if possible (e. g., a pleural flap). In large defects, plastic repair may become necessary. Only in the less frequent cervical fistulas can the approach be made through the neck.

Chapter 16

Injuries to the Heart by Blunt Trauma

I. Basic Considerations

As in the great textbooks, the impressive, severe cardiac injuries caused by blunt force will also be described in this book: cardiac ruptures, traumatic septal defects, heart valve lesions, and injuries to the coronary arteries. However, this should not obscure the fact that the clinical significance of such injuries is quite modest. The few cases that come into question for treatment represent decided **rarities.**
In contrast to these rare injuries, **cardiac contusion,** in the framework of blunt thoracic trauma, is **very frequent.** The diagnosis of this injury is often not established [2]. The pathologic picture is not well-known; furthermore, in the majority of cases the diagnosis is not simple.
There are **two situations** in which cardiac injury is overlooked:

1. In **very severe thoracic trauma,** the surgeon is so overwhelmed by multiple rib fractures, paradoxical respiration, hemothorax, pneumothorax, or subcutaneous emphysema that the heart is often not considered. Table 22 shows the companion injuries that often accompany cardiac contusion.

2. The second situation is almost the opposite of the one previously described. If there are **no rib fractures,** the force of the external impact is underestimated. In the youthful, elastic thorax, the heart can be injured between the sternum and spinal column without fracture of the ribs. On occasion, contusion marks will then point to the severity of the thoracic trauma (Fig. 91). Heart injuries without rib fractures are not at all uncommon: among our patients, rib fractures were not present in 25% of all heart injuries caused by blunt force.

In clinical reports, the **frequency** of cardiac damage in closed thoracic trauma is given at 10% [411, 450, 464]; we observed cardiac trauma in 16% of patients hospitalized for blunt thoracic injuries.

Table 22. Frequent companion injuries to the thorax in cardiac injuries

Suspicion of cardiac injuries especially in	
	Sternal fractures
	Parasternal multiple rib fractures
	Multiple rib fractures on the left side with mobile thoracic wall
	Traumatic asphyxia
	Mediastinal hematoma

Basic Considerations

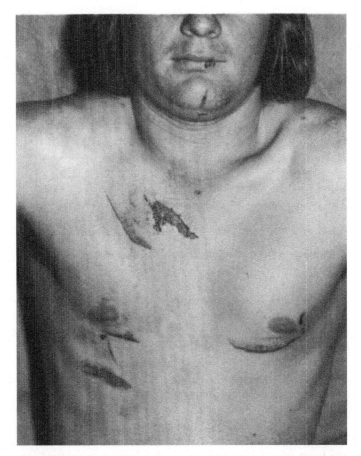

Fig. 91. Contusion marks on a 22-year-old male patient with severe cardiac contusion without rib fracture in a steering wheel injury

Who is to treat patients with cardiac injuries? In most cases, the accident victim is brought to a general surgical department or trauma center. Only rarely is an operation urgent, for instance, in cases of **cardiac tamponade, luxation of the heart,** or **cardiac rupture.** Transfer to a center for cardiac surgery then cannot be considered. I am of the opinion that the surgeon should also take over the treatment of **cardiac contusion,** because of the frequent companion injuries in the thoracic area, if necessary in cooperation with the internist.

Other — less frequent — cardiac injuries due to blunt force require clarification by means of heart catheterization and angiocardiography and belong in the hands of a **cardiac surgeon.**

Mechanism of Injury

In most cases, the heart is damaged by frontal **compression** force. The typical accident mechanism is the steering wheel injury of automobile drivers. The functional condition of the heart at the moment of impact plays an important role. Powerful compression during the filling phase of the heart chambers can cause rupture of the heart wall or valvular lesions [418].

In second place, **deceleration injuries** are a source of cardiac damage, e. g., a plunge from a great height. Thus, 80% of all victims of airplane crashes exhibit injuries to the heart [428].

II. Pericardial Injuries, Luxation of the Heart

Two forms of pericardial injury can be distinguished:

1. **Lacerations in the pleuropericardium.**

2. **Rupture of the diaphragmatic part of the pericardium.** This rare injury is described in Chap. 19.

Lacerations in the pleuropericardium caused by the impact of blunt force usually run longitudinally in front of or behind the phrenic nerve, more often on the left than on the right side of the thorax. They are often combined with cardiac contusion.

No doubt most of the pericardial lacerations follow an **asymptomatic pattern of development.** If there is a pneumothorax at the same time, air can show up on the roentgenogram as a **pneumopericardium.** Small lacerations and minor bleeding that does not develop into cardiac tamponade are of no clinical significance and heal spontaneously.

If the pericardial laceration is large, there is a threat of a partial or total **luxation of the heart** into the pleural cavity. This leads to manifestations of entrapment of the heart in the pericardial tear with resultant mechanical impairment, and occasionally with compression of the coronary arteries or torsion of the heart. Luxation of the heart is not always present immediately after trauma. Occasionally, luxation into the pleural cavity does not occur until several days later [395, 437].

Diagnosis

Luxation of the heart usually results in a life-threatening condition with tachycardia and hypotension. There can be venous congestion. Heart sounds can become weakened. On the basis of clinical findings, a differential diagnosis of cardiac tamponade will have to be made. Diagnosis is especially difficult if there are additional injuries in the thoracic area [437].

The most important examination, the chest **roentgenogram,** will indicate the displaced position of the heart, occasionally only an unusual cardiac silhouette (Fig. 92). The interpretation of the radiologic findings seems to be particularly difficult in differentiating from atelectasis formation, a hemopericardium, and an aneurysm of the heart wall [402]. The presence of a pneumopericardium makes the diagnosis easier.

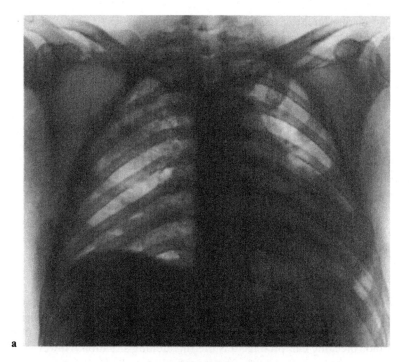

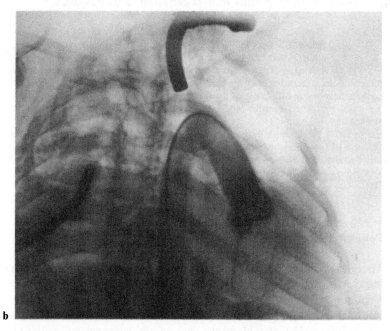

Fig. 92. a Roentgenogram of the thorax with luxation of the heart through a pericardial rupture on the left side. **b** In the aortogram, the luxation of the heart into the left thorax can be visualized very clearly

The displacement of the heart may be shown in the **ECG** by a shift of the cardiac electric axis [425]. Along with this, ST-T wave changes and a bundle-branch block are common. With successful therapy, the ECG variations are reversible [402, 437].

Therapy

Treatment consists of a thoracotomy with repositioning of the heart. The pericardium is closed, leaving openings for drainage, or if the pericardium is torn anteriorly to the phrenic nerve, a drainage window is created behind the nerve. Minor pericardial lacerations or a pneumopericardium without symptoms do not require treatment.

III. Hemopericardium, Cardiac Tamponade

In blunt trauma, the following **causes** of bleeding into the pericardial cavity and of cardiac tamponade are considered: ruptures of the heart wall, injuries to coronary vessels, or bleeding from the pericardium. Also, foci of contusion of the heart with minor bleeding can produce this life-threatening situation. However, cardic tamponade results more frequently from **penetrating cardiac injuries.**

The first reports and also the recognition of the threat to life posed by the accumulation of blood in the pericardium are therefore based on the experiences with open heart injuries. In the sixteenth century, Ambroise Paré [494] described the first case of cardiac tamponade. As early as 1679, Riolanus suggested pericardiocentesis as treatment for heart wounds [432]. Morgagni [440] also recognized the significance of cardiac tamponade as a cause of death in cardiac injuries. His theory about the compression of the heart by the effusion of blood, published in 1761, has maintained its validity up to the present day.
Larrey [431], Napoleon's field surgeon, reported in 1829 on the successful drainage of the pericardium in hemopericardium developing after a stab wound. However, as late as 1882, Billroth still designated the "paracentesis of the hydropic pericardium" as an operation that "comes very close to what some surgeons call the prostitution of the surgical art, others a surgical frivolity."

Pathophysiology

The elasticity of the pericardium is very slight. An acute accumulation of fluid in the intrapericardial space up to approximately 120 ml can easily be diverted into the anatomic cavities. A larger amount of fluid that rapidly accumulates, however, will result in significant hemodynamic effects: in an acute formation of a hemopericardium, as little as **150 ml of blood** can cause a life-endangering cardiac tamponade. In a chronic development (e. g., in a uremic pericardial effusion), the pericardial tissue will yield in response to the rising pressure and much larger amounts of fluid — up to several liters — can be tolerated.

The intrapericardial rise in pressure caused by the fluid brings about a compression of the intrapericardial structures that have a lower internal pressure. It is not the obstruction of veins and auricles that is responsible for the functional consequences but the prevention of ventricle dilatation during diastole. This supposition, advanced already by Starling, was proved by Isaacs in 1954 and is in opposition to the academic opinions of long standing [446].

The filling up of a ventricle is dependent upon the pressure gradient between venous pressure and the diastolic pressure of the ventricle. In cardiac tamponade, the intrapericardial pressure also causes a rise in the diastolic pressure in the ventricles. By lowering the pressure gradient, less blood flows in, the stroke volume falls, and the venous pressure rises.

In the process, special significance is also due the pulmonary circulation: the lowering of the pressure gradient between the left auricle and left ventricle during diastole is of special importance because of the slight difference in pressure in the pulmonary circulation [407].

Interestingly, the evacuation of a small amount of blood is more effective in lowering the intrapericardial pressure than the amount of additional fluid necessary is in raising the pressure to the same extent [446].

This explains two observations important for the treatment of acute cardiac tamponade:

1. The removal of small amounts of fluid from the pericardium, even without complete evacuation, can temporarily improve the hemodynamic situation very decisively.

2. The infusion of volume raises the venous pressure and thereby the pressure gradient during the ventricle diastole and thus temporarily raises the stroke volume.

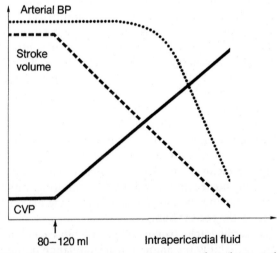

Fig. 93. Schematic representation of the course of central venous pressure, stroke volume, and arterial blood pressure in increasing cardiac tamponade. The central venous pressure rises continuously, while the arterial blood pressure does not begin to fall until the late phase. The reduction of stroke volume can be counterbalanced for some time by increasing the heart rate (based on the investigations of Martin and Schenk [436] and other authors)

Compensatory mechanisms attempt in this situation to maintain adequate cardiac function: an increase in the heart rate temporarily prevents a fall in the cardiac output. Peripheral vasoconstriction can temporarily maintain a normal arterial blood pressure in spite of a falling stroke volume [436]. In this way, cardiac tamponade exerts an **earlier effect on the venous pressure** and a **later effect on the arterial blood pressure** (Fig. 93). This has essential significance for diagnosis and therapy: (1) the change in venous pressure and not arterial blood pressure is important for early diagnosis and (2) if arterial blood pressure is already beginning to fall, there is only a little time left for treatment.

Diagnosis

The **classic triad** of cardiac tamponade (high venous pressure, distant heart sounds, arterial hypotension) is found among trauma patients in only 35% – 40% of the cases [457, 507, 508].
The **measurement of central venous pressure** is the most important criterion for the diagnosis of a cardiac tamponade. The signs of venous congestion with distended neck veins are the clinical correlate of an elevated venous pressure. However, in massive hypovolemia, the venous pressure can be normal until complete circulatory collapse has occurred. Obviously, only a single measurement is not sufficient and repeated venous pressure readings should be made.
The **drop in arterial blood pressure** is already a very late sign. **Distant heart sounds** are seldom found.
Paradoxical pulse is likewise a classic, but uncharacteristic sign of cardiac tamponade. Involved is a marked decrease of arterial blood pressure and therefore of pulse during inspiration. A slight fall in pressure during inspiration is normal. The term "paradoxical pulse" is therefore misleading and only describes an exaggerated form of a physiologic phenomenon.* A paradoxical pulse can quite often be determined by palpation or through measurements also in traumatic cardiac tamponade. It must be pointed out emphatically that in contrast to chronic forms of cardiac tamponade, the **roentgenogram** as well as the **ECG** offer no significant help in the diagnosis; since it takes only very little blood to cause an acute tamponade, the heart silhouette usually has not widened and low voltage is almost never present [447].
If the patient's condition permits performance of **fluoroscopy,** it reveals an almost complete lack of cardiac pulsations.
Pericardiocentesis is not only therapeutic but also an important diagnostic tool. Its technique will be presented below. Fear of using it is unfounded. Even an unintentional puncture of the right ventricle usually has no aftereffects and can be avoided by using the technique with ECG monitoring, which is described below. However, it can sometimes be unsuccessful despite the existence of tamponade if blood coagulates in the pericardium.
Echocardiography (sonography) with **ultrasound** makes it possible to determine with great reliability the amount of accumulation of fluid in the pericardium. **Radioisotopic scanning** is less sensitive.

---
* Kussmaul, who coined the phrase in 1873, meant by it that with this respiratory change in pressure, paradoxically no respiratory changes could be palpated in the region of the heart.

Therapy

Therapy in the **rapid development** of cardiac tamponade in closed trauma, as is generally the case in penetrating heart injuries, is basically **operative.** Only by immediate intervention can the infrequent cardiac rupture be dealt with. In these cases pericardiocentesis, besides confirming the diagnosis, serves only as temporary relief and does not exempt one from the operation immediately following. Also, in this situation, no time should be lost in attempting to install drainage by way of a closed insertion of a plastic catheter.

If the cardiac tamponade resulting from blunt trauma develops **slowly,** over a period of hours, or if a hemorrhagic pericardial effusion does not occur until later, the treatment after pericardiocentesis can be put on a wait-and-see basis. Under good supervision, any new tamponade symptoms will be recognized early. The number of additional punctures and the length of the interval between them, taking the general situation into account, will determine whether operative intervention is necessary.

In these late cases, therapy consists more in the drainage of the pericardium than in the control of the hemorrhage. In general, entry is made by an anterolateral thoracotomy on the left. After opening up the pericardium in front of the phrenic nerve, the blood or effusion is evacuated, the heart inspected, and possible sources of bleeding eliminated. Behind the phrenic nerve, a drainage opening from the pericardium into the left side of the thorax is made, which is in turn emptied by means of a chest tube. The incision in the pericardium in front of the phrenic nerve is closed to avoid luxation of the heart.

Technique of Pericardiocentesis

With the patient in a supine position, entrance is made at the angle formed by the xyphoid process of the sternum and the left costal arch (Fig. 94). A parasternal ap-

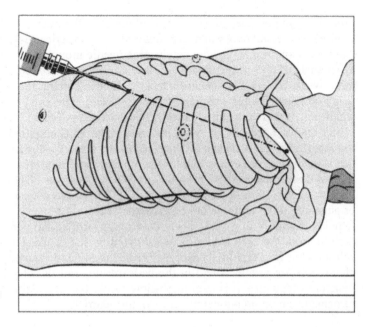

Fig. 94. Technique of pericardiocentesis (see text)

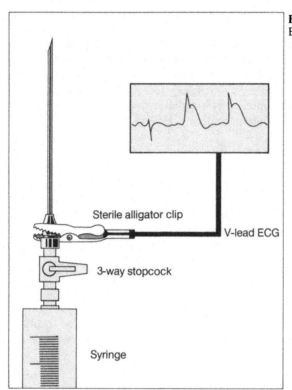

Fig. 95. Pericardiocentesis under ECG control (see text)

proach is also possible, but the danger of injury to the heart is greater, and the procedure is successful only when large amounts of intrapericardial fluid are present.

After local anesthesia, an adequately large needle mounted on a syringe is inserted at an angle of 30° to the anterior surface and in the direction of the middle of the left clavicle, toward the pericardium; in a slender patient, the pericardium will already be reached after a short distance (2 – 5 cm). The entry into the pericardium will be felt, if there is a tamponade, by the abatement of resistance.

If time allows, I prefer making the **puncture under ECG monitoring.** Using an alligator clip, the puncture needle is connected to the V lead of the ECG monitor. If contact is made with the epicardium in the puncture attempt, the lead in the epicardial ECG differs unmistakeably from the previously observed ECG by its characteristic massive upward shift of the ST segment (Fig. 95). In this way, an injury to the heart or puncture of the ventricle can be avoided.

It holds true only in a very slowly developing cardiac tamponade that the blood derived from the pericardium is defibrinated by the contractions of the heart and will not clot. In a rapidly developing cardiac tamponade caused by hemorrhaging, blood clots are usually found in the pericardium, and the blood rushing out after puncture coagulates. It is then impossible to use the coagulability of the blood for recognizing an unintentional puncture of the ventricle.

IV. Posttraumatic Pericarditis

After blunt thoracic trauma, symptoms of pericarditis can appear days or even months later.

In 1665, De Marchettis provided the first description of pericarditis that appeared after an injury [479]. In 1764, Akenside [394] reported on a 14-year-old boy who complained of pains in the heart region after a powerful blow to the chest. In the autopsy after his death 6 months later, the pericardium was discovered to have adhered completely to the heart.

A **traumatic hemopericardium** will usually cause symptoms only if the amount of blood causes a cardiac tamponade. Hemorrhages in the pericardium of a lesser degree will be absorbed by the pericardial lymphatic vessels [415]. In some cases (according to Tschirkov [463] in 6%), a **pericarditis** develops nevertheless. Three forms can be differentiated:

1. **Pericarditis without effusion formation**
2. **Pericarditis with effusion**
3. **Constrictive pericarditis**

Unless there is pericardial effusion, a classic pericardial friction rub can be observed. Fever, retrosternal pains, rise in the erythrocyte sedimentation rate, and possibly leukocytosis are other, though after trauma uncharacteristic findings.

In **effusion formation,** this can lead to cardiac tamponade with venous congestion, high venous pressure, paradoxical pulse, and later arterial hypotension. An excellent gauge of reduced cardiac output despite normal blood pressure values is limited kidney function demonstrated by oliguria. Since these cases involve a slowly developing effusion, the roentgenogram, in contrast to one of an acute cardiac tamponade, will show the characteristic tent-shaped enlargement of the cardiac silhouette. The ECG demonstrates low voltage and T wave inversions.

A **constrictive pericarditis** develops within a period of months or even years but has also been observed as early as 24 days after injury [448].

The origin of such pericardial alterations is not clear. Since steroid preparations can influence the development, an autoimmune reaction was discussed as a cause [463]. No proof of this theory was adduced, and since steroids affect every exudative process, there is no basis for this idea. A comparable syndrome exhibiting the same symptoms is the postcardiotomy syndrome after heart surgery.

Therapy

1. Posttraumatic **pericarditis without formation of effusion** requires only **symptomatic therapy** and will disappear spontaneously in a short time.

2. When **effusion forms,** the use of **steroids** is helpful. If the formation of effusion produces signs of **cardiac tamponade,** pericardiocentesis will be unavoidable. If there is renewed effusion formation, either repeated pericardiocenteses or a closed insertion of a thin plastic catheter into the pericardium for drainage will be necessary. If this is unsuccessful, an **operative drainage** of the pericardium into the left pleural cavity or by way of an inferior pericardiotomy is indicated.

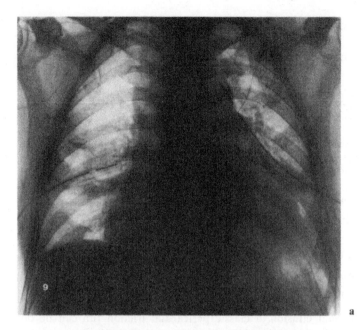

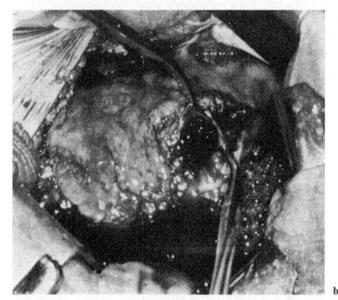

Fig. 96 a – c. Posttraumatic pericarditis with hemorrhagic pericardial effusion and cardiac tamponade. **a** Characteristic thoracic roentgenogram with pericardial effusion 9 days after the accident; **b** During the operation, the serosanguineous fluid pours out after opening of the thickened pericardium; **c** Postoperative roentgenogram after 4 months

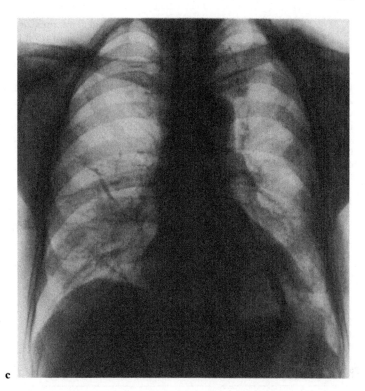

Fig. 96 c

3. If a **constrictive pericarditis** with significant limitation of function occurs, a **pericardiectomy** cannot be avoided.

Example: In a 60-year-old patient with other severe injuries, a cardiac contusion with multiple rib fractures on both sides was verified on the day of the accident. Nine days after the accident, a massive, profuse hemorrhagic effusion with pericardial tamponade developed. (Fig. 96a). Simultaneously, oliguria and an increase in urea were evident. Pericardiocentesis performed a total of four times improved the unfavorable hemodynamic situation only a day at a time. For this patient, we resorted to opening and draining the pericardium into the left chest by means of a small thoracotomy. During the operation, 300 ml of a serosanguineous fluid were found in the thickened pericardium (Fig. 96b). Subsequently, the patient recovered completely (Fig. 96c).

V. Cardiac Contusion

Every cardiac injury caused by blunt force that is not accompanied by a primary rupture of a heart chamber or an injury to intracardiac structures is designated as a cardiac contusion.*

---

* Formerly, functional disturbances of the heart "without proof of morphologic substrate" were designated **commotio cordis.** Since it can be assumed that pathoanatomic changes of the heart wall also occur in these cases, that the observed clinical developments cannot be explained as pure functional damage, and that a clinical differentiation is impossible anyway, it is justifiable that this term is hardly ever used today.

Although stab wounds have been on record since antiquity, it seems to have taken a long time before the possibility of heart damage from the effects of blunt force was discerned. The first description, going back to the year 1550, was made by Rota [479]. He found, upon the death of a patient after a long period of suffering, that the pericardium was expanded and the heart substance destroyed.

In the seventeenth century, Borch (1676), Blancard (1688), and Nebel (1696) reported on closed heart injuries [450, 479]. Borch described a massive enlargement of the right atrium, which contained blood clots resulting from cardiac contusion, in an 8-year-old boy who was injured in a fall. Blancard found ulcerations in the left ventricle and in the atria of a farmer who had been run over by a hay cart and died 11 days later. Nebel reported on a rupture of the right atrial appendage of the heart caused by a fall from a horse. Without external injury, death ensued immediately.

Pathoanatomic Findings

These vary widely and range from small subepicardial or subendocardial hemorrhages to extended foci of contusion (Fig. 97). Frequently, there are small epicardial

Table 23. Most important examinations in cardiac contusion

Clinical: auscultation, signs of heart failure
Roentgenograms of the thorax
Central venous pressure
ECG
Determinations of enzymes (CPK isoenzymes, LDH isoenzymes)
Cardiac output

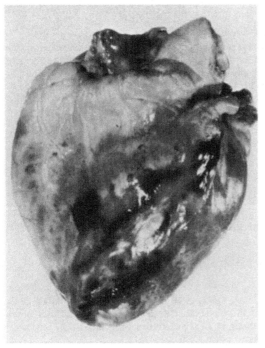

Fig. 97. Extensive hemorrhagic involvement of the anterior wall of the heart in a severe cardiac contusion

Fig. 98. Foci of contusion with hemorrhaging and edema formation in the myocardium of the left ventricle in severe cardiac contusion

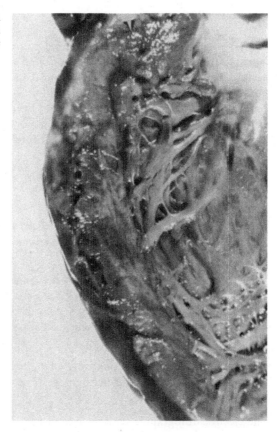

lacerations, particularly in the anterior wall of the right atrium, or lacerations of the endocardium. Occasionally, there is also formation of edema (Fig. 98). The histologic picture exhibits all levels of transition of muscle fiber damage up to necrosis and repair processes with leukocyte infiltrates and a buildup of scar tissue [411, 412, 413, 422].

Diagnosis

The diagnosis of cardiac contusion is not at all simple in many cases; diagnostic clues have to be sought (Table 23). This fact, together with an underestimation of the clinical significance of this injury, is the reason that many cases of cardiac contusion are overlooked or recognized belatedly. The frequency of the disease in clinical statistics is proportionate to the zeal with which it is sought.

Furthermore, we must remember that in cardiac contusion there is characteristically a **sequence of developments** in the clinical picture. Some symptoms and pathologic conditions do not show up until some time after the accident, brought on by hematoma and edema formation in the myocardium. The entire picture is very irregular.

Clinical Findings

Many patients complain about precordial pains. In contrast to the pains caused by injury to the thoracic wall, they are not affected by breathing. **Auscultation of the heart** provides no pathologic information if there are no injuries to cardiac structures; in exceptional cases, a pericardial friction rub may occasionally be audible. Among our patients, there was right or left heart failure in about one-fourth, which led to an increase in central venous pressure or to a drop in blood pressure without hypovolemia, which necessitated the use of catecholamines.

Electrocardiogram

Every possible variation of ECG can be observed [408, 434]. **There is no typical ECG pattern for cardiac contusion.** Furthermore, electrocardiographic patterns change very rapidly. Even a normal ECG does not obviate the possibility of cardiac contusion.

1. **Disturbances in cardiac rhythm and the conduction system:** frequently, there are arrhythmias of the atrium and ventricular extrasystoles; less frequently, the picture develops into one of a bundle-branch block or of an atrioventricular conduction disturbance that can result in total heart block and possibly requires the implantation of a pacemaker [460] (Fig. 99).

2. **Disturbances in repolarization:** very often, there are unspecified ST-T wave changes and findings of subepicardial damage (Fig. 100). There is seldom an actual infarct picture (Fig. 101).

The electrocardiographic patterns established among our patients are listed in Table 24. Since the ECG findings play a leading role in the diagnosis of cardiac contusion, the ECG belongs in the routine evaluation of every severe thoracic trauma. In the absence of pathologic findings, it serves as a basis of comparison to subsequent electrocardiograms.

Radiologic Examination

An acute dilatation of the heart in the roentgenogram will naturally lead to the conclusion that a cardiac contusion exists. In contrast to the rather frequent description in the literature [435], we were able to make these observations only very rarely among our patients. We found that the thoracic roentgenograms were seldom helpful in the diagnosis because, among other reasons, they were usually taken of patients in a recumbent position. For all cases of left-sided heart failure, however, it is important for the diagnosis of lung congestion or edema (Fig. 102).

Enzyme Determinations

Inasmuch as enzyme investigations are of great importance for the diagnosis of a myocardial infarction, it was logical to rely on enzyme changes also for the diagno-

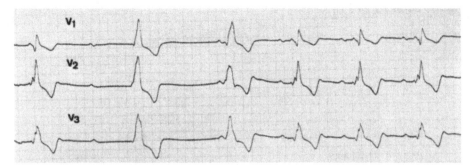

Fig. 99. Transient total atrioventricular block with a ventricular escape beat, fusion beat, and ensuing sinus rhythm with a right bundle-branch block pattern in a 47-year-old male patient with cardiac contusion

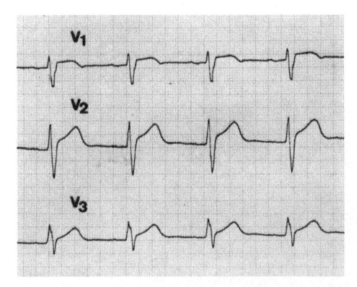

Fig. 100. Subepicardial damage on right side in cardiac contusion (35-year-old patient)

Table 24. Main ECG patterns in cardiac contusion (108 patients)

Normal ECG		13
Disturbances in rhythm, primarily ventricular	24	59
Other rhythm and conduction-system disturbances	35	
Repolarization disturbances (subepicardial damage, unspecified ST-T wave changes)		66
Infarct patterns		3

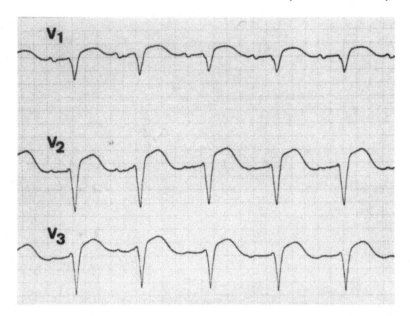

Fig. 101. ECG infarct pattern in cardiac contusion (same 19-year-old male patient as in Fig. 97)

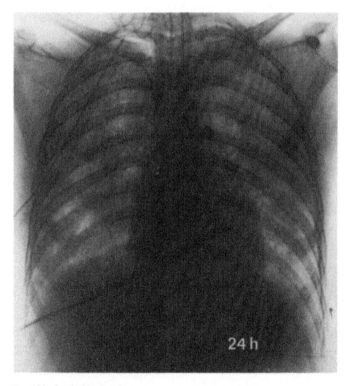

Fig. 102. Lethal lung edema in severe cardiac contusion

sis of cardiac contusion. However, it must be pointed out that for the diagnosis of cardiac contusion, the usual enzyme determinations (CPK, GOT, LDH) are totally useless since they are unspecific and since injuries to other organs or to the skeletal musculature likewise lead to an increase of these enzymes.

1. Creatinine Phosphokinase (CPK)

In all patients, there is a significant elevation of CPK; we found values of over 3000 – 4000 IU (where values up to 50 IU are normal) (Fig. 103). These are values that far exceed those observed in myocardial infarction. The damage to the heart muscle alone could never be the cause of such a high enzyme increase.

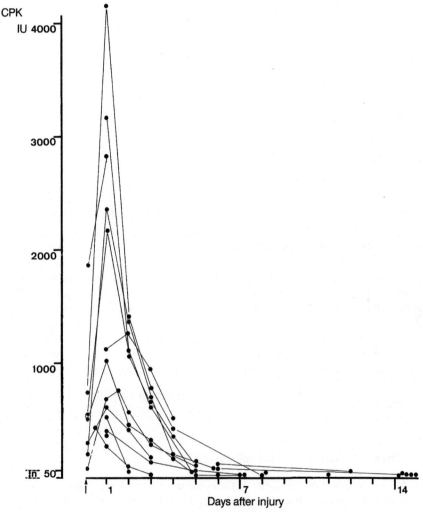

Fig. 103. The massive elevation of the total creatinine phosphokinase is essentially caused not by cardiac contusion but by trauma to the skeletal muscles

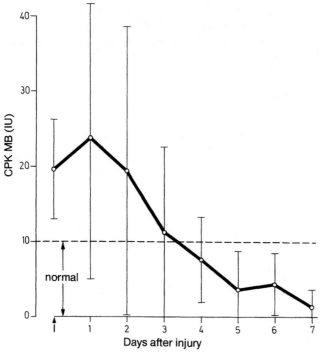

Fig. 104. Increase in level of isoenzyme MB of creatinine phosphokinase during 3 days in cardiac contusion (n = 12) (see text)

Every injury to the peripheral musculature, indeed even the intramuscular injection of certain medications, results in a CPK increase [465]. In a comparable group of thoracic injuries without cardiac contusion, we likewise found a CPK rise in every case.

The determination of the **CPK isoenzymes** is more authoritative for the diagnosis of cardiac injury. Since we began using this method, we have found among all patients with cardiac contusion that there is an increase of the isoenzyme MB already on the day of the accident (Fig. 104). The decrease to normal values occurs between the 3rd and 4th days after trauma. Since small amounts of isoenzyme MB are released also in injuries to the skeletal musculature, the proportional amount of isoenzyme MB in the total CPK is significant for the diagnosis of myocardial damage: a $\frac{\text{CPK MB}}{\text{Total CPK}}$ of over 8% provides a very significant suspicion of a cardiac contusion.

2. Glutamic-Oxaloacetic Transaminase (GOT)

According to our investigations, this enzyme is only moderately and uncharacteristically elevated in a cardiac contusion; a massive GOT rise points in the direction of liver damage. This enzyme is also so nonspecific for cardiac muscle damage that its determination is of no practical significance.

3. Lactate Dehydrogenase (LDH)

The same is true for the determination of total LDH. Also in this enzyme group, **isoenzymes** can now be delineated (Fig. 105). The LDH_1 and LDH_2 isoenzymes are quite specific for cardiac injuries. Damage to erythrocytes (through hemolysis) and certain kidney diseases likewise increase this enzyme fraction. Injuries to the skeletal musculature do not cause a rise of LDH.
In all patients with cardiac contusion, we found an unequivocal increase in LDH_1 and LDH_2 isoenzymes. The enzyme increase was evident in every case already on the day of the accident and remained for a long time (about 2 weeks), a fact that makes this determination especially significant (Fig. 106).

Measurement of Cardiac Output

Not all cardiac contusions result in a restriction of cardiac output. Nevertheless, its determination can be important for the diagnosis and evaluation of the disease picture since a decrease in cardiac output often cannot be recognized clinically. In the classic work of Pomerantz and colleagues [445], a diminished cardiac output was discovered in 11 of 17 patients. Among our patients, we undertook a determination of cardiac output only in selected cases and verified 4 of 19 patients with cardiac contusion as having a diminished cardiac output. Measurements of patients who were assumed to be hypovolemic were not included.

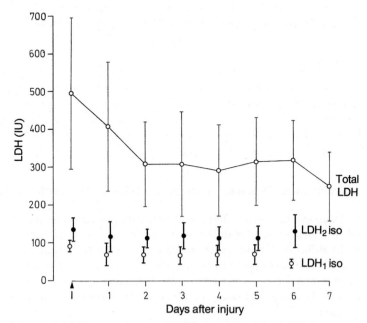

Fig. 105. Behavior of the total LDH (normal up to 195 IU) (n=52), of the LDH_1 isoenzyme (normal up to 48 IU), and of the LDH_2 isoenzyme (normal up to 76 IU) (n=21) in cardiac contusion

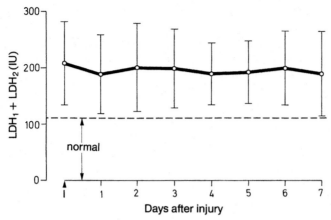

Fig. 106. Prolonged elevation of cardiac-specific LDH_1 and LDH_2 isoenzymes in cardiac contusion (n = 25)

Coronary Angiography

Tracings resembling those of a myocardial infarction on an ECG are almost always produced by contused musculature and not by injury or traumatic occlusion of a coronary artery. Among our patients, we found none in whom there was reason to conduct coronary angiography. In view of the rarity of injury to coronary arteries by blunt thoracic trauma, I find, in accord with other authors [429], the only real indication for coronary angiography to be posttraumatic angina pectoris.

Scintigraphy

Individual reports have been made [412, 432, 461, 466] on the application of radioisotopic methods in cardiac contusions. Although the experience provided by animal research is convincing, still little is known about the diagnostic possibilities in the clinic. Further developments will show whether scintigraphy can make an essential contribution to the diagnosis of cardiac contusion.

Differentiation of Cardiac Contusion and Degenerative Cardiac Diseases

In older patients with a history of preexisting arteriosclerotic cardiac disorders or other heart diseases, the differentiation of traumatic heart damage can be extraordinarily difficult. A damaged heart can also be further traumatized. For the clinical treatment of such injured persons, the distinction is academic since therapy is the same in either case; nevertheless, the differentiation may be important for forensic reasons. In individual cases, the course of developments will possibly provide essential clues.

To sum up, it must be kept firmly in mind that in some cases it is not until the **total findings** have been evaluated that a diagnosis of cardiac contusion can be made. A normal ECG does not rule out the possibility of a cardiac contusion. The determination of the **CPK MB** as well as the **LDH$_1$** and **LDH$_2$** isoenzymes is very helpful.

Clinical Course

Cardiac contusion is actually a benign injury for the most part but can subsequently lead to threatening situations, which if promptly recognized can usually be dealt with effectively (Table 25).
Of particular importance here are the **disturbances in heart rhythm.** In the first few days, they can appear unexpectedly. If disturbances of rhythm or the conduction system of the heart have not developed by the 5th day after the accident, then according to my experience this complication will no longer have to be taken into account. Rhythm disturbances, however, once occurring can endure for weeks.

Table 25. Clinical course in cardiac contusion

	108 patients who survived the day of their accident Therapy required by:
Frequent:	
Cardiac rhythm disturbances	40
Acute cardiac insufficiency	17
Infrequent:	
Cardiac tamponade with traumatic pericarditis	2
Secondary cardiac rupture	0
Heart wall aneurysm	0

Example: A truck driver was lying under his vehicle changing the oil when suddenly the jack failed and the patient was squeezed between the truck and the ground. The roentgenogram of the thorax showed no pathologic condition; there were no rib fractures. The ECG of the patient was kept under surveillance on the monitor in the intensive care unit. On the evening of the accident there was suddenly a temporary AV block; after 2 days, a massive life-threatening ventricular tachycardia developed unexpectedly from a sinus rhythm (Fig. 107). With infusion of lidocaine, the normal sinus rhythm returned. For 5 days, sporadic rhythm disturbances were still observed. Two weeks after the accident, the patient left the hospital free of complaints.

Example: A 27-year-old patient was pressed against a wooden wall by a power shovel at a construction site and suffered severe thoracic contusion with traumatic asphyxia. There were no rib fractures. On the day of the accident, supraventricular extrasystoles occurred. At the same time, tachycardia with a rate up to 200 developed, which was reduced by verapamil. Cardiac failure with a fall in blood pressure later required treatment with epinephrine for 2 days. Subsequently, there was a constant alternation between atrial fibrillation, atrial flutter, and sinus rhythm, and the use of beta blockers was repeatedly necessary. After a hospital stay of 2 months, this patient was released home.

Symptoms of **cardiac failure** are less common; however, they are often so pronounced that cardiac shock occurs and the use of catecholamines becomes necessary.
Occasionally during the patient's course, a **pericardial effusion** is observed. Especially dreaded are **belated ruptures** in the area of the contusion after cardiac contusion.

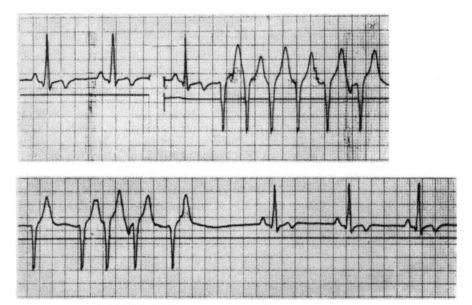

Fig. 107. Sudden development of a ventricular tachycardia from a sinus rhythm; lidocaine in a dosage of 1.5 mg/min restored the sinus rhythm (see text)

Table 26. Therapy of cardiac rhythm disturbances in cardiac contusion

General	Remedy hypoxia
Ventricular extrasystoles	1. In hypokalemia, potassium infusion (maximally 40 mEq KCl in 45 min)
	2. Lidocaine
	Direct IV 50 – 100 mg
	In infusion 1 – 4 mg/min
	3. Ajmaline
	Direct IV 25 – 50 mg, slowly
	In infusion 500 mg/24 h
	4. Procainamide
	Direct IV 100 mg
	In infusion 3 g/24 h
	5. In digitalis-related arrhythmia
	Diphenylhydantoin
	Direct IV 125 mg
Supraventricular extrasystoles with tachycardia	1. Verapamil
	Direct IV 5 – 10 mg
	In infusion 200 mg/24 h
Atrial fibrillation with tachycardia	1. Digitalis
	2. Verapamil
Tachycardias without resorting to verapamil	Beta antagonists
Bradycardias	1. Orciprenaline
	If necessary, atropine
	If necessary, pacemaker

They usually affect a ventricle and are then generally fatal. Such ruptures have been described as occurring from 9 days to 7 weeks after the heart injury [421]. An even less frequent consequence is the formation of a **left ventricular aneurysm** of the cardiac wall.

Among our patients, we have witnessed acutely threatening situations in 35% of the patients caused by disturbances of cardiac rhythm or by cardiac failure with cardiogenic shock.

Therapy

The indispensable prerequisite for optimal therapy is **admission to an intensive care unit** with continuous **ECG monitoring.** This procedure should be followed even when there is only a **suspicion** of cardiac contusion.
Obviously, hypovolemia and hypoxia must be corrected. The volume infusion should be given cautiously; excessive transfusion should be avoided. The measurement of central venous and possibly of pulmonary artery pressure helps in the regulation of volume infusion.
Therapy corresponds essentially to that of myocardial infarction. The use of antiarrhythmic medications is governed by the usual principles of cardiac care (Table 26). Special attention must be given to an adequate and very generous potassium infusion inasmuch as the serum potassium concentration is usually low after severe trauma (in emergency admissions of 100 patients with chest injuries, the serum potassium level averaged 3.4 mEq/liter with individual values as low as 2.3 mEq/liter).
The use of digitalis preparations is generally indicated only when there are signs of cardiac failure. When blood pressure drops, there should be no hesitation in the early use of epinephrine, dopamine, or isoproterenol.
The rare occurrence of a pericardial effusion with symptoms of cardiac tamponade makes a single or repeated pericardiocentesis and, in exceptional cases, also the operative drainage of the pericardium necessary.

Prognosis

In the severely injured who dies a short time after admission to the hospital, the significance of cardiac contusion as a cause of death usually cannot be established.
If the patient survives the first 24 h, the **prognosis** of the cardiac contusion under **treatment in an intensive care unit is good.** Mortality is determined largely by the companion injuries. In our series of 108 patients with cardiac contusions who survived the 1st day, only 2 died due to the heart injury: a young man in pulmonary edema and a 60-year-old patient with very severe preexisting coronary atherosclerosis. Seventeen others died due to the consequences of other injuries.
There have been descriptions of **ongoing residual rhythm disturbances** [433, 411]. In a follow-up of 22 patients 1 – 3 years after the accident, we found 6 cases with continuing pathologic ECG variations, mostly repolarization disturbances. Five patients complained of paroxysmal tachycardia.
As a curiosity, I would like to mention one case of posttraumatic bone formation in the myocardium, confirmed by autopsy 3½ years after the accident [419].

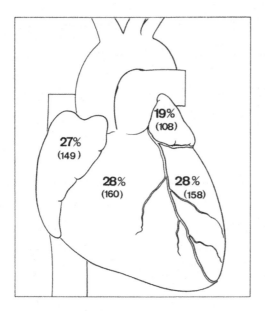

Fig. 108. Location of cardiac wall ruptures at autopsy: collective statistics of 575 cardiac wall ruptures

VI. Heart Wall Ruptures

The diagnosis of a cardiac wall rupture is usually made by autopsy. Both ventricles and the left atrium are affected equally often; the left atrium ruptures somewhat less frequently (Fig. 108). The patient bleeds to death only when there is significant injury to the pericardium. In most cases, death occurs as the result of a rapidly developing **cardiac tamponade.**

Prognosis is naturally the worst in cases of ventricular laceration. A rupture of the left ventricle as the result of blunt trauma always causes death within a few minutes. Patients with a rupture of the right ventricle can survive somewhat longer, but practically all of them die within the first 30 min [444]. If the laceration is in the area of an atrium, the likelihood is greater that the patient will reach the hospital alive. In these cases, there is a real possibility of saving the life by means of an immediate thoracotomy [443, 447].

There are known cases of heart wall ruptures that do not manifest themselves until days or even weeks after trauma [421, 438]. Such cases are ruptures that were temporarily closed by a thrombus or are delayed ruptures due to cardiac contusion.

Diagnosis

The **symptoms of acute cardiac tamponade** indicate a cardiac wall rupture.

Therapy

Only an **immediate operation** gives promise of success; in this situation, even the general surgeon should not hesitate to undertake it. The access is made by an antero-

VII. Traumatic Septal Defects

Of the septal defects caused by blunt trauma, those of the **atrial septum** are not clinically significant. There is no report in the literature of an operation for such a lesion. A compression of the filled atrium will apparently cause a tear in the thin atrial wall rather than in the septum. The traumatic atrial septal defect shows up only as a companion injury to other severe injuries of the heart.

Patients with ruptures of the **ventricular septum** can survive the accident for months or even years, as long as the lesion is not combined with other intracardiac injuries. The defect can be hemodynamically insignificant, or if there is a large shunt, can be quickly fatal. At times, a delay in development is observed in which the perforation of a damaged septal area occurs 3 – 5 days after the accident.

 In 1847, Hewett [424] reported for the first time on a ventricular septal defect in a boy who had been run over by a heavy wagon and died 30 min later of injury to his heart. In 1955, the first successful operation of such a lesion from blunt trauma was performed by Campbell [406]. Reports of other operations are no longer uncommon in recent years.

Diagnosis

The leading sign is the appearance of a **systolic murmur** with its point of maximum intensity at the left parasternal area. Occasionally, there is a systolic thrill. In addition to the uncharacteristic symptoms, such as precordial pains, dyspnea, and cyanosis, there can also be signs of acute heart failure.

Also in patients in poor general condition, a cardiac dye curve can support a clinical suspicion; definitive diagnosis is provided by catheterization of the heart.

Therapy

In a severe, therapy-resistant cardiac failure, all that is left is prompt operation. In the rest of the cases, the indication for an operation is similar to a congenital ventricular septal defect. Spontaneous closures months after trauma are known to have occurred [417, 452]. If possible, the operation should be scheduled at least 8 weeks after trauma since by then the synthetic patch that is usually necessary can be better anchored in the fibrotically altered tissue.

VIII. Heart Valve Injuries

Of the heart valves, the most frequently injured by **blunt force** are the aortic valve, followed by the tricuspid and mitral valves, while the pulmonary valve is almost never damaged. In the aortic valve, the valvular apparatus itself is injured or torn, whereas in the atrioventricular valves, more frequently the papillary muscles or the tendinous cords are detached. The lesion naturally always results in valvular insufficiency and never in stenosis.

In general, valve injuries on the high pressure side of the heart quickly lead to cardiac decompensation, but there are various reports ranging from severe, dramatic insufficiency to cases with a nearly subclinical course. Ruptures of the tendinous cords of the mitral valve appear to lead more slowly to cardiac insufficiency.

In contrast, tricuspid insufficiency is usually tolerated quite well, and typically an extended lapse of time, often one of years, passes before an operation is performed. Thus, the case of Brandenburg was not treated operatively until 24 years and that of Astorri not until 23 years after the accident [397, 404].

The trauma causing the injury is not always judged to be severe. Thus, in both of the cases of Bailey [398], steering wheel injuries were involved in which mitral tendinous cords were avulsed. The injuries were adjudged to be so slight, however, that at first the patients were not hospitalized.

Diagnosis and Therapy

Heart valve injuries caused by blunt trauma are always first recognized during the **subsequent course.** This has no implications for treatment because an operative intervention would not be undertaken until symptoms of heart failure had been noted.

One should be alert to the appearance of heart murmurs and right or left heart failure during the subsequent course after a contusion. If these key signs are in evidence, cardiac catheterization together with a cardioangiogram will confirm the diagnosis and simultaneously provide the necessary information about the hemodynamic effects and, through them, the indication for an operation. From the reports in the literature to date, there is an apparent tendency not to attempt a reconstruction of the valve but to replace it with an artificial prosthesis.

IX. Injuries to the Coronary Arteries

A **healthy coronary artery** is extraordinarily resistant to the effects of blunt trauma. It is more likely that the adjacent myocardium will incur damage, as Moritz [441] was able to demonstrate in animal experiments. Infarction patterns on the ECG after blunt trauma can therefore almost always be attributed to extended heart contusions and not to the occlusion of a coronary artery, if there is no preexistent degenerative disease of the coronary vessels [444].

For a long time, it was assumed that an occlusion of a coronary artery caused by blunt trauma occurred only as a result of arteriosclerotic changes. Individual observations [401, 459] provide evidence, however, that this is not the case; yet these exceptions continue to be rare. There have also been descriptions of ruptures of the coronary arteries [423] that need not lead to cardiac tamponade.

When signs of a cardiac infarction appear on the ECG after blunt trauma, coronary angiography is justified in the acute phase only if, in the special situation of an occlusion, operative intervention would be necessary and possible. At a later point in time, coronary angiography will be considered in a patient with a posttraumatic angina pectoris, increasing heart failure with an infarction pattern on the ECG, or a cardiac aneurysm.

X. Traumatic Cardiac Aneurysm

While false aneurysms can be formed in the left ventricular wall after penetrating heart injuries, they are mostly **true mural aneurysms** when they occur after blunt trauma. They are caused by necrosis in the myocardium resulting from a cardiac contusion or, very rarely, from occlusion of a coronary artery. Such aneurysms are observed almost exclusively in the **left ventricle.** Depending upon the amount of myocardial damage, they can develop already within days after trauma.

The suspected diagnosis is first provided by the **roentgenogram,** since the **clinical signs** are totally uncharacteristic: disturbances in the heart rhythm and cardiac insufficiency. Proof is furnished by the **left-sided cardiogram.** The **coronary angiography,** which is always to be conducted at the same time, answers the question as to the occurrence of a coronary occlusion. Even if there has been no occlusion of these vessels, however, the blood flow in the coronary arteries can be impeded when the ventricular wall itself bulges out, as Hasper [420] has observed.

If there are no serious contraindications, the **treatment** of a cardiac aneurysm should in principle be surgical since rupture or an arterial embolism are a constant threat. The indication for operation, once the diagnosis has been confirmed, should not be made dependent upon the complaints. Thus, there have been operations performed in cases that were totally free of any symptoms.

The operative intervention with the use of extracorporeal circulation, which consists in excising the aneurysmal protrusion and directly suturing the ventricle, has a very good prognosis because there is generally no further concurrent myocardial damage.

Chapter 17

Penetrating Wounds of the Heart

I. Penetrating Cardiac Injuries

Basic Considerations

Penetrating cardiac injuries are fatal in 62% – 84% of the cases before admission to a hospital [488, 501, 503]. If such a patient survives to receive hospital treatment, however, with optimal treatment the further **prognosis** is astonishingly **good**. This is especially true of stab wounds. Of 52 patients reported by Viikari in 1976 [506], as many as 98% survived, whereas other recent publications indicate a survival of 80% – 90%. In gunshot injuries, the chances of survival under optimal conditions is still as high as 60% [471, 483, 491, 503].

These favorable outcomes are obtainable only under one condition: **immediate thoracotomy**. When confronted by an injury of this kind, the general surgeon will recognize that a transfer to a center for cardiac surgery is out of the question and that he therefore must perform the operation himself. Rehn, who performed the first successful suture repair of a heart wound, was also not a cardiac surgeon. Beach [471] and Trinkle [505] have reported very good results of larger series in hospitals that have no special divisions for cardiac surgery.

This general principle of immediate operation also applies particularly to situations that are apparently hopeless. Even the actual occurrence of cardiac arrest is not a contraindication for operative intervention.

Example: In a suicidal attempt, a 45-year-old man shot himself in the cardiac area with an automatic rifle. He was brought to the hospital 45 min after the injury. In the emergency room cardiac arrest occurred. There was a large entry wound with ragged edges precordially on the left side. The physician on duty evaluated the situation as unfavorable on the basis of the wound and the "doubtlessly severe" heart injury and dispensed with therapeutic procedures.
In the autopsy, a hemopericardium of 250 ml was found with only slight, superficial contusion of the right ventricle as the source of bleeding. There was no perforating cardiac injury and no other life-threatening lesions.
Comment: The patient's survival time of 45 min makes severe cardiac injury unlikely. The patient died of a cardiac tamponade. Operative intervention immediately upon arrival at the emergency room would have saved the life of the patient.

Example: A 29-year-old patient arrived at the emergency ward with a gunshot wound in the thorax caused by an automatic rifle. He was in cardiac arrest and not breathing. An immediate thoracotomy revealed a large amount of coagulated blood in the pericardium. His heart, initially inactive, soon displayed strong pulsations. There was a bullet penetration of the right ventricle. The gunshot wounds of entry and exit were sutured. The patient recovered without aftereffects.

The conviction that a therapeutic attempt should be made even in an apparently hopeless situation was confirmed by the remarkable work of Mattox et al. [488]. These authors examined the fate of 37 patients with cardiac injuries who were already in cardiac arrest when brought to the hospital but still showed some signs of reflex activity or suffered cardiac arrest upon admission. Twenty-two of the cases involved gunshot wounds. By means of immediate thoracotomy, 67% of these patients survived.

Up to the nineteenth century, mankind was helpless in the face of injuries of the heart. Wounds of this central organ occupied the thoughts of the poet more than the physician. Homer [484] in the *Iliad* lets Alkathoos die of a stab wound to the heart made by a lance: "... and the spear stuck in his heart, which, still twitching, caused the shaft end of the lance to tremble."
Patroclus strikes the heart of Sarpedon with a spear, who, after making a brief speech, dies [479].

All early physicians regarded cardiac wounds to be fatal, among them Hippocrates, Aristotle, Celsus, and also Galen, who not infrequently saw heart injuries among the gladiators. Hollerius (1498 – 1562) was the first to maintain that heart wounds could be healed, a view that had still not gained acceptance by the last century [479].
Even Ambroise Paré, who in 1594 in his *Opera Chirurgica* was the first to describe a penetrating heart wound that had been verified by means of an autopsy, regarded all cardiac injuries as fatal. In his case, during a duel a nobleman in Turin had received a stab wound just under the left nipple from a sword, had pursued his opponent, and then collapsed and died. Discovered was "... a wound so large that a finger could be thrust into his heart."
Fernel († 1598) and Tourby autopsied patients who had survived a heart wound and discovered scar formation in the heart, in Tourby's case, 4 years after a sword injury [479].
Fischer [479], in his extended survey of the literature in 1868, found among 452 cases with cardiac injuries 72 recoveries, of which 36 were verified by autopsy.
Even leading surgeons showed an almost superstitious awe of the heart. Billroth's saying is well-known: "A surgeon who would attempt to suture a heart wound should certainly lose the respect of his colleagues."
In 1895 Cappelen attempted a cardiac suture repair. The patient died 2½ days later, however [501]. In 1896 Rehn [496] made the first successful attempt at heart suturing by closing a hemorrhaging wound of the right ventricle. This decisive step in cardiac surgery occurred in the same year that Stephen Paget [493] was still of the opinion "that no new method and no new discovery can overcome the natural difficulties that attend a wound of the heart."
But as early as 1906, a mere 10 years after the first successful heart suturing, Rehn was able to assemble a list of 124 cases of cardiac injuries that had been operated on with an astonishing survival rate of 40% [497].

Mechanism of Injury and Location of Cardiac Wounds

In addition to **stab** and **gunshot injuries** and wounds of the heart caused by **flying objects,** there has recently been an increase in **iatrogenic** cardiac injuries, especially those caused by intracardiac catheters used to diagnose cardiac defects, by pacemaker electrodes, and by central venous and pulmonary catheters. A variety of other medical measures can lead to cardiac injuries, more recently even acupuncture [492].
The **frequency** of injury to individual chambers of the heart is to a large extent related to the **area** bordering the anterior thoracic wall. Furthermore, wounds of the left ventricle are more likely to cause death before arrival at the hospital than those of the right ventricle because of the former's higher interior pressure.

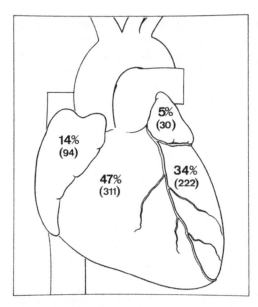

Fig. 109. Location of penetrating cardiac injuries (cumulative statistics of 657 penetrating cardiac injuries from 22 clinical publications since 1968)

Among clinical patients, of all the heart chambers it is the right ventricle that is affected in almost half the cases (47%), followed by the left ventricle and by the right atrium. Injuries to the left atrium are rare exceptions (Fig. 109), and there are seldom injuries to intracardiac structures or the coronary arteries.

Clinical Picture

Small penetrating heart wounds can seal themselves and heal spontaneously. This is possible especially in the region of the right ventricle with its muscularly strong wall and its low interior pressure.

Two different clinical situations characterize the picture in significant heart wounds:

1. If the injury of the pericardium has created a sufficiently large opening into the pleural cavity to allow for the drainage of blood, the blood will flow out into the thoracic cavity: the result will be **hypovolemic shock** and **death from loss of blood.**

2. If the injury of the pericardium does not permit drainage, **hemopericardium** and **cardiac tamponade** will result. By causing a rise in the intrapericardial pressure, the tamponade temporarily impedes hemorrhagic death. The cardiac tamponade is a "two-edged sword: both lethal and lifesaving" (Naclerio [150]) since in a short time it results in collapse of the circulatory system.

Of special importance clinically are cases with **delayed symptoms.** Cardiac tamponade can develop hours later, sometimes even after weeks. This is the case, for example, when a thrombus formed at the site of the injury dislodges.

Diagnosis

The **wound, shock,** and **cardiac tamponade** all point toward cardiac injury. Heart murmurs are heard in valvular injuries, in injuries of the septum, and in the forma-

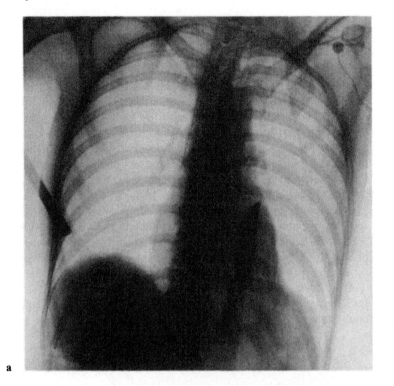

Fig. 110 a, b. Stab wound of the right ventricle made with a knife

tion of an aortovenous fistula into the right ventricle. Extreme bradycardia and heart block can occur with involvement of the conduction system.

The wound: in gunshot injuries, cardiac involvement should be considered not only in precordial wounds but also in every wound in the thoracic area. Embedded knives and other perforating objects plug the heart wound; the roentgenogram will document their exact location in relation to the cardiac shadow (Fig. 110).

Shock: a state of shock can be caused by loss of blood or cardiac tamponade. In hemorrhagic shock, there is usually a significant **hemothorax.** Also in cardiac tamponade, volume infusion, by raising the venous pressure, produces a better filling of the ventricle and a rise in arterial pressure.

Cardiac tamponade: the pathophysiology, diagnosis, and treatment of cardiac tamponade are described in detail in Chap. 16.

The complete classic triad (increased venous pressure, muffled and distant heart sounds, and arterial hypotension) is found in only 35% [508] to 40% [507] of the cases of cardiac tamponade caused by penetrating injuries. Repeated measurements of central venous pressure are of significant importance for early diagnosis since the arterial pressure does not fall until a later stage (see Fig. 93). A paradoxical pulse if often observable.

In 60% of patients with cardiac tamponade caused by a penetrating injury, **coagulated blood** is found in the pericardium [508]. It is therefore understandable that

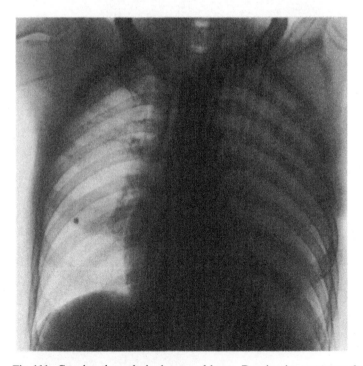

Fig. 111. Gunshot through the heart and lungs. Despite the presence of a severe cardiac tamponade, the cardiac silhouette has not become enlarged. The left-sided hemothorax developed from the injury to the lung. The projectile is embedded in the right side of the thorax

in 15% [508] to 25% [432] **pericardiocentesis** turns out to be negative despite the presence of a tamponade.

Radiologic examination: in an acute cardiac tamponade, there is often no widening of the cardiac silhouette (Fig. 111). The roentgenogram of the chest will provide information, however, about companion injuries of the lung, a hemothorax, or a pneumothorax and about the location of intrathoracic foreign bodies.

Electrocardiogram: the changes in the ECG are varied and totally uncharacteristic. The classic low voltage is seldom present in acute cardiac tamponade. Even a normal ECG in no way precludes the possibility of a cardiac injury.

When a patient is in critical condition, no diagnostic procedure must be allowed to cause a postponement of the only possible therapy, namely, an immediate thoracotomy with exposure of the heart.

Therapy

After the first era of resignation and the second era of the first successful operative interventions, there followed a third era during the 1940s of differentiated, hesitant operative intervention. Griswold [481] as well as Blalock and Ravitch [473] had publicized a restrained approach to operative treatment and suggested that pericardiocentesis first be performed and operation only after repeated pericardiocentesis had been unsuccessful. Until the recent past, this strategy had been widely accepted in the United States and in South Africa.

Today, it has become clear that this tactic was **on the wrong course** and preference should instead be given to an **aggressive, early operative approach.** We cannot enter into a discussion of the whole series of reasons in favor of an immediate operation; however, it is obvious that one should not leave a patient hovering between life and death for hours with all the problems of supervision and the limited therapeutic potential of pericardiocentesis in the face of a coagulated hematoma if the injury can be taken care of definitively and with good results by a primary operation.

The improvement of prognosis by the change from differentiated wait-and-see to an aggressive operative procedure is impressive: between two comparable series, Sugg [501] was able to lower the mortality from 37% to 14% and Symbas [502] from 17% to 5%. In larger series, Beall [472], Harvey [483], and Neville [491] reported similar experiences.

The **therapeutic treatment** embraces:

1. Shock treatment

2. Insertion of chest tubes

3. Possibly pericardiocentesis

4. Operation

Obviously, attention will also be paid to whatever **associated injuries** exist.

Shock Treatment

This goes parallel to the diagnostic and other therapeutic measures and may never be a reason for postponement of an operation.

Thoracic Drainage

Unless a thoracic cavity is opened by an immediate operation, thoracic drains are installed when there is a pneumothorax or hemothorax. They prevent a tension pneumothorax and provide information about blood loss in the pleural cavity.

Pericardiocentesis (for technique, see p. 187)

Pericardiocentesis, prior to the opening of the pericardium, can bring about a noticeable improvement of the hemodynamic situation even though very little blood is evacuated. The use of anesthesia with mechanical ventilation, which tends to reinforce the detrimental aspects of cardiac tamponade even more, is thereby better tolerated.

Indication for Operation

In consideration of the opinions expressed above, the indication for an operation can be defined as follows:

1. A penetrating cardiac injury with cardiac tamponade or massive hemorrhage requires an immediate operation, possibly after a preceding pericardiocentesis. If circulatory arrest has already occurred or if the poor condition of the patient does not permit transfer to the operating room, the immediate thoracotomy is performed in the emergency room.

2. Other patients are examined carefully and operated on if there is a significant lesion, particularly when there are signs of tamponade or a hemorrhagic fall in blood pressure.

Foreign bodies stuck in the heart but protruding (e. g., knives) are left in and not removed until the operative opening of the pericardium. If there are doubts about the location with regard to the heart, they are removed on the operating table in the prepared operating room.

Operative Approach

The approach is made by a left-sided anterolateral thoracotomy in the fifth intercostal space. If the exposure is insufficient, the approach can be extended by cutting across the sternum to the right. The median sternotomy has several disadvantages: it takes longer and, more importantly, makes it more difficult to expose additional injuries in the mediastinum or thoracic areas and to evaluate the posterior surface of the heart.

Operative Tactics

The operation, apart from the approach, takes place in four phases:

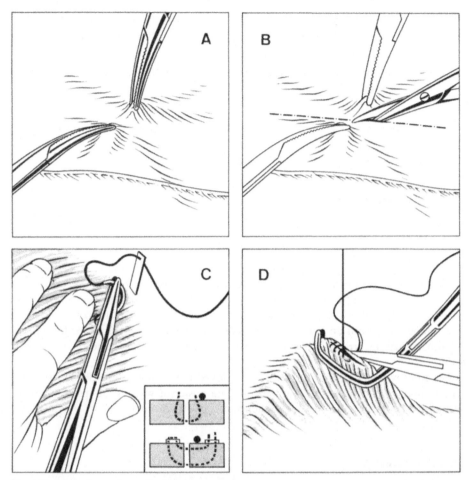

Fig. 112 A – D. Operative procedure in penetrating heart injuries. **A** Lifting the pericardium with two clamps in front of the phrenic nerve; **B** Opening the pericardium lengthwise and at a safe distance from the nerve; **C** Suturing of a ventricular wound under digital hemostasis; a coronary artery lies outside the suture or the suture is placed underneath; **D** Continuous suturing of an injury of the atrium

1. **Evacuation of blood from the pericardium.** The pericardium is opened with a large longitudinal incision in front of the phrenic nerve (Fig. 112 A and B). This is a decisive and dangerous moment in the operation because massive hemorrhage can occur when the tamponade is relieved. Before proceeding with the opening of the pericardium, the approach must be sufficiently large and blood or a blood substitute must be available. Suction facilities and an irrigating solution should be at hand.

2. **Provisional hemostasis:** it is essential, in the sea of blood, to locate the source of bleeding. On the ventricle, the provisional hemostasis is always accomplished by compression with the finger. On the atrium, it is usually possible to apply an atraumatic clamp (e. g., Satinsky clamp). If not, digital compression is also employed

there (in case of large damage, if necessary, by introduction of the index finger bent at the middle joint) (Fig. 112 C and D).

3. **Waiting:** the cardiac tamponade has been relieved and the bleeding temporarily stopped. Definitive closure will cause blood loss. It is worthwhile in this phase to give the anesthesiologist time to stabilize the circulation and replace the blood volume.

4. Without pressure of time, the **definitive treatment** of injured structures now proceeds.

Treating the Heart Wound

1. Ventricular Wall

While slowly withdrawing digital compression, the closure of the ventricle is made with interrupted sutures, which on the left ventricle can be placed through a pledget of Teflon felt to prevent cutting through the musculature. Suture material: right ventricle, 2-0 or 3-0 silk; left ventricle, 1-0 or 2-0 silk. The sutures go as far as the endocardium but do not touch it because of the danger of thrombus formation. Coronary arteries are avoided and, if necessary, the suture is placed underneath (Fig. 112 C).

In gunshot wounds, devitalized tissue is removed before the suture closure to avoid the formation of a false mural aneurysm. The posterior wall of the heart is always examined to exclude the possible existence of any other injury.

2. Atrial Wounds

Injuries in the area of the atria can almost always be grasped with an angled vascular clamp (Satinsky clamp) and taken care of with a continuous suture with 4-0 or 5-0 silk (Fig. 112D). The atrial wall is very fragile. In the area of the right atrioventricular junction, caution is advised because of the closely adjacent coronary arteries. For technical reasons, wounds on the posterior wall of the left atrium can hardly be sutured; it is better to tamponade them [e. g., with Tabotamp (Surgicel)] (Senning, personal communication).

Wounds of the atria usually bleed very profusely because the thin muscle wall hardly impedes the exit of blood.

3. Injuries of the Intrapericardial Vena Cava

These can for the most part be clamped off tangentially and sutured. If this is impossible, an internal shunt can be inserted through the right atrial appendage of the heart (see Chap. 18).

4. Injuries of the Coronary Arteries

Occasionally, an epicardial branch will be injured, very seldom the coronary artery itself. Ligatures of the main trunks are not tolerated [495]. If a direct suture is impossible, the techniques of coronary artery surgery, particularly those of aortocoronary bypass, are applied.

From among a large series of penetrating cardiac injuries, Espada et al. [478] reported on nine injuries of coronary arteries. Of these, eight were ligated and in only one case was an aortocoronary bypass performed. Although all patients with ligated coronary arteries showed postoperative changes in the ECG, none of them exhibited any clinical manifestations of coronary insufficiency. The enzyme values became normalized.

5. Injuries of Intracardiac Structures

After definitive hemostasis has been implemented, attention should be turned to any clues of a possible septal injury or lesion of the valvular apparatus. A palpable thrill is an indication.

In these cases, a precise clarification is arrived at postoperatively by means of cardiac catheterization and an angiocardiogram. Additional injuries are taken care of later as a planned operation with the use of extracorporeal circulation.

In departments of cardiac surgery, the immediate treatment of intracardiac companion injuries, using extracorporeal circulation, will be considered on a case-by-case basis [432].

The **closure of the pericardium** will not be undertaken until a normal systolic blood pressure reading is attained to determine with certainty whether or not the cardiac suture line is tight. Behind the phrenic nerve, a wide drainage window is created into the left pleural cavity, and the longitudinal incision of the pericardium in front of the nerve is closed to avoid cardiac dislocation.

II. Late Sequelae of Penetrating Cardiac Injuries

There are several known characteristic pathologic alterations resulting from penetrating cardiac injuries that confirm the necessity of **postoperative follow-up** in these patients.

Cardiac Aneurysm

False aneurysms of the heart wall are caused almost exclusively by penetrating cardiac injuries. As in the case of closed heart injuries, they are formed in the area of the left ventricle because of the higher interior pressure.

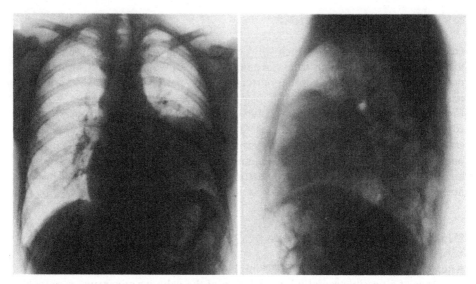

Fig. 113. False cardiac aneurysm of the left ventricle. Gunshot injury from a Flobert rifle, primary suturing. Operation on the aneurysm 5 weeks after the injury

This complication is not infrequent when such patients are seen in regular postoperative follow-up. Symbas [502] found ventricular aneurysms in 5 of 56 patients surviving penetrating cardiac injuries, i. e., in almost 10%. Of the cases reported in the literature, approximately half were asymptomatic.

The main finding for diagnostic purposes is a **bulge on the border of the left ventricle** on an **otherwise normal roentgenogram** (Fig. 113). Frequently, there are an apical systolic ejection murmur and signs of myocardial infarction on the ECG. Precordial pains, arrhythmias, and arterial emboli can occur. The diagnosis is confirmed by a left-sided ventriculogram.

Formation of an aneurysm can appear soon after the trauma.

Example: In one of the cases we observed, an aneurysm formed within 3 weeks after a gunshot passed through the left ventricle. Because of its rapid growth and threatened rupture, the operation was required 5 weeks after the accident (Fig. 113).

As reported in the literature, operations for posttraumatic cardiac aneurysms were performed between 20 days and 24 years after the accident [489]. In general, because of the danger of a rupture and the possibility of an arterial embolism, the resection of such aneurysms is recommended even when the patient is asymptomatic. The prognosis of these operations is excellent since most of them involve younger patients with an otherwise healthy myocardium without coronary damage.

Arteriovenous Coronary Fistula

Arteriovenous fistulas are known to have occurred in every part of the body after penetrating injuries. Most of the fistulas involving a coronary artery and the venous side of the circulatory system, as mentioned in the literature, are those between the

right coronary artery and the **right atrium.** However, fistula linkages to the right ventricle and to the accompanying vein have also been described [498].

Many of these fistulas are clinically silent. If they produce symptoms, the latter are very uncharacteristic. The most significant and most frequent finding of cases reported was the occurrence of a loud "machinery murmur" over the heart. Cardiac insufficiency caused by the left-to-right shunt is rare. Clinically, the diagnosis can only be suspected.

In an examination by cardiac catheterization, the pressure values in the heart chambers are usually normal. **Coronary angiography** provides definitive diagnosis.

Since this is an unusual clinical picture, the indication for an operation is controversial. Decompensated cardiac failure and signs of an increasing shunt or an enlargement of the fistula call for an operation using extracorporeal circulation. However, there has also been favorable progress reported with conservative treatment carried out for over 20 years [476].

Coronary Artery Aneurysms

This is seen as an extremely rare consequence of injury. Operative treatment with the possibilities offered by today's coronary surgery is recommended because of the danger of rupture or the possibility of a thrombotic closure [485].

III. Foreign Bodies in the Heart

Foreign bodies can reach the heart by **penetrating the heart wall** or by **embolization** into the right side of the heart, seldom into the left, from a distant venous entrance site.

1. By direct route into the heart wall or through it, the overwhelming majority are penetrating cardiac injuries, mainly caused by gunshot or shrapnel, etc. The slow migration and later penetration of Kirschner wires used in internal fixation in the thoracic area [480] or of needles is unexpected. The penetration of pointed bone fragments or fish bones from the esophagus is also known to have occurred.

2. It is mostly bullet projectiles that embolize into the heart, but more recently there has been an increase in the number of detached venous catheters.

 In 1815 Latour reported the story of a soldier who was considered dead and carried off after a bullet injury in the chest with severe hemorrhaging. He recovered from the injury and died 6 years later from another disease. During the autopsy, the bullet was found encapsulated in the right ventricle [479]. In 1818 Hennen reported on a needle in the heart with no explanation as to how it got there. The patient died of carditis.

If we assume that the needle reached the heart, not by way of embolism but, what is more likely, via the esophagus, the report of Davis in 1834 must be regarded as the first about a foreign body embolism reaching the heart: a 10-year-old boy died 5 weeks after a small piece of wood penetrated into his chest. It was found in the right ventricle, though there was no sign of a wound in his heart [479].

It is a known fact that foreign bodies **lodged** in the **heart wall** can often be tolerated without impairment. In the medical literature, there is a report [470] of such a case lasting 29 years. Recently, there was a newspaper report of the death of a French veteran with an intracardiac foreign body obtained during World War I. He died of the consequences of old age. Bland and Beebe [474] examined 40 patients with intracardiac foreign bodies from World War II 20 years after injury, and in many of them, apart from the psychic stress of a projectile in the heart, they found no disturbance. However, 25% of them had suffered pericardial effusion.

The (slight) danger of a foreign body in the cardiac musculature consists in the possibility of its **migration** into the heart chamber or pericardium, which can cause a delayed cardiac tamponade.

More dangerous, however, are **free** foreign bodies in the heart chamber. There, particularly, the danger of an **embolism** exists, from the right side into the lung or, rarely, as a crossover embolism into the arterial circulation, or from the left side of the heart as an arterial embolism. The foreign body itself need not embolize, but thrombi generated by the foreign body can be carried off by the blood stream. The second great danger of free foreign bodies within the heart is the possibility of **endocarditis** and **septicemia.**

Diagnosis

Opaque foreign bodies can be localized fairly accurately by roentgenograms taken in two planes. Freely moving fragments can attract attention by their change of position.

Harken [482], in a series of patients from World War II, established the fact that in half of the cases referred as having "intracardiac foreign bodies," careful radiologic screening demonstrated an extracardiac location. Of the remaining 50%, the operation revealed that an additional one-third of the foreign objects were outside the myocardium.

In many cases, therefore, **angiocardiography** is necessary for exact localization. Occasionally, coronary angiography can also be helpful [487].

Therapy

There are still differences of opinion about **indications for the removal** of intracardiac foreign bodies. From a peace-loving Switzerland, I can contribute little from my own experience.

Obviously, in treating a penetrating heart wound the primary attempt will be to extract a foreign body, provided this is possible without additional damage and no vital hazard to the patient results.

There are specific situations in which the **clear indication is given** for later removal of the foreign body: all infected foreign bodies, all freely moving foreign bodies, and those that lead secondarily to a hemopericardium. If the patient's symptoms indicate embolization into the periphery, a local approach will naturally be made there.

An elegant method was successfully employed by Schott [500] in a gunshot embolism in the right side of the heart involving a fully mobile, round free body. By positioning of the patient under fluoroscopic control, he succeeded in displacing it, with the help of the force of gravity, into a pelvic vein from where it could be removed.

If the **indication for an operation is not clear,** the dangers of leaving things as they are will have to be weighed against the operative morbidity in each individual case. The potential of modern cardiac surgery with its use of extracorporeal circulation certainly allows for much broader indications than in earlier years. In an older person, foreign bodies that are firmly embedded and show no clinical symptoms should be left alone.

Chapter 18
Injuries of the Great Intrathoracic Vessels

I. Rupture of the Aorta

Basic Considerations

The main problem of this injury in the clinic lies in **timely diagnosis.** Though in what follows I report in detail on questions of practical procedure and operations, it must be kept in mind that many more patients die of an overlooked rupture of the aorta than of operative difficulties or postoperative complications.
The rupture of the aorta is not a rare injury by any means. The statistical evidence is extremely varied, but one can assume that today there is a rupture of the aorta involved in 15% of fatal traffic accidents [545, 532, 533]. Nevertheless, 10% – 20% of the injured survive the accident and receive hospital treatment [538, 550, 562, 565]. Of this still quite considerable number of patients, only individual cases are operated on. There are no statistics for the number of cases in which a timely diagnosis, in view of general circumstances and clinical findings, might actually have been possible.
It must be emphasized here that there is no such thing as a "characteristic accident anamnesis." The accident mechanisms cited below are diverse. What is more, they are the same accident circumstances that are responsible for most of the severe thoracic injuries anyway. Often, patients suffer multiple injuries; sometimes, injuries of other parts of the body are completely in the forefront and apparently there is no thoracic trauma.

 In 1557 Vesal [557] was the first to describe an aneurysm of the thoracic aorta as the result of a traumatic aortic rupture. Nevertheless, closed injury of the aorta was long regarded as a rare occurrence. It was not until 1959 that Passaro and Pace [551] reported on the first successful suture repair of an acute rupture of the aorta, after a patient of Ellis had died after the operation 1 year previously. The aorta was clamped for 17 min without bypass to treat a 3-mm tear in the area of the isthmus. The patient survived with no ill effects even though during the operation there was an acute dilatation of the left ventricle with severe ECG changes and a rise in arterial pressure of over 200 mmHg.

Mechanism of Injury

The following is a description of several typical accident mechanisms that cause rupture of the aorta [570]:

1. **A combined deceleration and compression effect.** The primary examples are thoracic compression suffered by automobile drivers hitting the steering wheel and rupture of the aorta in airplane accidents.

2. **Vertical deceleration:** a fall from a height above 10 m.

3. **Direct thoracic compression or contusion.**

4. **Falling flat on the back,** mostly observed in older patients.

Zehnder [569, 570] has called attention to the fact that a horizontal deceleration **alone,** without thoracic compression, does not cause rupture of the aorta and that as has been proved, a deceleration of 45 g can be tolerated. The rupture of the aorta in a pedestrian accident is likewise explained by Beier [513] as being caused by a mechanism analogous to vertical deceleration: the pedestrian who was hit topples forward and the heart is forced in a cranial direction.

Compression of the thorax and deceleration cause a **flexure burst** at the convexity of the aortic arch because of its fluid content and the left-sided hilar structures.

Numerically speaking, traffic accidents of automobile drivers far outnumber other causes. Among our patients, this was the case in 10 of 18 with acute ruptures of the aorta. Of the other accident causes, it seems noteworthy to me that two patients (50 and 59 years of age) underwent a fall on their back at home and two patients suffered a ski accident. At the Winter Olympics in 1964, there were two accident fatalities in which rupture of the aorta was involved [519].

Location

Reports from the first half of the current century consistently assign the **preferred location** for aortic rupture to the ascending aorta [560]. Today, the situation is altogether different. This astonishing change is explained by the fact that impairment of

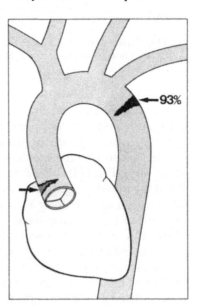

Fig. 114. Location of aortic rupture: 361 of 387 acute ruptures of the aorta that came under clinical observation occurred in the isthmus area and 12 in the ascending aorta (compiled statistics)

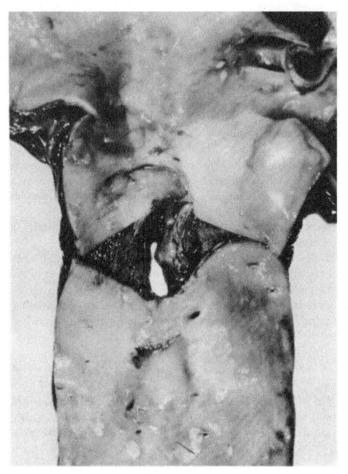

Fig. 115. Typical transverse tear of the descending aorta in the isthmus area; perforation into the left hemithorax 7 days after the accident

the vessel's wall, especially by syphilitic mesaortitis, which predisposes the area of the ascending aorta to rupture, has become very rare.

Today, aortic ruptures take place **primarily in the isthmus area,** i. e., at the insertion of the ligament of Botalli, so that this predilected site can be called its classic location. In patients who come under clinical care, the rupture occurs at this spot in 93% of the cases (Fig. 114): of 387 traumatic ruptures of the thoracic aorta, there were 361 at the isthmus, 12 at the ascending aorta, 6 at the aortic arch, and 7 in the area of the remaining descending aorta (statistics compiled from recent literature).

The rupture is always **transverse** (Fig. 115), and usually a large part of the circumference is torn. It can be **completely** torn, in which case a brief survival is possible in rare exceptions if it is covered by the mediastinal pleura. In almost all patients who receive clinical treatment it is **partial:** the adventitia temporarily prevents extravasation of blood and ruptures later or enables a false aneurysm to form. It is also possible that only a **lesion of the intima** occurs.

Symptoms and Diagnosis

The clinical picture is basically determined by which wall layers are ruptured and at which site the rupture occurs.

In a rupture of the **ascending aorta,** which for the most part occurs intrapericardially, the symptoms are those of **cardiac tamponade with venous congestion.**

The symptoms and findings of a rupture of the descending aorta are presented in Table 27. An important symptom is **back pain** radiating toward the shoulder, which occurs in one-third of the patients [461]. The patients are often **in shock** as a result of the severe general trauma; occasionally, there is **hypertension** in the **upper extremities.**

Compression caused by the mediastinal hematoma occasionally leads to shortness of breath, dysphagia, Horner's syndrome, or through pressure on the recurrent laryngeal nerve to hoarseness.

A **systolic murmur,** precordial or infraclavicular, is found in roughly one-fourth of the cases [461]. It is difficult to hear from the dorsal side.

If the hematoma extends to the origin of the left subclavian artery, a **pulse difference** between the right and left arms can be detected. Of special significance is a **difference in blood pressure** between the upper extremities and the arteries of the lower half of the body ("pseudocoarctation syndrome") since this symptom verifies the presence of an aortic rupture.

With diminished blood supply in the spinal area, **paraplegia** can occur, and if in the renal area, **oliguria.**

Diagnosis would be simple if the numerous symptoms were present with great regularity. Actually, in the early phase, there are often only some symptoms or none at all. It is the **roentgenogram** that should arouse suspicion.

Table 27. Symptoms and findings in a traumatic rupture of the aorta in the classic location

Pains, possibly radiating in the back			
Systolic murmurs			
Compression	Of left subclavian artery	→	Pulse difference of left and right radial arteries
	Of trachea	→	Dyspnea
	Of left main bronchus	→	Atelectasis
	Of esophagus	→	Dysphagia
	Of recurrent nerve	→	Hoarseness
	Of stellate ganglion	→	Horner's syndrome
Distal ischemia			Pseudocoarctation syndrome
	Spinal	→	Paraplegia
	Renal	→	Oliguria
Perforation	Into thorax	→	Left hemothorax
	Into esophagus	→	Hematemesis
	Into bronchus	→	Hemoptysis
Radiologic findings	Widened mediastinum		
	Trachea displaced to the right		
	Dislocation of left main bronchus downward		
	Abnormal aortic contour, fuzzy definition of aortic arch toward the left		
	Possible hemothorax on the left side		

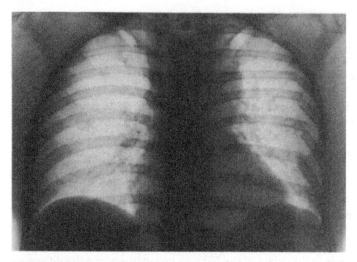

Fig. 116. Widened mediastinum in rupture of the aorta. No attention was paid to this finding until there was a perforation with fatal results

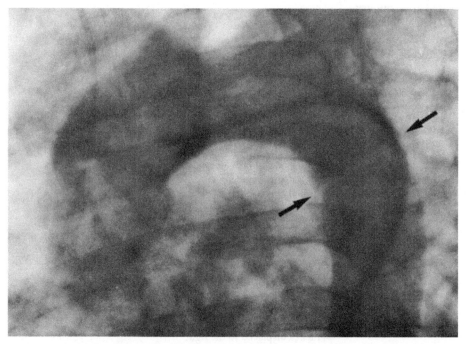

Fig. 117. Transverse intimal tear of the descending aorta at the typical site without extravasation of contrast medium during angiography, confirmed intraoperatively. The patient with multiple injuries survived despite delayed rupture of the spleen and a gallbladder empyema during the further course

The most common and most easily recognizable radiologic finding is the **widened mediastinum** (Fig. 116). This mediastinal widening can be discreet, but also very impressive. It should be kept in mind that in many cases this finding is not caused by extravasated blood from the rupture site on the aorta but by a **mediastinal hematoma** that develops in the vicinity of the aorta from the laceration of smaller vessels. If as a consequence of this mediastinal hematoma aortography is performed, a rupture of the aorta can be recognized before a dissection and development of a false aneurysm has occurred. This was the case in the pure intimal lesion of the aorta shown in Fig. 117.

Hematoma formation in the mediastinum can lead to the dislocation of the intrathoracic trachea to the right and to the downward displacement of the left main bronchus. If bleeding has already occurred in the thoracic area, a hemothorax on the left side will also be found.

A thoracic roentgenogram is taken of every severely injured patient. Many aortic ruptures have been overlooked because these pictures were examined only superficially or were evaluated improperly. In Chap. 3 we described in detail the difficulties of making an assessment of the mediastinum when the patient is in a recumbent position and the further procedures for a widened mediastinum.

Only aortography can provide clarification. Some authors disagree about which approach for the aortic catheter is most favorable. In a severely injured person, an examination with a **femoral** catheter is faster and less cumbersome than going in through the arm; the danger of perforation is minimal if no force is used when there is resistance in the isthmus area. An examination through the **right brachial artery** is, however, a good alternative. Since the intervention should be as simple, quick, and gentle as possible, I refrain from applying a transseptal procedure. A **venous injection of a contrast medium** is inadequate and cannot provide detailed visualization of the aorta (Fig. 117).

Although a widened mediastinum is the most frequent and most important diagnostic sign of a rupture of the aorta, it is not present in every case (see p. 28).

Therapy

Indication for Operation

The indication for operation is provided by the diagnosis. Fatal perforation does not always occur, though it may do so within minutes, hours, or days, **at any time.** Every unnecessary delay exposes the patient to this risk.

Example: A 22-year-old female patient fell while skiing. The only sign of a thoracic injury was a hematoma above the sternum. She was hospitalized because of a minor concussion of the brain. The roentgenogram of the thorax revealed a moderate left upper mediastinal widening with a clear boarder (Fig. 118 a). No significance was attached to this finding in view of the minor trauma and healthy condition of the patient.

Ten days later she felt pains in her back. On the following day, she also experienced shortness of breath. A roentgenogram taken 12 days after the accident showed a diffuse opacity of the entire left half of the thorax (Fig. 118 b). Rupture of the aorta was then suspected and the patient was flown to the medical center by helicopter.

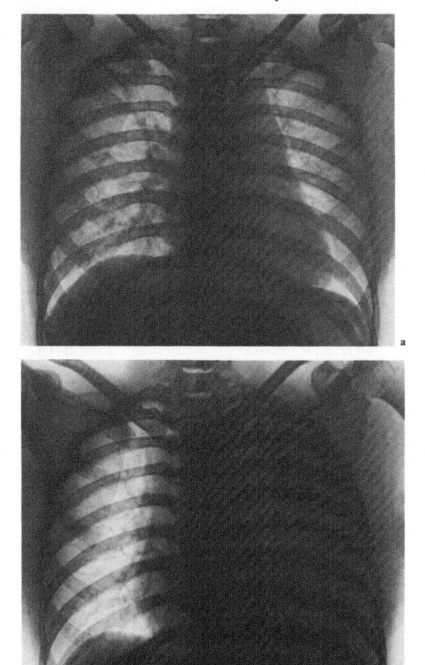

Fig. 118 a, b. Rupture of the aorta of a 22-year-old female patient who fell while skiing (see text). **a** Roentgenogram taken the day of the accident showing moderate widening of the upper mediastinum. **b** Hemothorax on the left side after perforation 10 days after the accident

Upon admission to the emergency room, the patient was still in excellent general condition with normal blood pressure and unconcerned. Several minutes later she was dead. A thoracotomy was too late to be successful. An autopsy revealed a tear of the entire aorta at its typical site except for a small bridge of tissue 5 mm in length.

Pharmacologic hypotensive treatment is to be resolutely rejected and preference given to an immediate operation. A lowering of the blood pressure is only indicated if an operation cannot be performed.

Tactical Procedure (Table 28)

The determination of the diagnosis and localization of the rupture by **preoperative aortography** should be striven for. In certain situations, however, this will have to be dispensed with:

1. When there is a hemothorax, which is assumed to have developed from bleeding from the aorta. Of special importance here is the appearance of an unexpected hemothorax days or weeks after trauma. The hemorrhaging into the thorax can ensue at two different times, as the case described above and another case under our care have unfortunately shown. The appearance of a hemothorax proves that perforation has already occurred and that exsanguination will most certainly follow.

2. When there is a pseudocoarctation syndrome with hemothorax or with a mediastinal hematoma, which is of considerable size already a short time after the accident or is growing rapidly. In that case, the diagnosis can be regarded as confirmed.

Table 28. Procedure when an acute aortic rupture is suspected

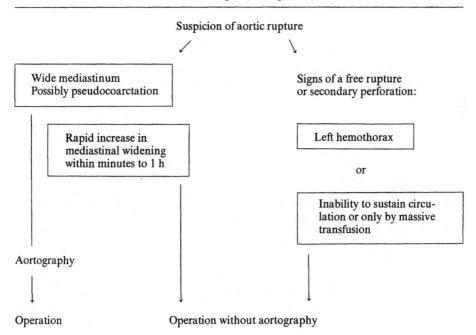

3. In patients with a falling blood pressure in whom the blood pressure cannot be maintained or can be maintained only with massive volume infusion.

In exceptional cases, an operation, even after there has been massive bleeding into the pleural cavity and even cardiac arrest, can still rescue the patient [537]; there is nothing to lose.

In the primary treatment of a patient with **multiple injuries** and with an incomplete or covered aortic rupture, other injuries **more acutely threatening to life** take **precedence.** Thus, a pneumothorax or tension pneumothorax will be drained, a significant intra-abdominal hemorrhage will be taken care of operatively, a craniotomy performed if there is an intracranial hemorrhage, and a cardiac tamponade drained before an aortic rupture is clarified by aortography.

If there are companion injuries that demand a prompt operation but are **not an immediate threat to life** (e. g., rupture of the bladder, closed peripheral arterial injuries, open fractures), the aortography is performed first. This helps in making a judgment as to whether or not a perforation is imminent. If it is negative, the surgeon can concentrate totally on the other injuries.

If a patient with an aortic rupture is **suspected of having an intra-abdominal injury,** it is worthwhile, **before** performing a thoracotomy, to check for bleeding in the abdomen: the **peritoneal lavage** as a simple, quickly performed intervention with a high degree of success has proved its worth for this. If this is positive, the abdominal bleeding is dealt with before the operation on an incomplete or covered aortic rupture is performed. In a very pronounced coarctation syndrome, the intra-abdominal hemorrhage can be only very minor; after restoration of blood flow to the abdomen, it can suddenly increase to life-threatening proportions. For this reason, in a negative or questionably positive peritoneal lavage, it is advantageous to leave the lavage catheter in place in the abdomen until after the operation on the aortic rupture.

If warranted, simultaneous with the radiologic representation of the aortic arch, the **angiography of other vessels** (carotid angiogram, intra-abdominal vessels, kidney arteries) can be undertaken with the same catheter without any substantial additional stress to the patient and with only a small extra sacrifice of time.

Example: A 27-year-old motorcycle rider ran into a streetcar. At the time of emergency admission, he was in hypovolemic shock with multiple skull and limb fractures and bilateral multiple rib fractures. The peritoneal lavage was negative. There was severe hematuria. The thoracic roentgenogram showed a mediastinal hematoma (Fig. 119 a).
Satisfactory blood pressure readings were obtained during continuous transfusion. After excluding the possibility of a vesical rupture by means of cystography, an **aortogram** was performed through the femoral artery, showing an aortic rupture at the typical site with extravasation of contrast medium (Fig. 119 b). **Renal arteriography** was then conducted on both sides with the same catheter. In the left kidney, there was considerable arterial bleeding with extravasation of contrast medium (Fig. 119 c). On the basis of the angiogram, the kidney injury was regarded as the source of bleeding. Therefore, the next step was a laparotomy with exposure of the left kidney, which revealed a massive rupture into the hilar area. A nephrectomy was performed.
After stabilization of the circulation, another angiogram of the aortic arch was performed by means of a catheter from the right arm since in the aortography by way of the femoral artery the catheter could not be advanced proximally beyond the origin of the subclavian artery. Again the aortic rupture was demonstrated at the classic site, this time without extravasation of the contrast medium (Fig. 119 d). The aortic arch and ascending aorta were intact.

Immediately thereafter, the operation on the aortic rupture was performed (Surgical Clinic A in Zurich). The aorta had been torn off transversely more than three-fourths of its circumference. The end-to-end suturing of the aortic rupture was performed during an occlusion time of 15 min.
The patient died of septicemia 23 days after the accident.

Operation

The operative **approach** in injuries of the descending aorta consists of a posterolateral thoracotomy in the fourth intercostal space.
Ruptures of the **ascending aorta** can be operated on only by using extracorporeal circulation.
In rupture of the **descending aorta,** circumstances are different. The necessary interruption of blood flow at the site of the rupture is fraught with two dangers:

1. Danger of distal ischemia, primarily in the spinal and renal areas.

2. Rise in blood pressure in the upper half of the body. If there is craniocerebral trauma, the cerebral excess of blood can lead to severe cerebral edema.

The second danger can be avoided by brief occlusion periods and a corresponding anesthesia technique, which — with medication to lower blood pressure, if necessary — will maintain normal arterial pressure.
Concerning the problem of distal ischemia, **various possibilities** exist (Fig. 120):

1. **Left heart bypass** [522, 531]: collateral circulation without oxygenation from the left atrium to the descending aorta or to the femoral artery. This was the procedure used most often in the past since it also prevents the flooding of the upper body with blood as well as decompensation of the left ventricle. For this, extracorporeal circulation must be available. Its great disadvantage, however, is the necessity of heparinization.

2. **Total femoral, venous-arterial bypass,** using extracorporeal circulation [541].

3. **Use of local external shunt:** without heparinization of the patient, collateral circulation can be carried out with a plastic shunt between the ascending aorta or, more simply, the left subclavian artery, to the descending aorta [539, 564, 567]. In 1970 Kirsh [540] reported on 12 operations with this device. Gott used a plastic shunt with heparin coating [548]. (The external shunt from the left ventricle to the descending aorta used by Molloy [546] is much more inconvenient.)

4. **No shunt, no extracorporeal circulation:** a series of individual reports has shown that a reconstruction of the aorta is also possible without negative consequences by a mere occlusion without the use of extracorporeal circulation or a shunt [521, 527, 537]. Recently, the tendency has prevailed more and more to treat the aortic rupture with this simple technique, and some authors today regard it as the **method of choice** [511, 523, 542].

The application of **external hypothermia at 30° C** is no longer in use today since the cooling off period is too long.

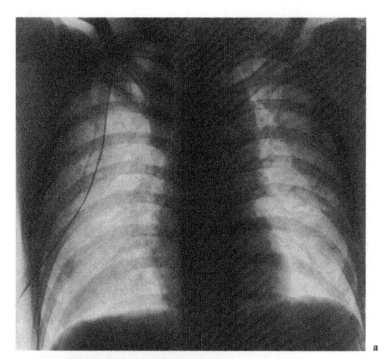
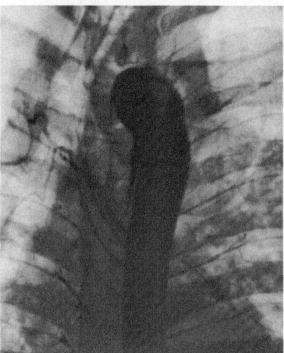

Fig. 119 a – d. A 27-year-old male patient severely wounded in a motorcycle accident (see text). **a Mediastinal hematoma** in the roentgenogram of the accident victim. Drainage of a tension pneumothorax on the side right. **b Rupture of the aorta** at the typical site with **aortography** showing extravasation of contrast medium; the catheter introduced from the **femoral** artery cannot be advanced any further into the aortic arch. **c Arteriogram of the kidneys** using the same catheter: arterial hemorrhage of left kidney in renal rupture. **d** After nephrectomy of the left kidney, **aortography** by means of a **brachial** catheter from the right, demonstrating the aortic rupture at the isthmus and an intact ascending aorta

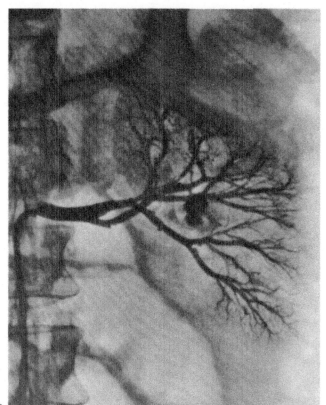

c

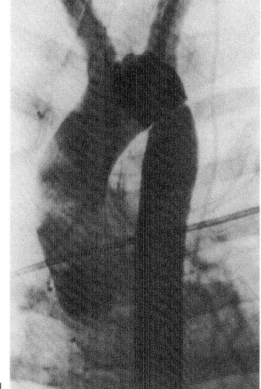

d

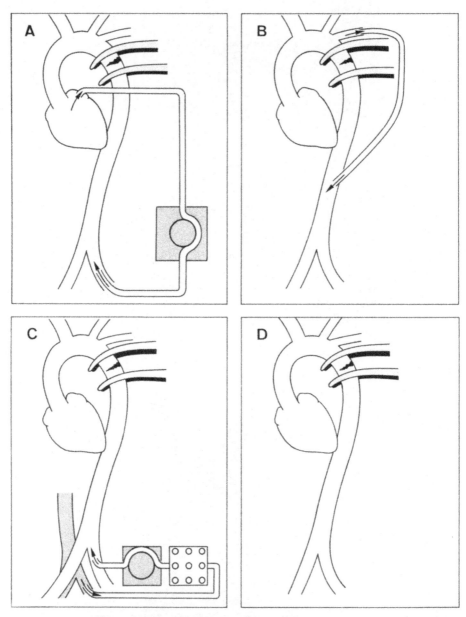

Fig. 120 A – D. Possible operative procedures when occluding a ruptured descending aorta (see text). **A** Left heart bypass; **B** Local external shunt from the left subclavian artery to the descending aorta; **C** Total femoral, venous-arterial bypass; **D** No shunt, no extracorporeal circulation

The most feared consequence of operations for aortic ruptures is the development of a **paraplegia** through ischemic damage to the spinal cord. The anterior spinal artery is served by the lower thoracic and upper lumbar segmental vessels from the aorta. Crawford [523] has shown that a paraplegia cannot be wholly avoided by any of the above-mentioned methods. He concluded that there are other factors, such as general hypotension, removal of a long section of the aorta in the operation on an aneurysm, or the intraoperative damage to collateral circulation, which play an essential role.

By refraining from using a bypass technique, such as extracorporeal circulation or local shunt, the number of episodes of paraplegia observed in his series was smaller than when these devices were used. Of greater importance seemed to be an operative procedure as conservative as possible with little dissection and with the shortest possible segment of the aorta occluded, and above all the avoidance and immediate treatment of intraoperative hypotension.

Summing up, for all practical purposes, it can be accepted as fact that:

1. Operation is possible and justifiable even without bypassing the occluded aortic segment.

2. Heparinization during use of extracorporeal circulation in a partial or total bypass is an additional danger to a person with multiple injuries and is prohibited in cases of craniocerebral trauma and multiple fractures. The use of an external shunt with or without heparin coating is a possible alternative.

3. Short operating time and simple technique without massive mobilization are decisive; a drop in blood pressure during the operation is to be avoided.

Operative procedure on the aorta: after exposing it proximally and distally from the point of rupture, the aorta and, if necessary, the subclavian artery are clamped. The pleura and adventitia are opened above the rupture and the hematoma is evacuated. As a rule, the end-to-end suturing is continuous with nonresorbable suture material; occasionally, a Dacron interposition graft is used.

Our Patients

We reviewed (including the cases of the Surgical Clinic A in Zurich) 16 cases of **acute** traumatic aortic ruptures. In five patients, the diagnosis was not determined: two of them died immediately upon arrival at the emergency room, three more during hospitalization. The rupture of the aorta was the cause of death only in one the last three: a perforation into the pleural cavity developed, causing the patient to bleed to death. In the two other patients, the diagnosis was verified at the autopsy as a secondary finding.

In 11 patients the diagnosis was established. One female adult died shortly after transfer from another hospital before she could be operated (the case was described above). Of the ten patients who were operated on six survived. The causes of death among the deceased patients were infection secondary to esophageal necrosis, massive bleeding, cerebral damage, and sepsis not connected with the aortic rupture.

II. Penetrating Injuries of the Aorta

Undoubtedly, almost all penetrating aortic injuries result in death by massive bleeding before surgical intervention is possible. In the past 10 years, however, patients with such injuries have been treated successfully and are no longer a rarity.

Already in 1922 Dshanelidze [528] successfully sutured, 1 cm above its origin, an injury of the ascending aorta 8 mm long.
It is interesting to note that up to the end of the 1950s, all successfully treated cases reported in the literature involved intrapericardial lesions of the ascending aorta. The wall of the ascending aorta is equipped with a surrounding connective tissue that can tamponade the injury [552]. In cardiac tamponade, the inelastic pericardium offers considerable resistance, which provides a longer survival time than is the case of hemorrhages into the open pleural cavity. A patient with a perforated injury to the ascending aorta survived even without treatment for 2 weeks until he died of cardiac tamponade [544]. The formation of an aortovenous fistula, either into the right ventricle, the pulmonary artery, or the right atrium can also, by the "autotransfusion" that develops, preserve the patient from bleeding to death.
The first successful operations on a penetrating injury of the extrapericardial aorta were not reported until 1958 by Perkins and Elchos [552] and Kleinert [541].
It is not surprising that stab injuries cause a lesser lesion and are therefore more amenable to treatment than gunshot injuries. Up to 1969, the ratio between these two kinds of injury in regard to successful treatment stood at 3 : 1 [566]. In the Vietnam War, the evacuation times were shortened substantially as compared to earlier wars. Because of that, Billy [515] was able to report in 1971 on a series of 39 penetrating shot and shrapnel injuries of the aorta (20 in the thoracic area) in which the mortality was 30%. In the Korean War, of 304 arterial injuries there was no aortic injury brought in for treatment [536]; in World War II, of 2451 there were only 3 [525]. However, in civilian life today, gunshot injuries are also in the vast majority, especially in the United States with its raucous customs [509].

Diagnosis

In an acute penetrating aortic injury, a precise preoperative diagnosis is never possible and should not be attempted. The symptomatology is determined by the location of the lesion. In **intrapericardial** injuries, the signs of cardiac tamponade are the most prominent. The picture is identical to that of a cardiac injury and only the intraoperative finding provides the diagnosis.

In the injury of the **extrapericardial portion** of the ascending aorta, of the aortic arch, and of the descending aorta, acute bleeding is prominent. The roentgenogram may show a widening of the mediastinum. The general condition and the amount of blood conveyed by the chest tube will provide a reference point for the urgency of an operation. In no case should additional examinations (e. g., aortography) delay an immediate thoracotomy. The exact diagnosis of this injury will also first be determined intraoperatively.

Therapy

The procedure with **intrapericardial aortic injuries** is the same as with penetrating cardiac injuries (see Chap. 17). If the left anterolateral thoracotomy is selected for the approach, the necessary exposure can be gained by extending the incision toward the other side of the thorax by cutting through the sternum.

Table 29. Operative approaches in injuries of the large vessels of the thoracic area

	Approach	Arteries	Veins
	Supraclavicular approach by splitting the clavicle	Right subclavian artery Distal left subclavian artery	Subclavian veins
	Trapdoor approach	Left subclavian artery (Right proximal subclavian artery) Innominate artery (carotid artery)	Brachiocephalic veins
	Median sternotomy If necessary, with supraclavicular extension	Ascending aorta and proximal aortic arch Pulmonary artery (mainstem) Innominate artery	Brachiocephalic veins
	Right thoracotomy	Right pulmonary artery (only anterolateral thoracotomy)	Vena cava (only anterolateral thoracotomy)
	Left thoracotomy	Descending aorta Left pulmonary artery (only anterolateral thoracotomy)	

The bleeding can be controlled by digital pressure. Tangential placement of an angled arterial clamp is often possible. The wound can usually be closed by direct suture. Obviously, one must be clear about the location of origin of the coronary arteries.

If the wounds of the ascending aorta cannot be treated as suggested, one will have to wait, maintaining digital compression all the while, until extracorporeal circulation can be utilized.

Injuries of the descending aorta are approached by a posterolateral thoracotomy. The attempt should be made to complete the suture with only partial clamping of the aorta or to limit the total occlusion time to a maximum of 30 min. If this appears to be impossible, the possibility of a local external shunt (see p. 231) should be kept in mind.

III. Closed Injuries of the Supra-aortic Arteries

Avulsion of the Innominate Artery

A pure compression injury with simultaneous hyperextension of the cervical spinal column can result in the typical injury pattern of an avulsion of the innominate artery from the aortic arch. As in aortic rupture, an intact adventitia may prevent exsanguination. In 1962 Binet [516] described the first case. Moreover, obviously less frequently, partial tears in the artery also occur [561].

The leading finding is the **widening of the upper mediastinum on the right.** A systolic murmur can be audible. It is interesting that only in less than half of the cases a difference in pulse in the radial artery or a lack of pulse in it was determined. A normal blood supply and normal peripheral pulse is therefore the rule and does not exclude the possibility of this lesion.

The radiologic finding in the upper mediastinum requires **angiographic clarification,** which verifies the diagnosis.

As in aortic rupture, **perforation** into the pleural cavity is a constant threat to the patient, which provides an ongoing indication for an operation. A synthetic prosthesis is almost always necessary. It may facilitate the operative procedure if the latter is implanted elsewhere in the aortic arch and the false aneurysm removed afterward [530].

The first cases reported were operated on with the aid of extracorporeal circulation. More recently, use of internal and external shunts has become more widespread. A series of cases, however, were also operated on by clamping the vessels with no other aids. Ciaravella [520] has suggested that the decision as to the necessity for bypass circulation be based on measurement of the pressure in the right common carotid artery after trial occlusion. He regards the collateral circulation as adequate if there is a pressure of over 50 mmHg in the distal stump.

Example: It is precisely with a patient with multiple injuries that such considerations, which may have validity for healthy persons, can hardly be relied upon. In the presence of craniocerebral trauma or preceding hypovolemic shock or hypoxia, the tendency toward cerebral edema formation can hardly be evaluated, and an additional diminution of perfusion can have deleterious consequences. We had such an experience with a female patient with partial avulsion of the innominate artery who had an occlusion time of only 2 min but had subsequent impairment of circulation caused by a free intimal flap that resulted in massive, cerebral edema that was therapeutically no longer controllable (operation in Surgical Clinic A).

Injuries of the Trunk of the Left Subclavian Artery

Even the infrequent injury to the trunk of the subclavian artery produces a typical pathologic picture [510]. In this case, a **contusion with localized thrombosis** is more frequent than rupture. The peripheral pulse is then no longer palpable although because of adequate collateral circulation the upper extremity appears to be hardly disturbed in its blood supply. A widened upper mediastinum is usually found and often a hemothorax too.

This injury must be taken into consideration particularly if there are **fractures of the clavicle** and, above all, of the **first rib.** Characteristic for this injury site, though not necessarily present in all cases, are **neurologic deficits.** In two-thirds of all aortograms, a reversal of flow in the vertebral artery, in other words a "subclavian steal," could be demonstrated in this injury. The discussion is still open as to whether the neurologic symptoms are caused by this subclavian steal or by emboli into the vertebral artery.

Of the three main trunks of the aortic arch, the **intrathoracic carotid artery** is the one least often injured in blunt trauma and then is often in combination with another supra-aortic branch [510].

IV. Injuries of the Great Veins and Pulmonary Vessels

Injuries of the **intrapericardial section** of the **vena cava** usually result in a **cardiac tamponade.** Preoperatively, they are indistinguishable from cardiac injuries.

All injuries of the vena cava are usually **perforating** injuries. Tears in the vena cava caused by **blunt trauma** seldom have clinical significance, although smaller tears can be tamponaded by the surrounding tissue and thus escape clinical verification.

If a connection to the pleural cavity has been created by penetrating injuries, the bleeding is usually profuse; however, it is usually assessed accurately by the bleeding from the chest tube and the **indication for an operation** is determined accordingly.

In the operation, total occlusion of the vessel will obviously be avoided. Satinsky clamps applied tangentially will usually suffice to achieve this goal. If not, an inner shunt can be installed by inserting a plastic tube through the right atrial appendage of the heart into the superior vena cava (Fig. 121).

Injuries of the **veins and arteries of the lungs** are almost always combined with cardiac or pulmonary injuries. Even though perforating injuries are the most common by far, lesions caused by blunt trauma are not infrequent. Their clinical pattern is characterized entirely by bleeding; in lesser injuries in the mediastinum, however, spontaneous hemostasis is possible.

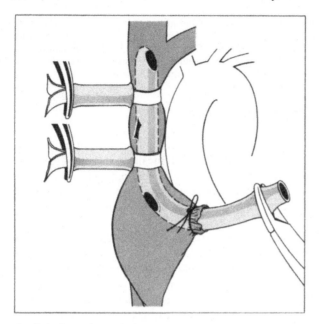

Fig. 121. Operative technique in large lesions of the superior vena cava: an internal shunt is inserted into the right atrial appendage of the heart [432]

In significant companion injuries of the bronchi and lungs, quite often no reconstruction will be attempted; a resection will be performed instead. This decision is made more easily in penetrating injuries than in blunt trauma since in closed injuries the other lung is often also involved.

V. Penetrating Injuries of the Vessels of the Superior Thoracic Aperture

Gunshot and stabbing injuries of the large vessels of the superior thoracic aperture that come into consideration for treatment make up only a small portion of all injuries of blood vessels [146] (according to the literature, 0.5% – 5%). They make great demands on the ability to promptly assess the patient's condition, on decisiveness, and on the technical skill of the attending surgeon. However, recent reports from clinics that have treated large series of such injuries indicate that with purposeful and competent procedures, many of these patients can be saved [146, 518, 534, 553, 563].
Arteries and veins are injured with equal frequency.

Diagnosis

Only a **prompt diagnosis** holds out the prospect of success. The rule applies that no patient with an external injury in the area of these vessels dare be released from the supervision of the attending surgeon before an injury of the vessel has been verified and treated or reliably excluded.

In addition to the nature, site, and direction of the wound, signs of massive blood loss, local hematoma, diminished or absent peripheral pulse, brachial plexus deficiencies, and bleeding into the thoracic cavity are suggestive factors.

A **roentgenogram of the thorax** is indispensable and not time-consuming. On the other hand, an angiographic examination is contraindicated in most cases because of the time lost. It should be performed only when there are no grounds for immediate operative intervention.

Therapy

The problem with these injuries is that they occur in an area where access for hemostasis is difficult. A clear plan for exposing the site of the injury quickly and effectively and for bringing the bleeding under control is absolutely necessary. Without such a plan, one should in no case be tempted to perform a "revision of the wound" when there is severe bleeding.

Thus, the **operative approaches** are of very special and decisive importance. They were presented in detail in Chap. 6. An inadequate approach in these dramatic situations often pronounces the death sentence of the patient. On the other hand, one should not accept the additional morbidity of splitting the sternum or a thoracotomy if it is unnecessary.

Based on these considerations, I should like to suggest the following **operative tactics:**

1. Adequate venous access, blood replacement, intubation.

2. Thoracic drainage when there is intrathoracic bleeding. In acute threat to life by noncompensable blood loss and massive bleeding from the thoracic chest tubes, a small anterolateral thoracotomy in the third intercostal space is made while still in the emergency room and blind compression of the bleeding site is applied through the thorax with towels or the hand.

3. In the operating room, the patient is positioned in an oblique position with the upper body turned 30°. The area is prepped and draped as widely as possible to allow all the variations of an operative approach to be considered. The approach should be suited to the existing situation; it will usually consist either of a trapdoor approach by splitting the sternum longitudinally as far as the third intercostal space or of a supraclavicular approach by splitting the clavicle. If difficulties of exposure are encountered, the approach is extended to a trapdoor incision. If an emergency thoracotomy in the third intercostal area has already been performed, the latter will likewise be extended to the trapdoor incision.

4. In special cases involving injuries on the right side, a total longitudinal incision of the sternum with supraclavicular extension also may be considered.

The treatment of the vessel injury is often possible by direct suturing; synthetic prostheses are seldom necessary. In injuries of the innominate artery and the common carotid artery, an inner shunt will be used if possible.

Also in venous injuries, reconstruction will be attempted. If the general situation renders this impossible, the brachiocephalic vein **or** the jugular or subclavian veins can be ligated unilaterally without negative consequences.

After reconstruction of the vessels, one should not forget to check other endangered structures in this region whose injuries can be easily overlooked: esophagus, trachea, thoracic duct, brachial plexus, and phrenic nerve.

VI. Posttraumatic Late Sequelae in the Great Vessels

Posttraumatic Aneurysms of the Aorta

The most favorable spontaneous course of development of a traumatic rupture of the aorta is the formation of a false aneurysm, which is gradually encapsulated by connective tissue.

Many of these patients are **asymptomatic.** According to Bennett [514], 41% of patients with a thoracic false aneurysm of the aorta exhibit no symptoms. This symptom-free state was even observed 47 years after the trauma [514]. The aneurysm is then discovered by radiologic examination as an incidental finding (Fig. 122).

In other patients, the increase in size of the aneurysm causes **compression symptoms** in the neighboring structures: compression of the trachea accompanied by dyspnea,

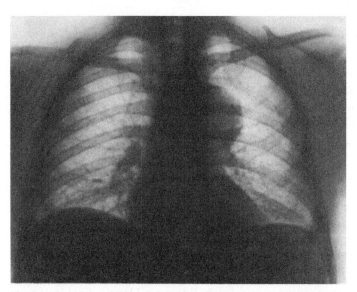

Fig. 122. Posttraumatic aneurysm of the aorta in a 29-year-old asymptomatic male patient. By fluoroscopic examination 6 years after the accident, a mediastinal bulge was detected. Thoracotomy was performed in Italy after the diagnosis of echinococcal cyst. In a subsequent resection of the aneurysm, a rupture of the entire circumference of the aorta with retraction of both sides was discovered. An uneventful postoperative course ensued after interposition of a Dacron graft

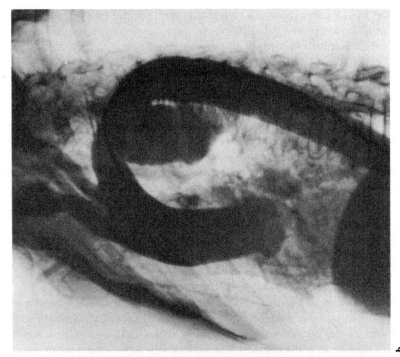
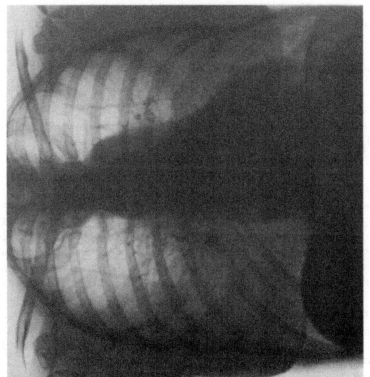

Fig. 123 a, b. Thoracic roentgenogram and aortography of a 66-year-old male patient: the diagnosis of a posttraumatic aortic aneurysm was made 3 years after the accident while seeking the cause of hoarseness and difficulty in swallowing

compression of the esophagus with dysphagia, compression of the main bronchus with formation of atelectasis, compression in the area of the stellate ganglion with development of Horner's syndrome, or pressure damage to the recurrent laryngeal nerve with concomitant hoarseness (Fig. 123).

The widening of the mediastinum is not always recognized as an aortic aneurysm (the case in Fig. 122); this possibility should be kept in mind in making a differential diagnosis of mediastinal tumors.

A traumatic aortic aneurysm should be **operated** on since rupture threatens at any time. A delayed rupture occurring 30 years after the accident has even been reported [562]. An operation may sometimes be ruled out in elderly patients if there are significant contraindications. A preceding **clarification by means of aortography** is indispensable.

The first operations on a posttraumatic aortic aneurysm were performed in 1950 by Weisel [568] and in 1951 by Hollingsworth [535]. Both surrounded the aneurysm with cellophane. The first excision of a posttraumatic aneurysm with tangential suturing of the aorta ensued in 1953 by Bahnson [512]. In 1955 Stranahan [564] reported the first resection of an aneurysm and bridging over of the defect in the aorta with a homologous aortic transplant.

Only in isolated cases of posttraumatic aneurysms is an end-to-end anastomosis of the aorta possible; in most instances, it will be necessary to insert a **synthetic graft.**

The **prognosis** of the operation on a chronic posttraumatic aneurysm is naturally much better than in an acute rupture. The mortality in large, recent series is around 5% [523, 533, 542]. The risk of paraplegia is slight, yet cannot be completely avoided by any method [523].

Posttraumatic Aortovenous Fistula

After penetrating injuries, arteriovenous fistulas can make their appearance between the aorta and the right ventricle, the pulmonary artery, the vena cava, or a brachiocephalic vein [517]. Their effects vary according to the shunt volume. They can lead to immediate cardiac failure right after their development or later to cardiac insufficiency, in cases of necessarily increased cardiac output. Because of increased pressure in the central venous system, venous congestion occurs in the upper half of the body.

A systolic-diastolic murmur over the fistula area points toward this consequence of the injury. In penetrating injuries of the cardiac and mediastinal regions, attention should be paid during the course of recovery to the appearance of a murmur. Congested neck veins are found if the fistula opening is in the area of the vena cava or a brachiocephalic vein. In a large shunt volume, the pressure amplitude increases. During the further course, all the signs of increasing cardiac insufficiency can appear.

On the **roentgenogram** an enlarged heart is commonly found and on occasion a widening of the mediastinum. An **aortogram** is indispensable for diagnosis and the planning of the operative procedure. **Cardiac catheterization** to evaluate the hemodynamic effects is also indicated, especially if an aortoventricular fistula is present, since the latter can be accompanied by aortic insufficiency.

The **therapy** of choice consists of **operative closure of the fistula.** In most cases, direct closure of the aorta and vein is possible. The indication for an operation is given not only because of progressive cardiac insufficiency but also due to the danger of rupture or the possibility of an infection; operation is not performed only when there are clear contraindications.

Among the cases reported in the literature, there were fistulas between the aorta and the right ventricle that were closed operatively within days to several months after trauma and fistulas between the aorta and brachiocephalic vein that usually were not closed for years (up to 20 years [517]) after the injury [566].

Posttraumatic Thoracic Outlet Syndrome

Fractures of the first rib and clavicle, but also other injuries of the superior thoracic aperture without fracture, can, through callous formations or fibrosis, later lead to a thoracic outlet syndrome. The most frequent **symptoms** in these cases are **neurologic:** severe radiating pains are the most prominent. Paresthesias and paresis occur frequently [547]. Less frequently, there are signs of **compression of the subclavian artery** with various stages of ischemia, which appear especially during provocative positioning of the shoulder girdle. In poststenotic dilatation of the subclavian artery, formation of thrombi and embolization to the periphery can occur. A **compression of the subclavian vein** is occasionally the cause of an acute venous thrombosis in this area.

It is important to differentiate pure scar tissue formation in or around the brachial plexus from an actual compression syndrome since in these cases therapy consists of extra- and interfascicular neurolysis. In thoracic outlet syndrome, on the other hand, in most cases an enlargement of the superior thoracic aperture is achieved by means of the relatively simple operative removal of the first rib through an axillary approach, as described by Roos [556]. This space-creating intervention is also indicated even when the first rib is not the cause of the compression syndrome.

Chapter 19
Injuries of the Diaphragm

I. Diaphragmatic Ruptures

Basic Considerations

Diaphragmatic ruptures caused by blunt trauma are not very frequent; however, they are not so rare that every surgeon would not on occasion be confronted by this injury. Among our patients, diaphragmatic ruptures were found in 3% of all severe thoracic injuries.

In many cases, the diaphragmatic rupture is not recognized initially, either because of the frequent companion injuries or often because of a misinterpretation of the thoracic roentgenogram. In every severe blunt abdominal or thoracic trauma, this injury must be considered.

The frequently used term "diaphragmatic hernia" is false since all three layers of the diaphragm (diaphragm, peritoneum, and pleura) are almost always torn. The result is a prolapse of the abdominal viscera into the chest cavity. Genuine traumatic diaphragmatic hernias have been observed but are very rare [581].

The first cases of traumatic diaphragmatic injuries along with their consequences were described by Ambroise Paré in 1579 [585]. One of his two patients had recovered from a severe gunshot injury but died 8 months later of incarceration of the colon displaced into the thorax; the little finger could barely be inserted into the opening of the diaphragm.

In 1853 Bowditch [573] called attention to the symptomatology of such injuries on the basis of a diagnosis made in a living person and the autopsy reports of other cases reported in the literature of that time.

Mechanism of Injury

It is always a considerable **broad-surfaced blow** that causes a diaphragmatic rupture. In most cases, it occurs against both body cavities, less often against the thorax alone, and still less frequently against the abdomen alone.

Today **traffic accidents** are the primary cause of diaphragmatic ruptures: of 739 cases in the recent literature in 76% and among our patients in 85%. Spontaneous diaphragmatic rupture is known, but very rare [572].

Location

It has been known for a long time that by far the majority of all injuries due to blunt force affect the **left side of the diaphragm**. In a compilation of 1845 cases described in the literature (Table 30), I found left-sided ruptures in 84.6% and right-sided diaphragmatic ruptures in 14.1%. The right side of the diaphragm is well protected by the broad adjacent liver. Sufficient impact results in injury to the liver rather than the diaphragm.

There are seldom multiple lacerations on the same side of the diaphragm and still less frequently a diaphragmatic rupture on both sides (1.3%).

The tear in the diaphragm in most cases runs radially in the area of the central tendon or at the transition from the latter to the muscular portion (Fig. 124). The avulsion of the diaphragm at the point of muscular attachment to the ribs is a much less frequent but also typical rupture location and is generally regarded as resulting from a single severe compression of the thorax [592]. An avulsion of the crura is considered a rarity. Andrus [571] has reported on one case.

An especially rare injury picture with its own symptomatology is found in a rupture in the pericardial area; this **pericardiophrenic rupture** results in a prolapse of the viscera into the pericardium (see below).

Table 30. Location of diaphragmatic ruptures

	1845 closed diaphragmatic ruptures (compiled statistics)	Our patients (26 cases)
Left	1561 (84.6%)	17
Right	260 (14.1%)	8
Both sides	24 (1.3%)	1

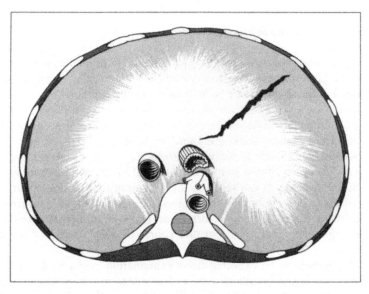

Fig. 124. Typical location of diaphragmatic rupture resulting from blunt trauma (diaphragm shown from below)

Pathophysiology

The difference in pressure between the negative intrapleural pressure and the positive intra-abdominal pressure results in increasing displacement of the contents of the abdomen into the thorax. With forced inspiration, this difference in pressure increases still more and can exceed 100 cm H_2O [577].

The negative pressure in the thoracic cavity disappears when mechanical ventilation is applied. It is understandable, therefore, that during the time a severely injured patient is being ventilated, a prolapse of the viscera into the thoracic cavity can be prevented and that the diaphragmatic rupture is not revealed until a roentgenogram is taken after weaning from mechanical to spontaneous breathing.

In a **left-sided diaphragmatic rupture,** the following order of frequency has been observed for organs that prolapse: stomach, left colon, spleen, omentum, small intestine, and left part of the liver. In a **rupture on the right side,** it is obviously the liver that is displaced most frequently into the thorax. There has also been a description of a case in which the left lung was displaced into the abdomen [571].

The **pathophysiologic effects** of a rupture on **respiration** and **circulation** are, to a large extent, determined by three mechanisms:

1. The function of the diaphragm is impeded since in this area a kind of paradoxical respiration appears.

2. By compression of the affected lung by the contents of the abdomen, the gas exchange surface is reduced.

3. The displacement of the mediastinum in advanced cases results in an impairment of the venous return to the heart.

Clinical Picture and Diagnosis

The clinical picture is very diverse. Often diaphragmatic ruptures exhibit few symptoms. Since there is usually a severe associated trauma, at first the **companion injuries** and the **shock** caused by them are most prominent.

Pains on the left side of the thorax that radiate toward the left shoulder are a sign of a diaphragmatic injury. In my experience, this symptom is quite often present. Frequently, contusion marks are found on the thoracic wall.

Shortness of breath can occur in various degrees. If eventration of the viscera causes significant mediastinal displacement, the dyspnea will be more marked, and cyanosis will develop. It can result in the formation of a tension situation analogous to a tension pneumothorax. In these cases, the central venous pressure rises.

In the early stages, there is almost never a sign of a gastrointestinal obstruction or strangulation. During the further course of developments, they may occasionally occur.

The **findings** to be expected upon **examination** might be a damping upon percussion, weakened breath sounds, and evidence of bowel sounds in the thorax upon auscultation. Shortly after the injury, however, these findings are hardly ascertainable. In place of damping, there is more likely to be a remarkable mixture of weak-

Table 31. Companion injuries in acute diaphragmatic ruptures caused by blunt trauma

	655 acute diaphragmatic ruptures in recent literature	Our patients (26 cases)
Rib fractures	297 (45%)	19 (73%)
Pelvic fractures	134 (20%)	13 (50%)
Fractures of extremities		10 (38%)
Craniocerebral injuries		8 (31%)
Spinal fractures		3 (12%)
Organ injuries in the abdomen:		
Spleen	195 (30%)	8 (31%)
Liver	89 (14%)	11 (42%)
Gastrointestinal tract	95 (15%)	5 (19%)
Kidneys	60 (9%)	5 (19%)

ened and hyperresonant percussion sounds since some of the displaced structures (stomach, colon) are heavily filled with air and, depending on their location, can influence the percussion findings. Because of intestinal paralysis, the bowel sounds after an accident are usually considerably reduced or are lacking altogether.

In the **blood gas analysis,** the arterial PO_2 is significantly reduced, partially because of the formation of local atelectasis by compression of the lung.

Other injuries can be helpful in establishing the diagnosis since there are typical **injury combinations** (Table 31). **Multiple rib fractures** are the most frequently associated injury. In 655 fresh diaphragmatic ruptures recorded in the recent literature, this combination was described in 25% of the cases; among our patients, 73% suffered multiple rib fractures. The combination with **pelvic fractures** is well-known as evidence for the severe trauma to the abdomen. The diagnosis of a pelvic fracture must raise the question of a diaphragmatic rupture and demands a chest roentgenogram. We found that this combination occurred in 20% of the cases listed in the literature mentioned above, and among our patients in half of all the cases.

Of the **intra-abdominal organ injuries,** diaphragmatic rupture is most frequently accompanied by rupture of the spleen (30%), followed by rupture of the liver (14%). In 15% there were other intra-abdominal injuries and in 9% injuries to the kidneys. The combination with injuries of the intra-abdominal organs has clinical significance inasmuch as the latter lead to a laparotomy and during the operation the diagnosis of a diaphragmatic rupture is established. The palpation of both diaphragmatic domes is a standard routine in every laparotomy following blunt trauma.

The **main complications** are incarceration or strangulation of prolapsed abdominal organs. In small diaphragmatic defects, such as occur in penetrating injuries, these complications are more frequent than in extended ruptures. Early diagnosis and early operation of the diaphragmatic rupture is the best prophylaxis.

Radiologic Examination

The roentgenogram of the chest is the key to diagnosis. Ruptures of the diaphragm are frequently overlooked, not because the roentgenogram fails to reveal any patho-

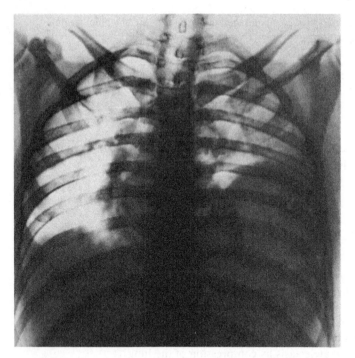

Fig. 125. Characteristic roentgenogram of a left-sided diaphragmatic rupture with a prolapsed stomach

logic findings, but because the latter are incorrectly interpreted. The following findings are characteristic:

1. Opacity in the thoracic area that is sharply delineated and not diffuse like a hemothorax in the roentgenogram of a recumbent patient (Fig. 125). This opacity is often homogeneous and not very dense and then corresponds to the magenblase, which is filled partially with fluid and partially with air.

2. Radiolucency in the thoracic area, either as large air-filled bubbles or as small, round radiolucent fields in a widespread opaque zone (Fig. 126).

3. An apparent elevated or undefinable diaphragmatic dome.

4. Displacement of the mediastinum and heart to the opposite side.

The interpretation of the roentgenogram presents difficulties especially when there is a significant simultaneous **hemothorax.** If a diaphragmatic rupture is suspected, the hemothorax is drained with a chest tube placed into the thorax atypically from a cranial entry site in a basal direction (see p. 138), attempting to avoid injuries to the prolapsed abdominal viscera.

For **confirmation** of the diagnosis when there are unclear findings in the plain roentgenogram, there are various possibilities available:

1. Introduction of a **nasogastric tube** and repetition of the roentgenogram: if the tube tip is seen in the thorax or if introduction into the stomach itself is impossible,

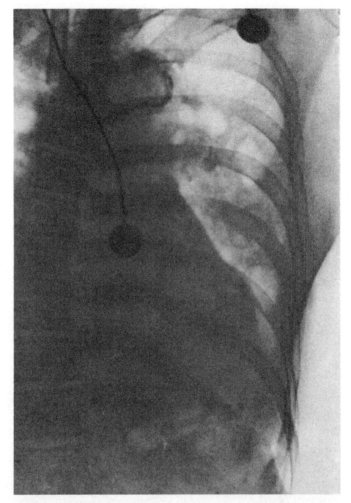

Fig. 126. Small, round radiolucent fields in the thorax: parts of the intestine within the thorax in a rupture of the left diaphragm

the stomach is prolapsed. A negative result of this examination naturally does not exclude the possibility of a diaphragmatic rupture.

2. During spontaneous breathing, 200 – 300 ml of **air** placed into the **abdomen** (e. g., by peritoneal lavage catheter) results in a pneumothorax if there is a diaphragmatic rupture. This simple examination is especially helpful in the diagnosis of a rupture of the right diaphragm.

3. In right-sided diaphragmatic ruptures with displacement of the liver into the thorax, the elevated position of the lower edge of the liver can frequently be observed in a **plain abdominal roentgenogram.**

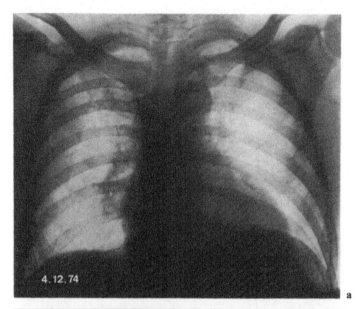

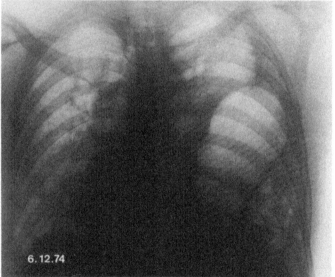

Fig. 127 a, b. A 24-year-old male patient with multiple injuries incurred in a fall from a scaffold 22 m high: brain concussion, basal skull fracture, fracture of the first rib on the right side, cardiac contusion, pelvic fracture, kidney contusion, fracture of the radius, diaphragmatic rupture. **a** Thoracic roentgenogram on day of accident with high, but apparently intact left diaphragm. **b** After prolapse of the viscera into the left thorax, the diagnosis of a diaphragmatic rupture is established. The diaphragmatic tear extended in the central tendon along the margin of the pericardium in a retropericardial direction. The stomach, the left colonic flexure, a convolution of the small intestine, and the greater omentum were found lying displaced in the thorax

4. **Contrast radiography.** After swallowing contrast medium or after its administration via nasogastric tube, the roentgenogram shows, in the head down position, the location of the stomach or the intestinal loops in the thoracic cavity. In my experience, this examination is seldom necessary. If it is, however, we always use barium sulfate and not a water-soluble contrast medium since a displacement of the loops of the small intestine or the colon can also be recognized in follow-up thoracic roentgenograms.

5. In fluoroscopic screening, a paradoxical movement or a diminished mobility in the area of the affected diaphragm is found. Occasionally, levels of fluid, which can change rapidly according to position, can also be observed in this way.

6. In right-sided diaphragmatic ruptures, a **liver scan** can provide information about the exact location of the liver.

7. **Angiography** of the celiac and superior mesenteric arteries [592] is a reliable but very demanding procedure. We never found its use necessary.

It is crucial that an unclear finding is not ignored and that all effort is made to determine the presence or absence of a diaphragmatic injury. The importance of serial roentgenograms must be emphasized. There are cases in which the diaphragm appears completely normal shortly after trauma (Fig. 127). The differences in pressure mentioned above, however, rapidly cause herniation of intra-abdominal organs into the thoracic cavity. An initially minor, inconclusive finding can evolve into a clear clinical picture due to progressive eventration.

Caution is advised in the use of exploratory puncture due to the danger of injury to the stomach or intestines.

Diagnostic Errors

1. The most frequent error in the diagnosis of a diaphragmatic rupture is to mistake it for a **hemothorax.** It can have serious consequences because in the process of inserting a chest tube the prolapsed contents of the abdomen can be injured. Also in our records, there were two patients in whom, under the diagnosis of a hemothorax, a chest tube was inserted and the stomach inadvertently drained. In retrospect, an accurate inspection of the roentgenogram would have made a correct diagnosis possible in both cases (see Fig. 4). For the differentiation of a right-sided hemothorax from that of a herniated liver, it may be necessary to perform a liver scan.

2. **Local pneumothorax** or **tension pneumothorax** [575] is another mistaken diagnosis, especially if this diagnosis is made solely on the basis of a clinical examination (Fig. 128).

3. **High diaphragm caused by a dilatated stomach.**

4. **High position of diaphragm caused by phrenic nerve paresis.** As in the case of the high diaphragmatic position caused by stomach dilatation, in contrast to a diaphragmatic rupture, the diaphragm itself is always recognizable as a thin, distinct structure above the magenblase.

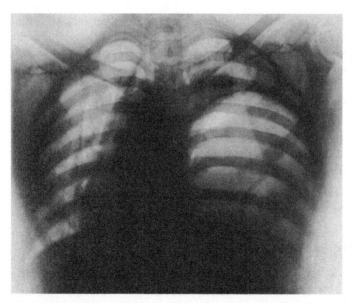

Fig. 128. The displacement of a large, air-filled magenblase into the left thorax in a diaphragmatic rupture can result in a situation comparable to a tension pneumothorax

5. **Atelectasis.** This is an unforgiveable error in diagnosis since atelectasis does not cause displacement of the mediastinal organs to the opposite side but a shift to the affected side.

Therapy

Indication for Operation

The indication for operation is provided by the diagnosis of a diaphragmatic rupture. The intervention should be made as soon as possible, less on account of the danger of incarceration but rather because of the constantly increasing **impairment to respiration.**
Injured patients with a diaphragmatic rupture usually have **multiple wounds.** The treatment of diaphragmatic injury without symptoms of incarceration and without serious cardiorespiratory effects can be postponed in favor of clarification and operation on life-threatening injuries (e. g., a craniotomy). In such cases, a nasogastric tube is always inserted.

Operative Approach

The left diaphragm can be sewn from the abdomen as well as from the chest. The exposure proves to be better from a thoracic approach. The question of approach, about which there are differences of opinion, seems to me to be clearly answerable:

Injuries in the thoracic area that require operative treatment are extremely rare. The chest roentgenogram provides information about the possible existence of other intrathoracic injuries. **Abdominal companion injuries,** on the other hand, are very common and difficult to evaluate, particularly after a thoracotomy has been performed. Even though the spleen can be removed by going through the thorax, a thorough abdominal inspection is impossible.

It seems to me, therefore, to be beyond discussion that the approach in an **acute left-sided** diaphragmatic rupture must as a rule be **abdominal.** Among other things, it restricts breathing less than a thoracotomy does. One exception to this is when there are severe intrathoracic injuries.

The suturing of the **acute right-sided** rupture from an abdominal approach is difficult: here I would go in through a **right-sided thoracotomy** in the fifth intercostal space if there are no abdominal symptoms.

In all **chronic ruptures,** the approach is definitely **thoracic** since there are often adhesions that cannot be dealt with from the abdominal side.

In every approach, the field of operation is draped in such a manner that an additional incision in the other body cavity is possible. A thoracoabdominal approach represents a greater morbidity than a laparotomy or thoracotomy and is usually unnecessary.

Operative Technique

The **reduction** of the prolapsed abdominal viscera is never difficult in an acute rupture. In the eventration of many abdominal organs, the small intestine is put back in place first, the stomach last.

The **closure of the diaphragm** is made with interrupted sutures with nonresorbable suture material. We use a single row of double sutures with silk. In an acute rupture, a direct closure is always possible. The branches of the phrenic nerve must be avoided.

In avulsions of the diaphragm from its origin on the thoracic wall, the **reinsertion** at the point of laceration may be difficult; it is then performed more cranially.

Intraoperatively, a **chest tube** is always put in; preoperatively, a **nasogastric tube.**

Prognosis

Spontaneous healing of a diaphragmatic rupture is known to occur, as confirmed by autopsy findings, but the prolapse of abdominal viscera, which almost always occurs, makes spontaneous healing impossible.

The simple, uncomplicated diaphragmatic rupture has a good prognosis when treated operatively. It is the **companion injuries** therefore that determine the fate of such a patient and cause considerable mortality among patients with diaphragmatic ruptures.

Rare Special Form: Pericardiophrenic Ruptures

Diaphragmatic ruptures in the area of the pericardium with prolapse of the abdominal viscera into the pericardium are well-known as isolated observations, and in exceptional cases also occur with luxation of the heart into the abdomen [580, 591].

 In 1937 Tixier [594] attempted an operation for this kind of ailment for the first time. The patient died 2 days later of a pneumothorax. In 1951 Santy [591] and in 1952 Crawshaw [574] treated such ruptures successfully.

The prolapse of the abdominal viscera into the pericardium can cause anginal pains, rhythm disturbances, or symptoms of cardiac tamponade. In the **roentgenogram,** the cardiac silhouette is enlarged; air-filled intestinal loops can show up in the heart area [578]. **Therapy** is always operative. However, virtually all pericardiophrenic ruptures that have been described were not operated on until already in the chronic final stage, as much as 23 years after trauma [587].

II. Penetrating Diaphragmatic Injuries

In contrast to closed diaphragmatic ruptures, penetrating diaphragmatic injuries can occur at any location. **Gunshot injuries** strike the left as well as the right diaphragm equally [597]. It is interesting that **stabbing injuries** occur twice as often to the left diaphragm as to the right, presumably because the attacker is usually right-handed and also possibly aiming at the left side where the heart is. The diaphragmatic injury is then usually anterolateral. In addition, **impalement injuries** or, in rare instances, **injury of the diaphragm** by a **fractured rib** also come into question [592].

Penetrating injuries of the diaphragm, unlike diaphragmatic ruptures caused by blunt force, are seldom overlooked. Since the examination is made operatively when a diaphragmatic or abdominal injury due to gunshot or stabbing is suspected, the diagnosis is established by the exploration. In evaluating stabbing injuries, it is easy to forget that the dome of the diaphragm during the expiratory phase can reach as high as the fourth rib.

Since a small defect in the diaphragm is usually all that is involved, the danger of an incarceration or strangulation of prolapsed intestines is especially great. Often only parts of the omentum lie in the defect to keep the way open, like a "foot in the door" (Rutherford [266]), for later entrance of the stomach or intestines.

A diaphragmatic injury without simultaneous lesion of intra-abdominal organs is rare. In the penetrating injury of the left diaphragm, the organs most frequently affected concomitantly are the stomach, then the spleen and the left colonic flexure. In lesions on the right side, it is the liver that is injured. A cholothorax is often the first indication of this lesion.

In the early phase after the injury, the **radiologic** examination still does not show any abdominal structures in the thoracic area; the diaphragm is usually normal in its configuration. There is often a hemothorax and a pneumothorax.

The **indication for operation** is usually given already by the other associated injuries. Every significant diaphragmatic wound should be closed.

When gunshot wounds cause severe damage, the closure of a diaphragmatic defect can create problems. In that case, when the injuries are on the edge of the diaphragm, it is reinserted at a level higher than the normal anatomic location. In a larger central defect, a plastic reconstruction must be attempted. Although synthetic tissues and synthetic nets have been implanted successfully, caution must be exercised in their use because of the danger of infection; consideration must be given to the possible use of endogenous structures, such as corium.

Chapter 20

Other Injury Patterns and Consequences of Injury in Thoracic Trauma

I. Traumatic Asphyxia

Synonyms

Druckstauung (Perthes, 1900 [629])
Stauungsblutungen (Braun, 1899 [604])
Traumatic apnea (Burrell, 1902 [605])
Stasis cyanosis (Alexander, 1909 [598])
Cervicofacial cutaneous asphyxia (Bolt, 1908)
Traumatic cyanosis (Hall, 1930)
Compressio thoracis
Masque ecchymotique (Ollivier d'Angers, 1837 [627])

In a severe compression of the thorax with sudden increase of pressure in the venous system, a **characteristic injury pattern** develops with, among other possible signs, small hemorrhages in the conjunctiva, the skin, and the mucous membranes of the throat and head and reddish-blue discoloration in the latter region. It is not at all uncommon, as might be assumed on the basis of the rather sparse accounts in the recent literature.

 Although in the German literature this condition bears his name, Perthes was by no means the first to report on it. He deserves the credit, however, for having discovered a clear interpretation for these findings in 1899 and 1900, which is still generally recognized today [628, 629].
In 1837 Ollivier d'Angers [627] was the first to describe this syndrome on the basis of results of autopsy on 23 patients who, as victims of a panic in Paris, had suffered thoracic compression. Other cases were observed by Tardieu (1855 and 1866), Willers (1873), and Hueter (1874) [612]. In 1899, i. e., in the same year as Perthes, Braun [604] reported on the same pathologic picture in connection with severe abdominal compression.

A severe **compression of the chest,** less frequently also of the abdomen [604, 624] — effective forces of up to 8 tons have been described — causes a sudden, massive **increase of intrathoracic pressure** and, through it, of the central venous pressure. Venous blood is pressed back into the veins of the head and neck and occasionally into the upper extremities. Since these veins have no valves or are provided with insufficient venous valves at best, it is understandable that the injury manifests itself primarily in the region of the head, and only in exceptional cases do symptoms appear in the lower extremities. The acute rise in pressure and the flooding of venules and capillaries results in numerous small hemorrhages.

Simultaneous closure of the glottis allows a better transfer of pressure into the thoracic cavities via the air-filled lungs and appears to play an important role in the development of the syndrome. Actually, in many cases the observation was made that the patients feared the threatened compression and presumably held their breath unconsciously, hence instituting a kind of Valsalva maneuver.

The same syndrome has also been described **without external violence,** for example, in an epileptic seizure [598], in pertussis, severe vomiting, bronchial asthma, and during childbirth [610].

The necessary impact force lasts from a few seconds up to several minutes. It is interesting to note that the violent but shorter effect of a pressure wave in "blast injuries" produces an altogether different injury pattern, namely, one of very severe contusions and ruptures of the lungs (Chap. 13).

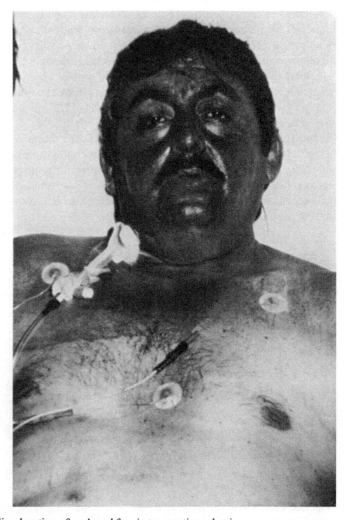

Fig. 129. Reddish-blue discoloration of neck and face in traumatic asphyxia

Clinical Picture and Diagnosis

The clinical picture is extraordinarily impressive and characteristic. If the patient's history is known, one glance is all that is necessary to make the diagnosis.

The head and neck are discolored a **reddish-blue** (Fig. 129). On the skin of this area, occasionally also of the upper (but almost never of the lower) extremities, **petechiae** are found (Fig. 130). If there was counterpressure supplied by a hatband or collar, the veins and capillaries of this region were protected against the overflow of blood; such pressure sites are clearly distinguishable as white blank spaces.

Frequently there are findings in the **eyes**: subconjunctival hemorrhages are never absent (Fig. 131). There can also be hemorrhages into the vitreous humor, the retina, or the optic nerve. Twenty percent of the patients show an exophthalmos [610]. Transient dilated pupils, scotomas, disturbances in bulbar motility, and temporary or permanent visual disorders up to the point of blindness have been recorded [613, 621].

One-third of the patients become **unconscious,** usually only for a short time [603]. States of confusion are frequent; occasionally, epileptic seizures are observed [610]. However, extensive cerebral hemorrhaging rarely ensues. Because of the sudden hyperemia in the brain, there is danger of cerebral edema.

Hemorrhages of the **mucosa** of the nose and mouth, otorrhagia, ruptures of the tympanic membranes, tinnitus, and temporary deafness can occur.

Paraplegias [624, 630] and even quadriplegias [632], usually with good prognosis, have been recorded.

Traumatic asphyxia can occur without significant thoracic injuries or rib fractures. There are, however, often **companion injuries** in the thoracic area; these are usually of greater significance than the traumatic asphyxia: multiple rib fractures, pneumothorax, hemothorax, and — often overlooked — spinal fractures. I should like to call attention particularly to cardiac contusion, which in our records was present in half of the patients with traumatic asphyxia.

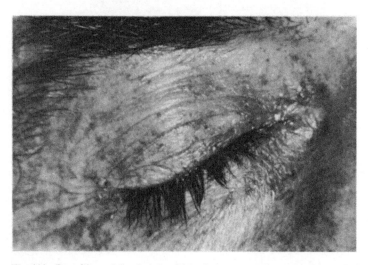

Fig. 130. Petechiae of the facial epidermis in traumatic asphyxia are found most often in the area of the eyelids

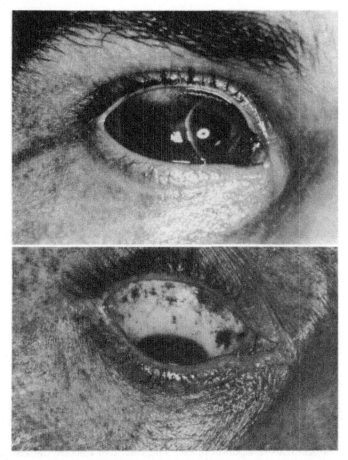

Fig. 131. In traumatic asphyxia, subconjunctival hemorrhages are never absent

Therapy

The **companion injuries** require therapy and usually not the traumatic asphyxia. Almost all the manifestations of the syndrome are reversible, and a specific therapy is unnecessary. In the other cases, e. g., in paresis, therapy cannot influence the course of the ailment. There is an exception when significant cerebral symptoms lead one to suspect cerebral edema: in that case, therapy for cerebral edema and restriction of fluid intake is important.

If the patient survives the severe accident situation and receives hospital treatment, the **prognosis** is usually good and is largely dependent upon the other injuries.

II. Injuries of the Thoracic Duct, Chylothorax

Injuries of the thoracic duct resulting in a chylothorax are occasionally observed. The frequency of this injury is probably greater than would be assumed from the somewhat more than 300 cases described in the literature since many cases are not published or are overshadowed by other injuries.

 It is not entirely clear as to who described the first case of a traumatic lesion of the thoracic duct since in many early cases it was probably an empyema and not a chylothorax that was involved. Most likely, the case observed in 1679 by Bonet [602] was caused by an injury of the thoracic duct: 14 days after a gunshot injury in the left side of the back, a large amount of whitish-yellow fluid began to flow out, which lasted for several months. The patient died from increasing cachexia. In 1895 Quinke described a chylothorax in blunt thoracic trauma with rib fractures [609].
As early as 1898, Cushing attempted to suture an injured thoracic duct [614]. In 1907 De Forest [607] demanded that the injured thoracic duct be ligated as if it were a bleeding vessel.

Mechanism of Injury and Clinical Picture

1. In **blunt trauma,** the injury of the thoracic duct occurs because of hyperextension of the spinal column (in one case, even by overextension of the spinal column while yawning [631]), by a fall from a great height, or because of severe thoracic compression. In one-fifth of all cases of closed injuries of the thoracic duct, there are also spinal fractures or fractures of the posterior parts of the ribs [609].

2. Thoracic duct injuries caused by **penetrating wounds** are very rare; the probability that the thoracic duct, which has a diameter of only 4 mm, might be injured without significant and usually fatal simultaneous injuries to the large vessels, is extremely unlikely. Thus, of the entire patient records from World War II, only one case has been described [635].

3. Today, the majority of all cases with chylothorax are due to **intraoperative** injuries to the thoracic duct, especially in operations in the left supraclavicular region: in removal of lymph nodes in the neck, scalenotomy, resection of malignant goiters, Blalock-Taussig operation, etc. The duct can also be injured through punctures of the subclavian or jugular veins. We experienced one case while performing a thoracic sympathectomy of a patient with intrathoracic adhesions as a result of former tuberculosis.

The thoracic duct, of which there are many anatomic varieties, usually arises from the cisterna chyli on the right side of the vertebral column and passes across to the left side at the level of the fifth thoracic vertebra. A **chylothorax** can develop on **both sides** if the injury occurs in the area of this intersection, i. e., between the third and sixth thoracic vertebrae [631] or if initially an extended mediastinal chyloma develops, which then breaks through on both sides.
A chylothorax occurring after injury to the thoracic duct classically appears **belatedly,** 2 – 10 days after trauma, though a lag of 22 days has also been observed [622]. During the often restricted nutrition following severe injuries, very little chyle flows through the duct; furthermore, there might at first be an extrapleural, mediastinal accumulation of lymph that would not pour out into the pleural cavity until later.
A **chylopericardium** is rarely found after intraoperative injuries of the duct [606], but has never been described as a consequence of an accident.
In the neck area, a **chylous fistula** can form after injuries to the thoracic duct.

The **danger** of a chylothorax lies, on the one hand, in the rapidly increasing filling of the pleural cavity with compression of the lung and mediastinum, and on the other, in the **loss of great amounts of fluid, rich in protein and, above all, rich in fat.** It must be kept in mind that in 24 h up to 2000 ml of lymph flow through the thoracic duct and that 75% of the fat is taken up into the circulatory system in this way. Thus, the untreated injury leads to a very severe clinical picture with increasing cachexia.

Infections are extraordinarily rare, a fact that is ascribed to the bacteriostatic characteristics of lymph [642].

Diagnosis

The diagnosis is never established until the drainage or puncture of a suspected hemothorax produces a **milky-white** or — to the extent that it is mixed with blood — cocoa-colored **fluid** (Fig. 132). It is then that the differential diagnosis from empyema must be made. The following properties differentiate lymph from pus:

1. Sterile
2. Odorless
3. Contains mostly lymphocytes
4. Alkaline reaction
5. Milky color disappears when shaken with ether
6. In a microscopic examination, fat droplets are found that take on coloration with Sudan III

Positive proof can also be produced by the ingestion of lipophilic food dyes that color the lymph but do not enter into other exudates [614].

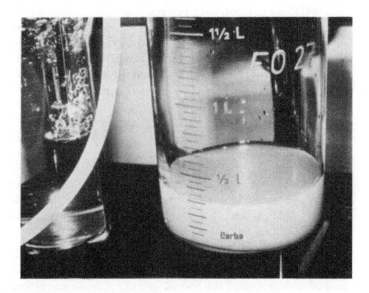

Fig. 132. The thoracic drainage withdraws milky fluid in a patient with chylothorax

The **roentgenogram** shows only the opacity of the hemithorax as in a pleural effusion, occasionally a widening of the mediastinum. The location of the lesion can be identified by means of lymphography [616]. The practical significance of this examination is very minimal, however, since no consequences for further treatment are produced.

Therapy

After a period of great optimism in the 1940s and early 1950s about operative treatment, today there is general agreement that the therapy for chylothorax should **initially** be **conservative** [150, 609, 622, 635, 641]. Most of the injuries of the thoracic duct can be healed in this way. A **chest tube** with continuous suction of 25 cm H_2O is installed. Peroral nutrition is discontinued and the patient is **fed parenterally.**
Total intravenous parenteral nutrition will reduce the flow of chyle in the duct decidedly and possibly make conservative therapy still more effective. In addition, the possibility of a comprehensive replacement of the dreaded losses of protein and fat has decreased the dangerous aspects of chylothorax today. Injury of the thoracic duct should no longer be a cause of death. An increasing cachexia may no longer be regarded as a reason for operating today and is rather the manifestation of inadequate treatment.
An **operative intervention** is indicated only if conservative treatment fails to achieve its goal in 3 – 4 weeks. It consists of the **ligation of the thoracic duct.** The preferred procedure is the exposure by means of a low right-sided posterolateral thoracotomy and ligation above the diaphragm. The one-sided distal ligature of the passage is adequate since competent valves prevent a return flow of chyle [614]. If the site of the injury is encountered intraoperatively, both parts of the duct are ligated. Preoperative ingestion of cream or intraoperative injections of dye into the distal esophagus [641] help to identify the thoracic duct.
Extensive animal experiments and clinical experience have shown that because of the great tendency of the lymphatics to create collateral systems, the ligature of the thoracic duct does not produce any deficit [601, 614, 617, 620, 622, 635, 641].
For the treatment of a **chylous fistula in the neck,** conservative therapy and the application of a pressure bandage are usually sufficient.

III. Cholothorax

The accumulation of bile in the pleural cavity (cholothorax) has clinical significance only in **penetrating injuries** of the right lower thorax that affect the diaphragm and the liver. Bile produces a much stronger pleural reaction than blood; the danger exists of a bilious pleuritis or of pleural empyema.

1. If as an exception it is not necessary to perform an operation in a liver and diaphragmatic injury because of its insignificance, a **chest tube** is inserted and placed to best advantage toward the bottom into the phrenicocostal sinus. Minor injuries will heal under drainage.

2. Consideration must be given to the fact that particularly in small diaphragmatic injuries, considerable amounts of blood mixed with bile can accumulate below the diaphragm. It is advantageous to remove them before they cause an infection. A substantial displacement of the diaphragm upward or evidence of a hematoma between the diaphragm and liver on a liver scan requires an operation.

IV. Traumatically Induced Hernias of the Chest Wall

By laceration of the intercostal soft tissue, occasionally combined with multiple rib fractures, a **hernia of the lung** or more frequently — because of simultaneous laceration of the parietal pleura — a **prolapse of the lung** can occur. This condition is rare. Interestingly enough, even a very slight injury can cause it: a herniated lung has even been observed after repeated thoracocenteses [638]. Such hernias usually first appear weeks or months after the accident.

Symptoms and Diagnosis

Hernias of the chest wall are often tolerated without inconvenience. Pleuritic symptoms, especially a chronic dry cough and occasionally also pains while breathing, can occur.
The **diagnosis** is established by **inspection:** the protrusion on the thoracic wall enlarges upon expiration, especially during a Valsalva maneuver, and decreases or completely disappears upon inspiration. The **roentgenogram,** taken during the expiration phase and tangential to the place of herniation, confirms the clinical diagnosis (Fig. 133).
Concerning the differential diagnosis, tumors, localized subcutaneous emphysema, and abscesses are usually easy to exclude [625].

Therapy

Since only in exceptional cases does improvement occur spontaneously or with conservative measures [634], the therapy is **operative** if treatment is necessary at all. Of the variety of operative methods proposed, that method will be selected that permits a secure closure using endogenous material as much as possible:

1. In contrast to defects caused operatively in tumor surgery, posttraumatic hernias are small for the most part. Therefore, simple methods will usually suffice: adaptation of two neighboring ribs [643] or closure by periosteal flaps of the two neighboring ribs in the manner of a swinging door, according to Doberer [615].

2. Larger defects can be covered by splitting a rib longitudinally and shifting one part of the rib over the defect (Vulpius) [615]. Corium transplants extended between the ribs can also be considered.

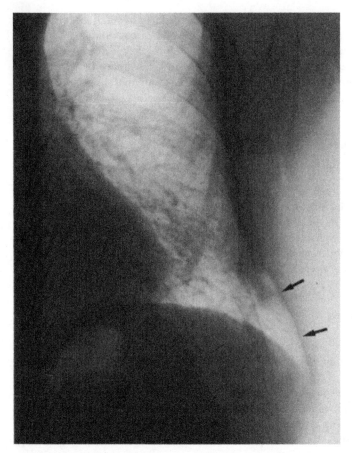

Fig. 133. Posttraumatic hernia of the lung after multiple basal rib fractures on the left side. Nine months after the accident, the breach in the thoracic wall was closed by internal fixation with plates of the divergent fractured ribs that had not healed

3. In hernias caused by dislocation of fractured ribs, the indication is given for internal fixation of the ribs, e. g., with small fragment plates.

V. Arterial Air Embolism

Arterial air embolism as a **complication of lung injuries** has hardly attracted any attention up to now, although it can be assumed that it occurs much more often than it is diagnosed, especially because of the increased use of **mechanical respirators.**
The pathologic pattern differs completely from venous air embolism. Through the entrance of air into the veins of the lung, whether directly from air-filled sections of the lung or from a pneumothorax, the air reaches the left side of the heart and the arterial circulation, where the embolization of air into the **coronary arteries** and into

the **brain** is of decisive importance. Even small amounts of air in the coronary arteries have a fatal effect. By injecting 0.1 – 0.2 ml of air into the left coronary artery of a dog, Goldfarb [611] was able to induce ventricular fibrillation. If there are connections between the right and left sides of the heart (open oval foramen, atrial septal defect, ventricular septal defect), an arterial air embolism can also develop from the supply of air into a peripheral vein (paradoxical air embolism).

Arterial air emboli are especially familiar as a complication of extracorporeal circulation, of a therapeutic pneumothorax, and of dialysis. The "pleura shock" of the older German literature was presumably caused, in most cases, by a cerebral air embolism, something that Brauer already suspected [599, 633]. In diving accidents, this pathologic pattern is of great significance.

Arterial air emboli can appear in **connection with thoracic injuries,** especially in **penetrating wounds** [637] and **blast injuries of the lung** (see Chap. 13). These complications are a threat also in connection with **therapeutic measures:** in thoracentesis [640], in surgical interventions in the lung, and above all in mechanical ventilation [618].

On the respirator, various circumstances favor the formation of a bronchovenous fistula: the lung is inflated with positive pressure, often positive end-expiratory pressure is used, and occasionally high ventilatory pressures are necessary. A decreased tensile strength of the lung tissues was demonstrated experimentally in the adult respiratory distress syndrome and in hypovolemic states [618]. The frequent occurrence of a pneumothorax or tension pneumothorax in a patient with thoracic injuries receiving mechanical ventilation leaves no doubt that air occasionally enters the arterial circulation through a tear in the lung tissue. Thus, this complication occurred during mechanical ventilation in all eight of Thomas' cases [637].

Symptoms and Diagnosis

Air embolism occurs suddenly and completely by surprise. Symptoms can, however, first appear sometime after embolization when the position of the patient is changed. The pathologic pattern is characterized by the embolization into the coronary arteries and into the cerebral circulation. The **coronary air embolism** leads to rhythm disturbances, ischemic pains, and ischemic ECG changes, occasionally also to ventricular fibrillation.

Well-known as **cerebral symptoms** are: attacks of dizziness and weakness, fear of death, headaches, cramps, unconsciousness, as well as every possible neurologic deficit, such as hemiplegia, paraplegia, hemianopsia, nystagmus, and loss of sight.

These are all **uncharacteristic symptoms** that are hard to interpret in a patient on a respirator. If such a complication comes into consideration at all, the **pathognomonic symptoms** should be sought, which will be present, however, only in a **very massive** air embolization and can therefore usually not be identified:

1. Ophthalmoscopic evidence of air bubbles in the vessels of the retina

2. Liebermeister's sign: sharply delineated zones of pallor on the tongue caused by embolic closure of the small arteries of the tongue [619]

3. Mottled skin

4. "Air hemorrhage": from a small incision in the superior area of the body, blood mixed with air can emerge [639]

Usually, all that remains is the **suspicion,** confirmed by the patient's history, the sudden appearance, and the uncharacteristic symptomatology. Additional diagnostic clarifications (ultrasound, angiography) remain illusory because of the urgency of time.

The diagnosis at **autopsy** can also be difficult, even when special attention is paid since even very small amounts of air can have a fatal effect. In a coronary artery air embolism, there is usually not enough time for a myocardial infarction to form [608, 637].

Prophylaxis

Among the prophylactic measures to be taken, **positioning** is significant [637]. Immediately after the accident and in the transport vehicle, patients with penetrating thoracic injuries should be laid on the **side of the injury.** In the dependent areas, the pulmonary venous pressure is greater, and therefore the danger of an air embolism is less. Furthermore, this position helps to avoid aspiration of blood into the healthy lung.

Based on the same considerations, we never perform **thoracocentesis** on a seated patient, but only when the patient is in a recumbent position.

Therapy

1. **Suspicion of an arterial air embolism during a thoracic operation:**
   — Trendelenburg's position to avoid further embolization into the brain.
   — The lung wound suspected to be responsible is excluded from the pulmonary circulation by two soft clamps. If this is not possible, the hilus is clamped for a short time.
   — Opening the pericardium and inspection of the coronary arteries: air bubbles in the coronary arteries can be massaged into the periphery or emptied by puncture with a fine needle.
   — Evacuation of air from the left ventricle through puncture at the apex.
   — Increasing arterial pressure by use of catecholamines.

2. **Arterial air embolism in the ward, e. g., on the respirator in the intensive care unit:**
   — Position with head down. A supine position is certain to favor embolization into the coronary arteries; however, the intermediary position recommended by Durant [608], midway between a prone position and lying on the left side, is certainly not practicable for a patient with severe cardiac disturbances because of air embolism.
   — Drug therapy of cardiac rhythm disturbances and arterial hypotension.
   — Treatment of brain edema if there is suspicion of a cerebral embolism.

— Resuscitation in case of cardiac arrest. If resuscitation is impossible and if there is a well-founded suspicion of air embolism, a thoracotomy with evacuation of air from the coronary arteries and possibly also from the left side of the heart is a courageous but decisive step. Less promising of success and technically more difficult is puncture of the left ventricle through the thoracic wall; the air is not removed from the coronary arteries by that procedure.

If possible, such a patient is treated by dispensing with positive end-expiratory pressure and by keeping the ventilation pressure as low as possible by appropriately setting the respirator.

Bibliography

Chapter 1 Initial Considerations in the Management of Severe Thoracic Injury

Chapter 2 The Patient with Additional Injuries in Other Parts of the Body

1. Allgöwer, M.: Beurteilung des Allgemeinzustandes und Schocktherapie beim Mehrfachverletzten. Langenbecks Arch. Chir. **322**, 230–241 (1968)
2. Blair, E., Topuzlu, C., Davis, J. H.: Delayed or missed diagnosis in blunt chest trauma. J. Trauma **11**, 129–145 (1971)
3. Buff, H. U.: Ergebnisse der Behandlung von Mehrfachverletzungen der Gliedmaßen. Langenbecks Arch. **322**, 1034–1040 (1968)
4. Den Otter, G., Krul, E. J.: Blunt thoracic trauma in multiple injuries. In: Buff, H. U., Glinz, W. (Hrsg.): Respiratorische Insuffizienz bei Mehrfachverletzten, S. 11–15. Erlangen: Perimed 1976
5. Heberer, G.: Beurteilung und Behandlung von Verletzungen des Brustkorbs und der Brustorgane im Rahmen von Mehrfachverletzungen. Langenbecks Arch. Chir. **322**, 268–284 (1968)
6. Key, G. F., Nance, F. C.: A time-management study of 25 patients with penetrating wounds of the chest and abdomen. J. Trauma **16**, 524–530 (1976)
7. Kremer, K.: Dringlichkeitsfragen bei der Erstversorgung kombinierter und Mehrfachverletzungen – Thoraxverletzungen –. Langenbecks Arch. Chir. **329**, 62–66 (1971)
8. Larena, A., Jussen, A., Reichmann, W.: Zeitpunkt der Osteosynthese bei Kombinationsverletzten. Chirurg **43**, 116–118 (1972)
9. Le Brigand, H., Dor, J.: Le traitement immédiat des traumatismes graves et fermés du thorax. 75e congrès chirurgie 1973, p. 138. Paris: Masson 1972
10. Lichtenauer, F., Schröder, H.: Thorakale Notzustände. Langenbecks Arch. Chir. **308**, 499–513 (1964)
11. Messmer, K., Lewis, D. H., Sunder-Plassman, L., Klöverkorn, W. P., Mendler, N., Holper, K.: Acute normovolemic hemodilution. Europ. Surg. Res. **4**, 55–70 (1972)
12. Oestern, H. J., Blömer, J., Muhr, G.: Thoraxverletzungen bei Polytrauma. Diagnostik, Therapie, Komplikationen und Prognose. In: Buff, H. U., Glinz, W. (Hrsg.): Respiratorische Insuffizienz bei Mehrfachverletzten, S. 17–22. Erlangen: Perimed 1976
13. Rüedi, Th., Wolff, G.: Vermeidung posttraumatischer Komplikationen durch frühe definitive Versorgung von Polytraumatisierten mit Frakturen des Bewegungsapparates. Helv. chir. Acta **42**, 507–512 (1975)
14. Schmit-Neuerburg, K. P.: Die Mehrfachverletzung – Besonderheiten der Indikationsstellung zur Knochenbruchbehandlung an den Extremitäten. Langenbecks Arch. Chir. **337**, 435–442 (1974)
15. Schriefers, K. H.: Dringlichkeitsfragen bei der Erstversorgung kombinierter und Mehrfachverletzungen. Langenbecks Arch. Chir. **329**, 53–62 (1971)
16. Vogel, W., Mittermayer, Ch., Buchardi, H., Birzle, H., Wiemers, K.: Spezielle respiratorische Probleme bei Polytraumatisierten. Langenbecks Arch. Chir. **329**, 491–503 (1971)
17. Wiemers, K., Vogel, W., Mittermayer, Ch., Birzle, H., Böttcher, D.: Lungenkomplikationen. Langenbecks Arch. Chir. **332**, 537–543 (1972)

Chapter 3 Interpretation of the Chest Roentgenogram

18. Attar, S., Ayelia, R. J., McLaughlin, J. S.: The widened mediastinum in trauma. Ann. thorac. Surg. **13**, 435–449 (1972)
19. Birzle, H., Bergleiter, R., Kuner, E. H.: Traumatologische Röntgendiagnostik. Lehrbuch und Atlas. Stuttgart: Thieme 1975
20. Flaherty, T. T., Wegner, G. P., Crummy, A. B., Francyk, W. P., Hipona, F. A.: Nonpenetrating injuries to the thoracic aorta. Radiology **92**, 541–546 (1969)
21. Greenway, B. A., Nicholls, B. A.: Traumatic rupture of the thoracic aorta – a radiological pitfall. Injury **7**, 11–13 (1975)
22. Hipona, F. A., Paredes, S.: The radiologic evaluation of patients with chest trauma. Cardiovascular system. Med. Clin. N. Amer. **59**, 65–93 (1975)
23. Kirsh, M. M., Crane, J. D., Kahn, D. R.: Roentgenographic evaluation of traumatic rupture of the aorta. Surg. Gynec. Obstet. **131**, 900–904 (1970)
24. Köhler, A., Zimmer, E. A.: Grenzen des Normalen und Anfänge des Pathologischen im Röntgenbild des Skelets. Stuttgart: Thieme 1967
25. Lernau, O., Bar-Maor, J. A., Nissan, S.: Traumatic diaphragmatic hernia simulating acute tension pneumothorax. J. Trauma **14**, 880–884 (1974)
26. Mathias, K., Beduhn, D., Wenz, W.: Angiographische Befunde bei Aortenverletzungen nach stumpfem Thoraxtrauma. Herz/Kreislauf **8**, 525–530 (1976)
27. Paredes, S., Hipona, F. A.: The radiologic evaluation of patients with chest trauma; respiratory system. Med. Clin. N. Amer. **59**, 37–63 (1975)
28. Sandor, F.: Incidence and significance of traumatic mediastinal hematoma. Thorax **22**, 43–62 (1967)
29. Schmitz, W., Storch, H. H., Roth, E., Beduhn, D., Hissen, W.: Die akute traumatische Ruptur der deszendierenden thorakalen Aorta. Dtsch. med. Wschr. **97**, 1–4 (1972)
30. Schmoller, H. J.: Lungen-, Herz- und Mediastinalverletzungen im Röntgenbild beim stumpfen Thoraxtrauma. Münch. med. Wschr. **115**, 991–997 (1973)
31. Wilson, R. F., Arbulu, A., Bassett, J. S., Walt, A. J.: Acute mediastinal widening following blunt chest trauma: Critical decisions. Arch. Surg. **104**, 551–558 (1972)

Chapter 4 Respiratory Insufficiency

32. Adams, C. B. T.: The retinal manifestation of fat embolism. Injury **2**, 221–224 (1971)
33. Anderhub, H. P., Keller, R., Herzog, H.: Spirometrische Untersuchungen der forcierten Vitalkapazität, Sekundenkapazität und maximalen Atemstromstärke bei 13798 Personen. Dtsch. med. Wschr. **99**, 33–38 (1974)
34. Ashbaugh, D. G., Bigelow, D. G., Petty, T. L., Levine, B. E.: Acute respiratory distress in adults. Lancet **1967 II**, 319–323
35. Aviado, D. M.: The pharmacology of the pulmonary circulation. Pharmacol. Rev. **12**, 159–239 (1960)
36. Aviado, D. M.: Adenosine diphosphate and vasoactive substances. J. Trauma **8**, 880–884 (1968)
37. Baltensweiler, J.: Fettemboliesyndrom. Bern: Huber 1977
38. Bendixen, H. H., Egbert, L. D., Hedley-Whyte, J., Laver, M. B., Pontoppidan, H.: Respiratory care. Saint Louis: Mosby 1965
39. Bergentz, S. E., Lewis, D., Ljungqvist, U.: Die Lunge im Schock: Thrombocytenanhäufung nach Trauma und intravasale Gerinnung. Langenbecks Arch. Chir. **329**, 658–664 (1971)
40. Berggren, S. M.: The oxygen deficit of arterial blood caused by nonventilating parts of the lung. Acta physiol. scand. **4**, Suppl. 11, 1–92 (1942)
41. Berman, J. R., Gutierrez, V. S., Boatright, R. D.: Intravascular microaggregation in young men with combat injuries. Surg. Forum **20**, 14–16 (1969)
42. Berman, J. R., Smulson, M. E., Pattengale, P., Sheinbach, S. F.: Pulmonary microembolism after soft tissue injury in primates. Surgery **70**, 246–253 (1971)
43. Berman, J. R., Iliescu, H., Ranson, J. H. C., Eng, K.: Pulmonary capillary permeability – a transfusion lesion. J. Trauma **16**, 471–480 (1976)

44. Berry, R. E. L., Sanislow, C. A.: Clinical manifestations and treatment of congestive atelectasis. Arch. Surg. **87**, 153–167 (1963)
45. Blaisdell, W., Schlobohm, R.: The respiratory distress syndrome: A review. Surgery **74**, 251–262 (1973)
46. Bredenberg, C. E.: Acute respiratory distress. Surg. Clin. N. Amer. **54**, 1043–1066 (1974)
47. Burford, T. H., Burbank, B.: Traumatic wet lung. J. thorac. Surg. **14**, 415–424 (1945)
48. Byrne, J. P., Jr., Dixon, J. A.: Pulmonary edema following blood transfusion reaction. Arch. Surg. **102**, 91–94 (1971)
49. Cahill, J. M., Jonasset-Strieder, D., Byrne, J. J.: Lung function in shock. Amer. J. Surg. **110**, 324–329 (1965)
50. Cameron, J. L., Sebor, J., Anderson, R. P.: Aspiration pneumonia: Results of treatment by positive pressure ventilation in dogs. J. surg. Res. **8**, 447–457 (1968)
51. Cameron, J. L., Reynolds, J., Zuidema, G. D.: Aspiration in patients with tracheotomies. Surg. Gynec. Obstet. **136**, 68–70 (1973)
52. Collins, J. A.: The causes of progressive pulmonary insufficiency in surgical patients. J. surg. Res. **9**, 685–704 (1969)
53. Conger, J. D.: A controlled evaluation of prophylactic dialysis in post-traumatic acute renal failure. J. Trauma **15**, 1056–1063 (1975)
54. Cloutier, C. T., Lowery, B. D., Carey, L. C.: The effect of hemodilutional resuscitation on serum protein levels in humans in hemorrhagic shock. J. Trauma **9**, 514–521 (1969)
55. Daniel, R. A., Jr., Cate, W. R., Jr.: Wet lung – an experimental study. Ann. Surg. **127**, 836–857 (1948)
56. Danielson, R. A.: Differential diagnosis and treatment of oliguria in post-traumatic and post-operative patients. Surg. Clin. N. Amer. **55**, 697–712 (1975)
57. Derks, Ch. M., Peters, R. M.: The role of shock and fat embolus in leakage from pulmonary capillaries. Surg. Gynec. Obstet. **137**, 945–948 (1973)
58. Di Vincenti, F. C., Pruitt, B. A., Reckler, J. M.: Inhalation injuries. J. Trauma **11**, 109–117 (1971)
59. Dressler, D. P., Skornik, W. A., Kupersmith, S.: Corticosteroid treatment of experimental smoke inhalation. Ann. Surg. **183**, 46–52 (1976)
60. Edelist, G.: Post-traumatic pulmonary insufficiency following chest trauma: Identification and prophylaxis. Canad. J. Surg. **18**, 323–327 (1975)
61. Enson, Y., Giuntini, C., Lewis, M. L., Morris, T. Q., Ferrer, M. E., Harvey, R. M.: The influence of hydrogen ion concentration and hypoxia on the pulmonary circulation. J. clin. Invest. **43**, 1146–1162 (1964)
62. Fisher, A. B., Hyde, R. W., Puy, J. R. M., Clarc, J. M., Lambertsen, C. J.: Effect of oxygen at 2 atmospheres in the pulmonary mechanics of normal man. J. appl. Physiol. **24**, 529–536 (1968)
63. Fleming, W. H., Bowen, J. C.: The use of diuretics in the treatment of early wet lung syndrome. Ann. Surg. **175**, 505–509 (1972)
64. Frey-Wettstein, M., Hoppler, R.: Mikroaggregate in Lagerblut. Schweiz. med. Wschr. **106**, 1436–1438 (1976)
65. Gaisford, W. D., Pandey, N., Jensen, G.: Pulmonary changes in treated hemorrhagic shock. Amer. J. Surg. **124**, 738–743 (1972)
66. Geiger, J. P., Gielchinsky, I.: Acute pulmonary insufficiency: treatment in Vietnam casualties. Arch. Surg. **102**, 400–405 (1971)
67. Giordano, J. M., Joseph, W. L., Klingenmaier, C. H., Adkins, P. C.: The management of interstitial pulmonary edema: Significance of hypoproteinemia. J. thorac. cardiovasc. Surg. **64**, 739–747 (1972)
68. Glinz, W.: Respiratorische Insuffizienz beim Mehrfachverletzten. Langenbecks Arch. Chir. **337**, 165–173 (1974)
69. Guiterrez, U. S., Berman, J. R., Soloway, H., Hamit, H. F.: Relationship of hypoproteinemia and prolonged mechanical ventilation to the development of pulmonary insufficiency in shock. Ann. Surg. **171**, 385–393 (1970)
70. Gump, F. E., Kinney, J. M., Iles, M.: Duration and significance of large fluid loads administered for circulatory support. J. Trauma **10**, 431–439 (1970)
71. Gump, F. E., Mashima, Y., Jorgensen, S., Kinney, J. M.: Simultaneous use of three indicators to evaluate pulmonary capillary damage in man. Surgery **70**, 262–270 (1971)

72. Gurd, A. R., Wilson, R. I.: The fat embolism syndrome. J. Bone Jt Surg. **56 B**, 408–416 (1974)
73. Haldemann, G., Reist, F.: Der Hyperoxygenationstest beim Schwerverletzten in der Beurteilung der posttraumatischen respiratorischen Insuffizienz. In: Buff, H. U., Glinz, W. (Hrsg.): Respiratorische Insuffizienz bei Mehrfachverletzten, S. 151–156, Erlangen: Perimed 1976
74. Hasse, J., Wolff, G., Grädel, E.: Die Bedeutung des Herzminutenvolumens für die Interpretation der arteriellen Sauerstoffspannung und des intrapulmonalen Rechts-Links-Shunt nach Thorakotomien. Anaesthesist **23**, 1–4 (1974)
75. Henry, J. N.: The effect of shock on pulmonary alveolar surfactant. J. Trauma **8**, 756–770 (1968)
76. Hill, D. J., Gerbode, F.: Prolonged extracorporeal circulation. In: Sabiston, D. C., Spencer, F. C. (Eds.): Gibbon's surgery of the chest, p. 867–877. Philadelphia-London-Toronto: Saunders 1976
77. Hossli, G., Haldemann, G.: Pulmonale Auswirkungen von Massivtransfusionen. In: Buff, H. U., Glinz, W. (Hrsg.): Respiratorische Insuffizienz bei Mehrfachverletzten, S. 91–94. Erlangen: Perimed 1976
78. Hutchin, P., Terzi, R. G., Hollandsworth, L. A., Johnson, G. Jr., Peters, R. M.: Pulmonary congestion following infusion of large fluid loads in thoracic surgical patients. Ann. thorac. Surg. **8**, 339–346 (1969)
79. James, P. M., Jr.: Shock lung. In: Oaks, W. W. (Ed.): Critical care medicine, pp. 3–11. New York-San Francisco-London: Grune & Stratton 1974
80. Jenkins, M. T., Jones, R. F., Wilson, B., Moyer, C. A.: Congestive atelectasis – a complication of the intravenous infusion of fluids. Ann. Surg. **132**, 327–347 (1950)
81. Johnson, G., Jr., Lambert, J.: Responses to rapid intravenous administration of an overload of fluid and electrolytes in dogs. Ann. Surg. **167**, 561–567 (1968)
82. Jones, R. L., King, E. G.: The effects of methylprednisolone on oxygenation in experimental hypoxemic respiratory failure. J. Trauma **15**, 297–303 (1975)
83. Kleinschmidt, F.: Lungentoxicität des Sauerstoffs. In: Podlesch, I. (Hrsg.): Sauerstoffüberdruckbehandlung, S. 27–30. Berlin-Heidelberg-New York: Springer 1972
84. Landis, E. M., Pappenheimer, J. R.: Exchange of substances through the capillary walls. In: Handbook of Physiology. Section 2: Circulation II, p. 961. Washington D. C.: American Physiological Society 1963
85. Lim, R. C., Blaisdell, F. W., Choy, S. H., Hall, A. D., Thomas, A. N.: Massive pulmonary microembolism in regional shock. Surg. Forum **17**, 13–15 (1966)
86. Ljungqvist, U., Bergentz, S. E., Lewis, D. H.: The distribution of platelets, fibrin and erythrocytes in various organs following experimental trauma. Europ. Surg. Res. **3**, 293–300 (1971)
87. Lowery, B. D., Mulder, D. S., Joyal, E. M., Palmer, W. H.: Effect of hemorrhagic shock on the lung of the pig. Surg. Forum **21**, 21–22 (1970)
88. Maloney, J. V.: Pulmonary effects of nonthoracic trauma: Means for better therapy suggested by the conference. J. Trauma **8**, 966–977 (1968)
89. Martin, A. M., Simmons, R. L., Heisterkamp, C. A.: Respiratory insufficiency in combat casualties: I. Pathologic changes in the lungs of patients dying of wounds. Ann. Surg. **170**, 30–38 (1969)
90. Mason, G., Hall, D. E., Lamoy, R. E., Wright, C. B.: Evaluation of blood filters: Dynamics of platelets and platelet aggregates. Surgery **77**, 235–240 (1975)
91. McAslan, T. C., Matjasko-chiu, J., Turney, S. Z., Cowley, R. A.: Influence of inhalation of 100% O_2 on intrapulmonary shunt in severely traumatized patients. J. Trauma **13**, 811–820 (1973)
92. McIlroy: Pulmonary shunts. In: Fenn, W. O., Rahn, H. (Eds.): Handbook of physiology. Respiration, Vol. II, Kap. 65, pp. 1519–1524. Washington D.C. 1964
93. McTaggart, D. M., Neubuerger, K. T.: Cerebral fat embolism. Acta neuropath. (Berl.) **15**, 183–187 (1970)
94. Mendelson, C. L.: The aspiration of stomach contents into the lungs during obstetric anesthesia. Amer. J. Obstet. Gynec. **52**, 191–204 (1946)

95. Meyers, J. R., Meyer, J. S., Bane, A. E.: Does hemorrhagic shock damage the lung? J. Trauma 13, 509–519 (1973)
96. Monaco, V., Burdge, R., Newell, J., Sardar, S., Leather, R. L., Powers, S. R., Dutton, R.: Pulmonary venous admixture in injured patients. J. Trauma 12, 15–23 (1972)
97. Moore, F. D., Dagher, F. J., Boyden, C. M., Lee, C. J., Lyons, J. H.: Hemorrhage in normal man: I. Distribution and dispersal of saline infusions following acute blood loss: Clinical kinetics of blood volume support. Ann. Surg. 163, 485–504 (1966)
98. Moore, F. D., Lyons, J. H., Pierce, E. C., Morgan, A. P., Drinker, Ph. A., McArthur, J. D., Dammin, G. J.: Post-traumatic pulmonary insufficiency. Philadelphia: Saunders 1969
99. Morgan, T. E., Finley, T. N., Huber, G. L., Fialkow, H.: Alterations in pulmonary surface active lipids during exposure to increased oxygen tension. J. clin. Invest. 44, 1737–1744 (1965)
100. Mosley, R., Doty, D.: Changes in filtration characteristics of stored blood. Ann. Surg. 171, 329–335 (1970)
101. Moss, G., Staunton, C., Stein, A. A.: Cerebral hypoxia as the primary event in the pathogenesis of the "shock lung syndrome". Surg. Forum 22, 211–213 (1971)
102. Moss, G. S., Das Gupta, T. K., Newson, B., Nyhus, L. M.: Morphologic changes in the primate lung after hemorrhagic shock. Surg. Gynec. Obstet. 134, 3–9 (1972)
103. Moss, G., Staunton, C., Stein, A. A.: The centrineurogenic etiology of the acute respiratory distress syndrome. Universal species independent phenomenon. Amer. J. Surg. 126, 37–41 (1973)
104. Moss, G. S., Stein, A. A.: The centrineurogenic etiology of the respiratory distress syndrome. Amer. J. Surg. 132, 352–357 (1976)
105. Murray, D. G., Racz, G. B.: Fat-embolism syndrome (respiratory-insufficiency syndrome). J. Bone Jt Surg. 56 A, 1338–1348 (1974)
106. Peltier, L.: A few remarks on fat embolism. J. Trauma 8, 812–841 (1968)
107. Petty, T. L., Ashbaugh, D. G.: The adult respiratory distress syndrome. Chest 60, 233–239 (1971)
108. Pontoppidan, H., Laver, M. B., Geffin, B.: Acute respiratory failure in the surgical patient. Advanc. Surg. 4, 163–254 (1970)
109. Pontoppidan, H., Geffin, B., Lowenstein, E.: Acute respiratory failure in the adult. New Engl. J. Med. 287, 690–698, 743–752, 799–806 (1972)
110. Proctor, H. J., Moss, G. S., Homer, L. D., Litt, B. D.: Changes in lung compliance in experimental hemorrhagic shock and resuscitation. Ann. Surg. 169, 82–92 (1969)
111. Powers, S. R., Mannal, R., Naclerio, M., English, M., Marr, C., Leather, R., Ueda, H., Williams, G., Custead, W., Dutton, R.: Physiologic consequences of positive end-expiratory pressure. Ann. Surg. 178, 265–272 (1973)
112. Remmele, W., Loew, D.: Pathophysiologie der Thrombocyten im Schock. Klin. Wschr. 51, 3–9 (1973)
113. Riedl, K., Wolff, G., Grädel, E., Hasse, J.: Der Aussagewert der arteriovenösen Sauerstoffdifferenz bei venöser Blutentnahme aus der V. cava superior oder dem rechten Vorhof. Helv. chir. Acta 39, 577–582 (1972)
114. Richman, H., Abramson, S. F.: Mendelson's syndrome: diagnosis, therapy, and prevention. Amer. J. Surg. 120, 531–536 (1972)
115. Rittmann, W. W., Gruber, U. F.: Die pathophysiologischen Veränderungen der Lunge im Schock. Langenbecks Arch. Chir. 329, 640–657 (1971)
116. Robertson, W. G., Hargreaves, J. J., Herlocher, J. E., Welch, B. E.: Physiologic responses to increased oxygen partial pressure. J. Aerospace Med. 36, 618 (1969)
117. Rodewald, G., Harms, H.: Pathophysiologie und Spätschäden nach Thoraxverletzungen. Thoraxchirurgie 12, 93–103 (1964)
118. Safar, P., Greuvik, A., Smith, J.: Progressive pulmonary consolidation: Review of cases and pathogenesis. J. Trauma 12, 955–967 (1972)
119. Sanders, C. A., Harthorne, J. W., Heitman, H., Laver, M. B.: Effect of vasopressor administration on blood-gas exchange in mitral disease. Clin. Res. 13, 351 (1965)
120. Schulz, H.: Elektronenmikroskopische Grundlagen bei Hyperoxie. Pneumologie 149, 181–192 (1973)

121. Smith, D. E., Virgilio, R. W., Trimble, C., Fosburg, R. G.: Comparison of venous sampling sites for intrapulmonary shunt determinations in the critically ill patient. J. surg. Res. **14**, 319–330 (1973)
122. Smith, J. L.: The pathological effects due to increased oxygen tension in the air breathed. J. Physiol. (Lond.) **24**, 19 (1899)
123. Starling, E. H.: On the absorption of fluids from the connective tissue spaces. J. Physiol. (Lond.) **19**, 312 (1896)
124. Steinbereithner, K., Kucher, R.: Schädel-Hirntrauma, Hirnödem, In: Kucher, R., Steinbereithner, K. (Hrsg.): Intensivstation, -pflege, -therapie, S. 424. Stuttgart: Thieme 1972
125. Stephenson, S. F.: The pathophysiology of smoke inhalation injury. Ann. Surg. **182**, 652–660 (1975)
126. Sugerman, H. J., Olofsson, K. B., Pollock, T. W., Agnew, R. F., Rogers, R. M., Miller, L. D.: Continuous positive end-expiratory pressure ventilation (PEEP) for the treatment of diffuse interstitial pulmonary edema. J. Trauma **12**, 263–274 (1972)
127. Sugerman, H. J., Rogers, R. M., Miller, L. D.: Positive end-expiratory pressure (PEEP). Indications and physiologic considerations. Chest **62**, 86–94 (1972)
128. Swank, R. L.: Alteration of blood on storage: Measurement of adhesiveness of "aging" platelets and leukocytes and their removal by filtration. New Engl. J. Med. **265**, 728–733 (1961)
129. Swank, R. L.: Pulmonary microembolism after blood transfusions: An electron microscopic study. Ann. Surg. **177**, 40–50 (1973)
130. Teplitz, C.: The ultrastructural basis for pulmonary pathophysiology following trauma. Pathogenesis of pulmonary edema. J. Trauma **8**, 700–713 (1968)
131. Uzawa, T., Ashbaugh, D. G.: Continuous positive-pressure breathing in acute hemorrhagic pulmonary edema. J. appl. Physiol. **26**, 427–432 (1969)
132. Van de Water, J. M., Sheh, J. M., O'Connor, N. E., Miller, I. T., Milne, E. N. C.: Pulmonary extravascular water volume: Measurement and significance in critically ill patients. J. Trauma **10**, 440–449 (1970)
133. Van de Water, J. M., Kagey, K S., Miller, I. T., Parker, D. A., O'Connor, N. E., Sheh, J. M., McArthur, J. D., Zollinger, R. M., Moore, F. D.: Response of the lung to 6–12 hours of 100 per cent oxygen inhalation in normal man. New Engl. J. Med. **283**, 621–626 (1970)
134. von Euler, U. S., Liljestrand, G.: Observations on the pulmonary arterial blood pressure in the cat. Acta physiol. scand. **12**, 301 (1946)
135. Ward, H. N., Lipscomb, T. S., Cowley, L. P.: Pulmonary hypersensitivity reaction after blood transfusion. Arch. intern. Med. **122**, 362–366 (1968)
136. Webb, W. R.: Pulmonary complications of nonthoracic trauma: Summary of the national research council conference. J. Trauma **9**, 700–711 (1969)
137. West, J. B.: Regional differences in blood flow and ventilation in the lung. In: C. G. Caro (Ed.): Advances in respiratory physiology, p. 198. London: Edward Arnold 1966
138. Wiemers, K., Scholler, K. L. (Hrsg.): Lungenveränderungen bei Langzeitbeatmung. Intern. Symposium Freiburg 1971. Stuttgart: Thieme 1973
139. Wilson, R. F., Kafi, A., Asuncion, Z., Walt, A. J.: Clinical respiratory failure after shock or trauma. Arch. Surg. **98**, 539–550 (1969)
140. Wilson, J. W.: Treatment or prevention of pulmonary cellular damage with pharmacologic doses of corticosteroid. Surg. Gynec. Obstet. **134**, 675–681 (1972)
141. Wolff, G., Dittmann, M., Claudi, B., Pochon, J. P.: Früherkennung von Gasaustauschstörungen. In: Buff, H. U., Glinz, W. (Hrsg.): Respiratorische Insuffizienz beim Mehrfachverletzten, S. 137–149. Erlangen: Perimed 1976
142. Zapol, W. M.: Membrane lung perfusion for acute respiratory failure. Surg. Clin. N. Amer. **55**, 603–612 (1975)
143. Zimmerman, J. E.: Respiratory failure complicating post-traumatic acute renal failure. Ann. Surg. **174**, 12–18 (1971)
144. Zimmermann, W. E., Walter, F., Vogel, W., Mittermayer, C.: Funktionell-klinische Untersuchungen der Lunge im Schock. Langenbecks Arch. Chir. **329**, 671–681 (1971)

Chapter 5 Indications for Operation in Blunt Thoracic Trauma

Chapter 6 Operative Approaches

145. Boyd, T. F., Strieder, J. W.: Immediate surgery for traumatic heart disease. J. thorac. cardiovasc. Surg. **50**, 305–315 (1965)
146. Bricker, D. L., Noon, G. P., Beall, A. C., Jr., De Bakey, M. E.: Vascular injuries of the thoracic outlet. J. Trauma **10**, 1–15 (1970)
147. Brigand, H. le: Evolution du traitement des traumatismes graves du thorax. J. Chir. (Paris) **110**, 451–476 (1975)
148. Dobell, A. R. C.: Thoracic incisions. In: Sabiston, D. C., Spencer, F. C. (Eds.): Gibbon's surgery of the chest, 3. Aufl., pp. 146–159. Philadelphia-London-Toronto: Saunders 1976
149. Dor, V., Ohresser, Ph., Leonardelli, M.: La place de la thoracotomie dans les grands traumatismes fermés du thorax. Lyon chir. **65**, 607–616 (1969)
150. Naclerio, E. A.: Chest injuries. New York-London: Grune and Stratton 1971
151. Steenburg, R. W., Ravitch, M. M.: Cervicothoracic approach for subclavian vessel injury from compound fracture of the clavicle; considerations of subclavian-axillary exposures. Ann. Surg. **157**, 839–846 (1963)
152. Webb, W. R.: Thoracic trauma. Surg. Clin. N. Amer. **54**, 1179–1192 (1974)

Chapter 7 Special Considerations in Penetrating Chest Injuries

153. Amato, J. J., Billy, L. J., Gruber, R. P., Rich, N. M.: Temporary cavitation in high-velocity pulmonary missile injury. Ann. thorac. Surg. **18**, 565–570 (1974)
154. Babichev, S. I., Briskin, B. S., Plaksin, L. N., Bryunin, V. G.: Civil penetrating chest wounds and their treatment. Chirurgia, Moskva **8**, 29–34 (1974)
155. Beall, A. C., Jr., Bricker, D. L., Crawford, H. W., De Bakey, M. E.: Surgical management of penetrating thoracic trauma. Dis. Chest **49**, 568–577 (1966)
156. Borja, A. R., Ransdell, H. T.: Treatment of penetrating gunshot wounds of the chest. Experience with one hundred forty-five cases. Amer. J. Surg. **122**, 81–84 (1971)
157. Borja, A. R., Ransdell, H. T.: Treatment of thoracoabdominal gunshot wounds in civilian practice. Experience with forty-four cases. Amer. J. Surg. **121**, 580–583 (1971)
158. Burke, J., Jacobs, Th. T.: Penetrating wounds of the chest. Ann. Surg. **123**, 363–376 (1946)
159. D'Abreu, A. L.: Experience of thoracic surgery gained in the central mediterranean theatre of war. In: Cope, Z. (Ed.): History of the second world war. Surgery. London: Her Majesty's Stationary Office 1953
160. Daniel, R. A., Jr.: Bullet wounds of the lungs: An experimental study. Surgery **15**, 744–782 (1944)
161. De Muth, W. E., Jr.: Bullet velocity as applied to military rifle wounding capacity. J. Trauma **9**, 27–38 (1969)
162. De Muth, W. E., Jr.: High velocity bullet wounds of the thorax. Amer. J. Surg. **115**, 616–625 (1968)
163. Fischer, R. P., Geiger, J. P., Guernsey, H.: Pulmonary resections for severe pulmonary contusions secondary to high-velocity missile wounds. J. Trauma **14**, 293–302 (1974)
164. Franke, H.: Dringliche Chirurgie der Brustwand- und Lungenschußverletzungen. Chirurg **14**, 428–432 (1942)
165. Ganzoni, N.: Die Schußverletzung im Krieg. Wesen, Behandlung, Prognose. Bern-Stuttgart-Wien: Huber 1975
166. Gray, A. R., Harrison, W. H., Couves, C. M., Howard, J. M.: Penetrating injuries to the chest. Clinical results in the management of 769 patients. Amer. J. Surg. **100**, 709–714 (1960)
167. Kirschner, M.: Die Steckschußverletzung. Chirurg **12**, 565–580 (1940)
168. Kolesov, A. P., Dyskin, E. A., Ozeretskovskii, L. B.: Mechanisms of injury in gunshot wounds of the lungs. Chirurgiya **5**, 54–59 (1975)
169. Levinsky, L., Vidne, B., Nudelman, I., Salomon, J., Kissin, L., Levy, M. J.: Thoracic injuries in the Yom Kippur war. Israel J. Med. Sci. **11**, 275–280 (1975)

170. Lichtmann, M. W.: The problem of contused lungs. J. Trauma **10**, 731–739 (1970)
171. McNamara, J. J., Messersmith, J. K., Dunn, R. A., Molot, M. D., Stremple, J. F.: Thoracic injuries in combat casualties in Vietnam. Ann. thorac. Surg. **10**, 389–401 (1970)
172. Mattila, S. P.: Penetrating chest injuries. Ann. Chir. Gynec. Fenn. **63**, 297–303 (1974)
173. Oglesby, J. E.: Twenty-two month's war surgery in Vietnam. Arch. Surg. **102**, 607–613 (1971)
174. Patterson, L. T., Schmitt, H. J., Armstrong, R. G.: Intermediate care of war wounds of the chest. J. thorac. cardiovasc. Surg. **55**, 16–23 (1968)
175. Robicsek, F., Sabbagh, A., Mullen, D. C., Daugherty, H. K., Perkins, R.: Immediate surgery in the management of penetrating chest injuries. A clinical experiment. J. cardiovasc. Surg. **13**, 156–159 (1972)
176. Rockey, E. E.: The case of thoracic and thoraco-abdominal wounds in the combat zone in Korea. J. thorac. cardiovasc. Surg. **24**, 436–456 (1952)
177. Romanoff, H.: Prevention of infections in war chest injuries. Ann. Surg. **182**, 144–149 (1975)
178. Valle, A. R.: An analysis of 2811 chest casualties of the Korean conflict. Dis. Chest **26**, 623–633 (1954)
179. Viikari, S., Mattila, S., Linna, M.: Stichverletzungen der Lunge und des Herzens. Zbl. Chir. **101**, 97–101 (1976)
180. Virgilio, R. W.: Intrathoracic wounds in battle casualties. Surg. Gynec. Obstet. **130**, 609–615 (1970)
181. Whelan, J. T., Burkhalter, W. E., Gomez, A.: Management of war wounds. Advanc. Surg. **3**, 227–350 (1968)
182. Winzeler, P.: Resultate der Behandlung von penetrierenden Thoraxverletzungen. Dissertation Zürich 1975
183. Zelder, O., Koch, H.: Schußverletzungen großer Körperhöhlen und des Schädels. Mschr. Unfallheilk. **75**, 168–179 (1972)
184. Zenker, R.: Die Erkennung und Behandlung der Schußverletzungen der Lunge und des Brustfells. Chirurg **14**, 129 (1942)
185. Zichner, L., Glinz, W.: Schußverletzungen im Thoraxbereich. Bruns' Beitr. klin. Chir. **221**, 25–34 (1974)

Chapter 8 Aspects of Intensive Care of Patients with Thoracic Injuries

186. Asbaugh, D. C., Peters, G. N., Halgrimson, C. G., Owens, J. C., Waddell, W. R.: Chest trauma: Analysis of 685 patients. Arch. Surg. **95**, 546–555 (1967)
187. Bendixen, H. H., Egbert, L. D., Hedley-Whyte, J., Laver, M. B., Pontoppidan, H.: Respiratory care. St. Louis: Mosby 1965
188. Boyd, D. R.: Monitoring patients with posttraumatic pulmonary insufficiency. Surg. Clin. N. Amer. **52**, 31–46 (1972)
189. Cloeren, S., Gigon, J. P., Hasse, J., Pusterla, C., Allgöwer, M.: Intensivtherapie bei Patienten mit Rippenserienfrakturen und Polytrauma. Thoraxchirurgie **20**, 1–11 (1972)
190. Dale, W. A., Rahn, H.: Rate of gas absorption during atelectasis. Amer. J. Physiol. **170**, 606–615 (1952)
191. Downs, J. B., Klein, E. F., Jr., Desautels, D.: Intermittent mandatory ventilation: A new approach to weaning patients from mechanical ventilators. Chest **64**, 331–335 (1973)
192. Glinz, W., Haldemann, G., Bronz, G.: Erfahrungen mit Dopamin beim Schwerverletzten. In: Hossli, G., Gattiker, R., Haldemann, G. (Hrsg.): Dopamin – Grundlagen und bisherige klinische Erfahrungen. Stuttgart: Thieme 1977
193. Gregory, G. A., Kitterman, J. A., Phibbs, R. H., Tooley, W. H., Hamilton, W. K.: Treatment of the idiopathic respiratory distress syndrome with continuous positive airway pressure. New Engl. J. Med. **284**, 1333–1340 (1971)
194. Horisberger, B.: Pulmonale Infekte nach Verletzungen. In: Buff, H. U., Glinz, W. (Hrsg.): Respiratorische Insuffizienz beim Mehrfachverletzten, S. 125–128. Erlangen: Perimed 1976
195. Hossli, G., Frey, P.: Beatmungsprobleme bei Thoraxverletzungen. Acta chir. Aust. **1**, 81–86 (1969)

196. Kanz, E.: Die Problematik der Intensivbehandlung aus der Sicht des Krankenhaushygienikers. In: Opderbecke, H. W. (Hrsg.): Planung, Organisation und Einrichtung von Intensivbehandlungseinheiten am Krankenhaus. Anaesthesiologie und Wiederbelebung, Bd. 33, S. 45–52. Berlin-Heidelberg-New York: Springer 1969
197. Kucher, R., Steinbereithner, K. (Hrsg.): Intensiv-Station, -Pflege, -Therapie. Stuttgart: Thieme 1972
198. Laver, M. B.: Kardiorespiratorische Probleme in der Intensivpflege. Langenbecks Arch. Chir. 342, 331–340 (1976)
199. Lawin, P. (Hrsg.): Praxis der Intensivbehandlung. Stuttgart: Thieme 1971
200. Lenaghan, R., Silva, Y. J., Walt, A. J.: Hemodynamic alterations associated with expansion rupture of the lung. Arch. Surg. 99, 339–343 (1969)
201. Simmendinger, H.-J., Packschies, P.: Komplikationen bei der Intensivbehandlung des Thoraxtraumas. Prakt. Anästh. 9, 343–351 (1974)
202. Steier, M., Ching, N., Roberts, E. B., Nealon, T. F.: Pneumothorax complicating continuous ventilatory support. J. thorac. cardiovasc. Surg. 67, 17–23 (1974)
203. Swan, H. J. C., Ganz, W.: Use of balloon flotation catheters in patients. Surg. Clin. N. Amer. 55, 501–520 (1975)
204. Tietjen, G. W., Gump, F. E., Kinney, J. M.: Cardiac output determinations in surgical patients. Surg. Clin. N. Amer. 55, 521–529 (1975)
205. Wolff, G.: Die künstliche Beatmung auf Intensivstationen. Berlin-Heidelberg-New York: Springer 1975
206. Zschoche, D. A. (Ed.): Comprehensive review of critical care. St. Louis: Mosby 1976
207. Zwillich, C. W., Pierson, D. J., Creagh, C. E., Sutton, F. D., Schatz, E., Petty, T. L.: Complications of assisted ventilation; a prospective study of 354 consecutive episodes. Amer. J. Med. 57, 161–170 (1974)

Chapter 9 Physiotherapy of Patients with Thoracic Injuries

208. Bartlett, R. H., Krop, R. H., Hanson, E. L.: Physiology of yawning and its application to postoperative care. Surg. Forum 21, 222–225 (1970)
209. Bartlett, R. H., Gazzaniga, A. B., Geraghty, T.: The yawn maneuver: Prevention and treatment of postoperative pulmonary complications. Surg. Forum 22, 196–198 (1971)
210. Baxter, W. D., Levine, R. S.: An evaluation of intermittent positive pressure breathing in the prevention of postoperative pulmonary complications. Arch. Surg. 98, 795–798 (1969)
211. Bendixen, H. H., Egbert, L. D., Hedley-Whyte, J., Laver, M. B., Pontoppidan, H.: Chest physical therapy. In: Respiratory care, pp. 93–103. St. Louis: Mosby 1965
212. Darin, J. C., Close, A. S., Ellison, E. H.: The value of a rebreathing tube in the prevention of postoperative atelectasis. Arch. Surg. 81, 263–268 (1960)
213. Fasol, P., Benzer, H., Haider, W., Lackner, F., Politzer, P., Stöger, A.: Die Therapie der Atemstörung beim schweren Thoraxtrauma. Anaesthesist 24, 367–371 (1975)
214. Giebel, P.: Der Einfluß künstlicher Totraumvergrößerung auf Ventilation und Blutgase. Langenbecks Arch. Chir. 301, 543–548 (1962)
215. Giebel, O., Horatz, K.: Die Anwendung künstlicher Totraumvergrößerung zur Behandlung von Atelektasen. Bruns' Beitr. klin. Chir. 214, 375–381 (1967)
216. Noehren, T. H., Lasry, J. E., Legters, L. J.: Intermittent positive pressure breathing (IPPB/I) for the prevention and management of postoperative pulmonary complications. Surgery 43, 658–665 (1958)
217. Rudy, N. E., Crepeau, J.: Role of intermittent positive pressure breathing postoperatively. J. Amer. med. Ass. 167, 1093–1096 (1958)
218. Schwartz, S. I., Dale, W. Z., Rahn, H.: Dead-space rebreathing tube for prevention of atelectasis. J. Amer. med. Ass. 163, 1248–1251 (1957)
219. Thoren, L.: Postoperative pulmonary complications. Observations on their prevention by means of physio-therapy. Acta chir. scand. 107, 193–205 (1954)
220. Van de Water, J. M., Watring, W. G., Linton, L. A., Murphy, A., Byron, R. L.: Prevention of postoperative pulmonary complications. Surg. Gynec. Obstet. 135, 229–233 (1972)

221. Ward, R. J., Danziger, F., Bonica, J. J., Allen, G. G., Bowers, J.: An evaluation of postoperative respiratory maneuvers. Surg. Gynec. Obstet. **123**, 51–54 (1966)

Chapter 10 Rib and Sternum Fractures

222. Aigner, P. W.: Rippenosteosynthese bei instabilem Thorax nach Trauma. Münch. med. Wschr. **118**, 171–172 (1976)
223. Adkins, P. C., Diller, M. D., Groff, B., Blades, B.: Experiences with metal struts for chest wall stabilization. Ann. thorac. Surg. **5**, 246–254 (1968)
224. Avery, E. E., Mörch, E. T., Benson, D. W.: Critically crushed chests; a new method of treatment and continuous mechanical hyperventilation to produce alkalotic apnea and internal pneumatic stabilization. J. thorac. Surg. **32**, 291–311 (1956)
225. Bartel, M., Wilde, J.: Klinische und differentialdiagnostische Betrachtungen bei Frakturen der ersten Rippe. Mschr. Unfallheilk. **70**, 248–257 (1967)
226. Brauer, L.: Erfahrungen und Überlegungen zur Lungenkollapstherapie. Beitr. Klin. Tuberk. **12**, 49–154 (1909)
227. Brunner, H., Hoffmeister, E., Koncz, J.: Stabilisierende Eingriffe am Thorax bei Trichterbrustkorrekturen und Verletzungen des knöchernen Brustkorbes. Med. Klin. **59**, 515–521 (1964)
228. Bryant, L. R., Trinkle, J. K., Wood, R. E.: A technique for intercostal nerve block after thoracotomy. Ann. thorac. Surg. **11**, 388–391 (1971)
229. Carlisle, B. B., Sutton, J. P., Stephenson, S. E.: New technic for stabilization for the flail chest. Amer. J. Surg. **112**, 133–135 (1966)
230. Chadenson, O., Cros, O., Liaras, A., Brunet, E., Tairraz, J. P., Neidhardt, J. H.: Reflexions sur le traitement de 102 volets thoraciques mobiles. Lyon méd. **225**, 425–435 (1971)
231. Constantinescu, O.: Zur Behandlung der Rippenserienfraktur. Zbl. Chir. **90**, 2160–2162 (1965)
232. Couraud, L., Bruneteau, A., Duraudeau A.: Volets thoraciques; Indication therapeutiques en fonction de leur siège et du contexte clinique. Ann. chir. thorac. cardio-vasc. **12**, 15–18 (1973)
233. Cullen, Ph., Modell, J. H., Kirby, R. R., Klein, E. F., Long, W.: Treatment of flail chest. Arch. Surg. **110**, 1099–1103 (1975)
234. Delaye, A., Mètras, D., Amoros, J. F., Malmejac, C.: Traitement des volets thoraciques. A propos de 53 observations. Ann. chir. **27**, 353–356 (1973)
235. Dittmann, M., Ferstl., A., Wolff, G.: Epidural analgesia for the treatment of multiple rib fractures. Europ. J. Intensive Care Med. **1**, 71–75 (1975)
236. Dor, V., Noirclerc, M., Chauvin, G., Mermet, B., Kreitmann, P., Leonardelli, M., Amoros, J. F.: Les traumatismes graves du thorax. Place de l'ostéosynthèse dans leur traitement. A propos de 100 cas. Nouv. presse méd. **1**, 519–524 (1972)
237. Drewes, J., Konrad, R. M., Schulte, H. D.: Rippenserienfrakturen und ihre Behandlung. Mschr. Unfallheilk. **70**, 110–124 (1967)
238. Duff, J. H., Goldstein, M., McLean, A. P., Agrawala, A. L.: Flail chest: A clinical review and physiological study. J. Trauma **8**, 63–74 (1968)
239. Ebbell, B.: Die alt-ägyptische Chirurgie. Die chirurgischen Abschnitte der Papyrus E. Smith und Papyrus Ebers. Skrifter Det Norske Videnskaps-Akademi, Oslo. Oslo: J. Dybwad 1939
240. Eschapasse, H., Gaillard, J.: Volets thoracic traumatiques. Rev. chir. orthop. **59**, suppl. 1, 302–311 (1973)
241. Gaillard, J. Henry, E., Fournial, G., Berthoumien, F., Eschapasse, H.: Indication de l'ostéosynthèse et de la suspension sternale dans les volets thoraciques mobiles. In: Buff, H. U., Glinz, W. (Hrsg.): Respiratorische Insuffizienz bei Mehrfachverletzten, S. 49–54. Erlangen: Perimed 1976
242. Garzon, A. A., Seltzer, B., Karlson, K. E.: Physiopathology of crushed chest injuries. Ann. Surg. **168**, 128–136 (1968)
243. Gibbons, J., James, O., Quail, A.: Management of 130 cases of chest injuries with respiratory failure. Brit. J. Anaesth. **45**, 1130–1135 (1973)

244. Gibbons, J., James, O., Quail, A.: Relief of pain in chest injury. Brit. J. Anaesth. **45**, 1136–1138 (1973)
245. Gibson, L. D., Carter, R., Hinshaw, D. B.: Surgical significance of sternal fracture. Surg. Gynec. Obstet. **114**, 443–448 (1962)
246. Handley, R. S.: A case of multiple thoracic injuries in Roman Britain. Brit. J. Surg. **25**, 461–464 (1938)
247. Holmes, T. W., Netterville, R. E.: Complications of first rib fracture. Including one case each of tracheooesophageal fistula and aortic arch aneurysm. J. thorac. Surg. **32**, 74–91 (1956)
248. Hoyer, J.: Rippenosteosynthese bei instabilem Thorax. Actuelle Chir. **8**, 87–94 (1973)
249. Jensen, N. K.: Recovery of pulmonary function after crushing injuries of the chest. Dis. Chest **22**, 319–343 (1952)
250. Jones, D.: Bilateral fracture of the first rib with bilateral pneumothorax. Injury **5**, 255–256 (1973)
251. Judet, R.: Ostéosynthèse costale. Rev. chir. orthop. **59**, suppl. 1, 334–335 (1973)
252. Keen, G.: Chest injuries. Bristol: Wright 1975
253. Kessler, E.: Eine einfache Operationsmethode zur Versorgung ausgedehnter Thoraxwandbrüche. Hefte Unfallheilk. **121**, 187–191 (1975)
254. Klammer, H.-L., Straaten, G., Aigner, P. W., Kliems, G.: Zuggurtungsosteosynthese des Sternums bei instabiler Thoraxwand. In: Buff, H. U., Glinz, W. (Hrsg.): Respiratorische Insuffizienz bei Mehrfachverletzten, S. 41–48. Erlangen: Perimed 1976
255. Kolb, E., Eckart, J., Tempel, G., Jelen, S.: Die Behandlung des traumatisch bedingten instabilen Thorax durch Dauerbeatmung. Mschr. Unfallheilk. **77**, 231–240 (1974)
256. Maloney, J. V., Jr., Schmutzer, K. J., Raschke, E.: Paradoxical respiration and "pendelluft". J. thorac. cardiovasc. Surg. **41**, 291–298 (1961)
257. Mattila, S. P., Kostianen, S., Korhola, O., Rilhimäki, E., Tähti, E.: Ventilation and pulmonary blood flow after blunt chest injury. Ann. Chir. Gynaec. Fenn. **63**, 292–396 (1974)
258. Moore, B. P.: Operative stabilization of nonpenetrating chest injuries. J. thorac. cardiovasc. Surg. **70**, 619–630 (1975)
259. Mulder, D. S., Greenwood, F. A. H., Brooks, C. E.: Posttraumatic thoracic outlet syndrome. J. Trauma **13**, 706–715 (1973)
260. Paris, F., Tarazona, V., Blasco, E., Canto, A., Casillas, M., Pastor, J., Paris, M., Montero, R.: Surgical stabilization of traumatic flail chest. Thorax **30**, 521–527 (1975)
261. Pierce, G. E., Maxwell, J. A., Boggan, M. D.: Special hazards of first rib fractures. J. Trauma **15**, 264–268 (1975)
262. Ransdell, H. T., McPherson, R. C., Haller, J. A., Williams, D. J., Conner, E. H.: Treatment of flail chest injuries with a piston respirator. Amer. J. Surg. **104**, 22–26 (1962)
263. Regensburger, D., Brunner, L., Hoffmeister, H. E., Stapenhorst, K.: Stabilisierende Eingriffe am Thorax nach schweren Thoraxtraumen. Mschr. Unfallheilk. **73**, 357–366 (1970)
264. Rehn, J., Hierholzer, G., Kayser, W.: Die Verletzungen der Brustwand und der Lunge. Mschr. Unfallheilk. **73**, 307–320 (1970)
265. Richardson, J. D., McElvein, R. B., Trinkle, J. K.: First rib fracture: A hallmark of severe trauma. Ann. Surg. **181**, 251–254 (1975)
266. Rutherford, R. B., Gott, V. L.: Thoracic injuries. In: Ballinger, W. F., Rutherford, R. B., Zuidema, G. D. (Eds.): The management of trauma, pp. 285–344. Philadelphia-London: Saunders 1968
267. Scholler, K. L., Vogel, W., Wiemers, K., Burchardi, H., Groh-Bruch, J.: Die Langzeitbeatmung in der Behandlung von Thoraxverletzten. Dtsch. med. Wschr. **93**, 747–753 (1968)
268. Schüpbach, P., Meier, P.: Indikationen zur Rekonstruktion des instabilen Thorax bei Rippenserienfrakturen und Ateminsuffizienz. Helv. chir. Acta **43**, 497–502 (1976)
269. Sinigaglia, C. M.: Il trattamento del volet costale. In: Staudacher, V. (Hrsg.): Chirurgia generale d'urgenza, pp. 242–243. Padova: Piccin 1975
270. Sladen, A., Aldredge, C. F., Albrarran, R.: PEEP vs. ZEEP in the treatment of flail chest injuries. Critical Care Med. **1**, 187–190 (1973)
271. Stoianov, I.: Neue Methode zur mechanischen Stabilisierung von Rippenfrakturen (Bulg.). Chirurgija (Sofia) **27**, 163–166 (1974)
272. Sulamaa, M., Wallgreen, E. I.: Trichterbrust. Operationsmethode und Spätergebnisse. Z. Kinderchir. **8**, 22–30 (1970)

273. Tiegel, M.: Behandlung mehrfacher Rippenbrüche mit einer anmodellierten Gipsplatte. Zbl. Chir. **63**, 242–244 (1936)
274. Trinkle, J. K., Richardson, J. D., Franz, J. L., Grover, F. L., Arom, K. V.: Management of flail chest without mechanical ventilation. Ann. thorac. Surg. **19**, 355–363 (1975)

Chapter 11 Pneumothorax and Hemothorax

275. Beall, A. C., Crawford, H. W., DeBakey, M. E.: Considerations in the management of acute traumatic hemothorax. J. thorac. cardiovasc. Surg. **52**, 351–360 (1966)
276. Brown, R. B., Boyd, S. A.: Thoracostomy versus thoracentesis for the initial drainage of traumatic hemothorax and hemopneumothorax. U.S. armed Forces med. J. **3**, 557–560 (1952)
277. Bülau, G.: Für die Heber-Drainage bei Behandlung des Empyems. Z. klin. Med. **18**, 31–45 (1891)
278. Burri, C., Gasser, D.: Der Vena-cava-Katheter. Berlin-Heidelberg-New York: Springer 1971
279. Carey, J. S., Hughes, R. K.: Hemodynamic studies in open pneumothorax. J. thorac. cardiovasc. Surg. **55**, 538–545 (1968)
280. Carlson, R. J., Klassen, K. L., Gollan, F., Gobbel, W. G., Jr., Sherman, D. E., Christensen, R. O.: Pulmonary oedema following the rapid re-expansion of a totally collapsed lung due to a pneumothorax: A clinical and experimental study. Surg. Forum. **9**, 367–371 (1958)
281. Cordice, J. W. V., Cabezon, J.: Chest trauma with pneumothorax and hemothorax. J. thorac. cardiovasc. Surg. **50**, 316–338 (1965)
282. Creech, O., Jr., DeBakey, M. E., Amspacher, W. H., Mahaffey, D. E.: The intrathoracic use of streptokinase-streptodornase. Amer. Surg. **19**, 128–147 (1953)
283. Culiner, M. M., Roe, B. B., Grimes, O. F.: The early elective surgical approach to the treatment of traumatic hemothorax. J. thorac. cardiovasc. Surg. **38**, 780–797 (1959)
284. Emerson, C. P.: Pneumothorax; a historical, clinical, and experimental study. Johns Hopk. Hosp. Rep. **11**, 1–450 (1903)
285. Fry, W. A., Adams, W. E.: Thoracic emergencies. Indications for closed tube drainage and early open thoracotomy. Arch. Surg. **94**, 532–538 (1967)
286. Heimlich, H. J.: Heimlich flutter valve: Effective replacement for drainage bottle. Hosp. Topics **43**, 122–123 (1965)
287. Humphreys, R. L., Berne, A. S.: Rapid re-expansion of pneumothorax a cause of unilateral pulmonary edema. Radiology **96**, 509–512 (1970)
288. Maloney, J. V.: The conservative management of traumatic hemothorax. Amer. J. Surg. **93**, 533–539 (1957)
289. Middendorp, U. G., Bachmann, O.: Zur Anwendung des Thoraxdrainageventils von H. J. Heimlich. Helv. chir. Acta **37**, 66–68 (1970)
290. Miller, W. C., Toon, R., Palat, H., Lacroix, J.: Experimental pulmonary edema following re-expansion of pneumothorax. Amer. Rev. resp. Dis. **108**, 664–666 (1973)
291. Nissen, R.: Erlebtes aus der Thoraxchirurgie. Stuttgart: Thieme 1955.
292. Rathke, L.: Die Erstversorgung des Hämatothorax und des offenen Pneumothorax. Chirurg **20**, 105–113 (1949)
293. Roy-Camille, R., Beurier, J., Martignon, M., Saillant, G., Berteaux, D.: Les épanchements intra-thoraciques associés aux fractures du rachis dorsal. In: Buff, H. U., Glinz, W. (Hrsg.): Respiratorische Insuffizienz bei Mehrfachverletzten, S. 37–39. Erlangen: Perimed 1976
294. Rutherford, R. B., Hurt, H. H., Brickman, R. D., Tubb, J. M.: The pathophysiology of progressive tension pneumothorax. J. Trauma **8**, 212–227 (1968)
295. Schulte am Esch, J., Vlajic, I., Pfeifer, G., Wappenschmidt, J.: Mediastinal- und Pleuraerguß als Folge frischer Frakturen der Brustwirbelsäule. Chirurg **46**, 36–40 (1975)
296. Schwander, D., Schwander, A., Senn, A.: Oedème pulmonaire aigu unilatéral après drainage d'un pneumothorax. Helv. chir. Acta **40**, 393–403 (1973)

297. Sturm, J. T.: Hemopneumothorax following blunt trauma of the thorax. Surg. Gynec. Obstet. **141**, 539–540 (1975)
298. Tillet, W. S., Sherry, S.: The effect in patients of streptococcal fibrinolysin (streptokinase) and streptococcal desoxyribonuclease on fibrinous, purulent and sanguineous pleural exudations. J. clin. Invest. **28**, 173–190 (1949)
299. Waqarudin, M., Bernstein, A.: Re-expansion pulmonary oedema. Thorax **30**, 54–60 (1975)
300. Whelan, Th. J., Jr., Burkhalter, W. E., Gomez, A.: Management of war wounds. Advanc. Surg. **3**, 227–350 (1968)

Chapter 12 Traumatic Emphysema

301. Hamman, L.: Mediastinal emphysema: The Frank Billings Lecture. J. Amer. med. Ass. **128**, 1–6 (1945)
302. Jehn, W., Nissen, R.: Pathologie und Klinik des Mediastinalemphysems. Dtsch. Z. Chir. **206**, 221–245 (1927)
303. Portmann, J., Mussgang, G.: Das traumatische Pneumomediastinum. Mschr. Unfallheilk. **66**, 244–247 (1963)
304. Munsell, W. P.: Pneumomediastinum. A report of 28 cases and review of the literature. J. Amer. med. Ass. **202**, 689–693 (1967)
305. Nissen, R.: Die chirurgische Behandlung des bedrohlichen Mediastinalemphysems. Zbl. Chir. **57**, 1023–1025 (1930)
306. Sauerbruch, F.: Die Bedeutung des Mediastinalemphysems in der Pathologie des Spannungspneumothorax. Bruns' Beitr. klin. Chir. **60**, 450–478 (1908)

Chapter 13 Lung Injuries from Blunt Trauma

307. Bernhard, A.: Das stumpfe Lungentrauma. Langenbecks Arch. Chir. **329**, 201–208 (1971)
308. Clemedson, C.-J., Hultman, H. I.: Air embolism and the cause of death in blast injury. Milit. Surg. **114**, 424–437 (1954)
309. Clemedson, C.-J.: Blast injury. Physiol. Rev. **36**, 336–354 (1956)
310. Clemedson, C.-J., Jönsson, A.: Dynamic response of chest wall and lung injuries in rabbits exposed to air shock waves of short duration. Acta physiol. scand. **62**, Suppl. 233 (1964)
311. Cooke, W. E.: Traumatic rupture of the lungs without signs of trauma in the chest wall. Brit. med. J. **1934 II**, 629–630
312. Chevrel, J. P., Arnalsteen, Ch.: Considérations sur le traitement des traumatismes graves du poumon et du pédicule pulmonaire. J. Chir. (Paris) **106**, 249–256 (1973)
313. De Muth, W. E., Jr., Smith, J. M.: Pulmonary contusion. Amer. J. Surg. **109**, 819–823 (1965)
314. Desaga, H.: Blast injuries. German aviation medicine, world war II. Vol. 2, p. 1274, Department of the Air Force 1950
315. Diller, W. F., Endrei, E.: Posttraumatische Rundherde der Lunge. Fortschr. Röntgenstr. **96**, 364–370 (1962)
316. Dingsør, N. G., Grønmark, T.: Traumatic cyst of the lung. Injury **6**, 241–243 (1975)
317. Errion, A. R., Houk, V. N., Kettering, D. L.: Pulmonary hematoma due to blunt nonpenetrating thoracic trauma. Amer. Rev. resp. Dis. **88**, 384–392 (1963)
318. Fallon, M.: Lung injury in the intact thorax. Brit. J. Surg. **28**, 39–49 (1970)
319. Fischer, E.: Lungenrupturen bei intaktem Thorax. Diss. Zürich 1912
320. Franz, J. L., Richardson, J. D., Grover, F. L., Trinkle, J. K.: Effect of methylprednisolone sodium succinate on experimental pulmonary contusion. J. thorac. cardiovasc. Surg. **68**, 842–844 (1974)
321. Fulton, R. L., Peter, E. T., Wilson, J. N.: The pathophysiology and treatment of pulmonary contusions. J. Trauma **10**, 719–730 (1970)

322. Fulton, R. L., Peter, E. T.: The progressive nature of pulmonary contusion. Surgery **67**, 499–506 (1970)
323. Fulton, R. L., Peter, E. T.: Compositional and histologic effects of fluid therapy following pulmonary contusion. J. Trauma **14**, 783–790 (1974)
324. Garzon, A. A., Becker, W. H., Lyons, H. A., Karlson, K. E.: Effect of chest trauma upon respiratory function. J. Trauma **5**, 404–410 (1965)
325. Gullotta, U., Wenzl, H.: Posttraumatische Lungenhämatome und Pneumatozelen. Fortschr. Röntgenstr. **121**, 35–42 (1974)
326. Hambach, R.: Nil nocere! Lungenschäden nach intensiver Infusions- und Sauerstoffbehandlung. Münch. med. Wschr. **108**, 424–426 (1966)
327. Hooker, D. R.: Physiological effects of air concussion. Amer. J. Physiol. **67**, 219–274 (1923–1924)
328. Huller, T., Bazini, Y.: Blast injuries of the chest and abdomen. Arch. Surg. **100**, 24–30 (1970)
329. Middendorp, U. G., Marty, A.: Traumatische Pneumatozele und zentrale Lungenruptur bei stumpfem Thoraxtrauma. Helv. chir. Acta **39**, 149–156 (1972)
330. Milne, E., Dick, A.: Circumscribed intrapulmonary hematoma. Brit. J. Radiol. **34**, 587–595 (1961)
331. Morgagni, G. B.: De sedibus et causis morborum. Venetiis 1761, Lib. IV: De morbis chirurgicis et universalibus. Epist. anatom. medica LIII: De vulneribus et ictibus colli, pectoris et dorsi. Artic. XXXI–XXXIII.
332. Nichols, R. T., Pearce, II. J., Greenfiel, L. J.: Effects of experimental pulmonary contusion on respiratory exchange and lung mechanics. Arch. Surg. **96**, 723–730 (1968)
333. Ratliff, J. L., Fletcher, J. R., Kopriva, Ch. J., Atkins, C., Aussem, J. W.: Pulmonary contusion. J. thorac. cardiovasc. Surg. **62**, 638–644 (1971)
334. Ribet, M.: Les lésions broncho-pulmonaires. Rev. Chir. orthop. **59**, 312–323 (1973)
335. Roscher, R.: Die stumpfe Lungenverletzung (Lungenkontusion). Dtsch. med. Wschr. **99**, 1013–1016 (1974)
336. Schardin, H.: The physical principles of the effects of detonation. In: German aviation medicine world war II. Vol. 2, pp. 1207–1224. Washington/DC: Government printing office 1950
337. Schwartz, A., Dreyfuss, P.: Des ruptures du poumon sans fracture de côte. Rev. chir. (Paris) **35**, 764–783 (1907)
338. Streicher, H. J.: Lungenverschattungen nach Thoraxkontusionen. H. Unfallheilk. **94**, 95–98 (1968)
339. Trinkle, J. K., Furman, R. W., Hinshaw, M. A., Bryant, L. R., Griffen, W. O.: Pulmonary contusion – pathogenesis and effect of various resuscitative measures. Ann. thorac. Surg. **16**, 568–573 (1973)
340. Valenta, J.: Respiratory insufficiency following lung contusion: An experimental study. Acta Univ. Carol. Med. (Praha) **19**, 295–341 (1973)
341. White, C. S., Richmond, D. R.: Blast biology. US Atomic Energy Commission Report, Tid –5764, 1959
342. Williams, J. R.: The vanishing lung tumor. Pulmonary hematoma. Amer. J. Roentgenol. **81**, 296–302 (1959)
343. Wilson, J. V., Turbridge, R. D.: Pathological findings in a series of blast injuries. Lancet **1943 I**, 257–261
344. Zuckerman, S.: Experimental study of blast injuries to the lungs. Lancet **1940 II**, 219–224
345. Zumtobel, V., Standfuss, H., Haffner, G.: Die Bedeutung der Lungenkontusion für die Prognose des Kombinationstraumas. Langenbecks Arch. Chir. **329**, 210 (1971)

Chapter 14 Tracheal and Bronchial Injuries

346. Biermer, A.: Casuistische Mitteilungen aus der medicinischen Klinik des Inselspitales. II. Über Pneumothorax. Schweiz. Z. Heilk. **2**, 150–162 (1863)
347. Bishop, C. O., Miller, A. C., Burch, B. H.: Fracture of the bronchial tree following blunt chest trauma. West. J. Surg. **68**, 345–349 (1960)

348. Burke, J. F.: Early diagnosis of traumatic rupture of the bronchus. J. Amer. med. Ass. **181**, 682–686 (1962)
349. Carter, R., Warsham, E. E., Brewer, L. A.: Rupture of the bronchus following closed chest trauma. Amer. J. Surg. **104**, 177–195 (1962)
350. Ecker, R. R., Libertini, R. V., Rea, W. J., Sugg, W. L., Webb, W. R.: Injuries of the trachea and bronchi. Ann. thorac. Surg. **11**, 289–298 (1971)
351. Eijgelaar, A., Homan van der Heide, J. N.: A reliable early symptom of bronchial or tracheal rupture. Thorax **25**, 116–125 (1970)
352. Gebhardt, Ch., Höhmann, H., Hoffmann, E.: Intrathorakale Rupturen des Tracheobronchialsystems bei stumpfen Thoraxtraumen. Dtsch. med. Wschr. **97**, 1689–1693 (1972)
353. Griffith, J. L.: Traumatic fracture of the left main bronchus. Thorax **4**, 105–109 (1949)
354. Hood, R. M., Sloan, H. E.: Injuries of the trachea and major bronchi. J. thorac. cardiovasc. Surg. **38**, 458 (1959)
355. Krauss, H., Zimmermann, E.: Bronchusabriß. In: Engel, St., Heilmeyer, L., Hein, J., Uehlinger, E. (Hrsg.): Ergebnisse der gesamten Lungen- und Tuberkuloseforschung, Bd. 15, S. 1–37. Stuttgart: Thieme 1967
356. Krinitzki, Sch. I.: Zur Kasuistik einer vollständigen Zerreißung des rechten Luftröhrenastes. Virchows Arch. path. Anat. **266**, 815–819 (1927)
357. Mahaffey, D. E., Creech, O., Jr., Boren, H. G., DeBakey, M. E.: Traumatic rupture of the left main stem bronchus successfully repaired eleven years after injury. J. thorac. Surg. **32**, 312–331 (1956)
358. Neugebauer, M. K., Fine, J. B., Hoyt, T. W.: Traumatic rupture of the trachea and right main stem bronchus. J. Trauma **14**, 265–269 (1974)
359. Olson, R. O., Johnson, J. T.: Diagnosis and management of intrathoracic tracheal rupture. J. Trauma **11**, 789–792 (1971)
360. Samson, P. C.: In: Disk. Richards, V., Cohn, R. B.: Rupture of the thoracic trachea and major bronchi following closed injury to the chest. Amer. J. Surg. **90**, 253–261 (1955)
361. Sanger, P. W.: Evacuation hospital experiences with war wounds and injuries of the chest. A preliminary report. Ann. Surg. **122**, 147–162 (1945)
362. Schönberg, S.: Bronchialrupturen bei Thoraxkompression. Berl. klin. Wschr. **49**, 2218–2221 (1912)
363. Seuvre, M.: Encrasement par une roue d'omnibus: Rupture de la bronche droite. Bull. mem. Soc. Anat. Paris **48**, 680 (1873)
364. Seybold, W. D.: Closed intrathoracic ruptures of the trachea and bronchi. Arch. Surg. **81**, 453–478 (1960)
365. Sommelet, J., Boileau, F., Friot, J. M., Préaut, J.: Rupture totale sous-cutanée de la trachée cervicale après traumatisme thoracique. J. Chir. (Paris) **108**, 423–434 (1974)
366. Sperling, E.: Beitrag zur traumatischen Bronchusruptur. Chirurg **35**, 3–10 (1964)
367. Streicher, H. J.: Bronchusrekonstruktionen nach totalem Abriß. Bruns' Beitr. klin. Chir. **204**, 246–256 (1962)
368. Urschel H. C., Razzuk, M. A.: Management of acute traumatic injuries of the tracheobronchial tree. Surg. Gynec. Obstet. **136**, 113–117 (1973)
369. Vossschulte, K., Bikfalvi, A.: Bronchusnaht und Bronchusresektion als organerhaltende Eingriffe. Dtsch. med. Wschr. **89**, 599–606 (1964)
370. Webb, A.: Patologia Indica. Calcutta 1848
371. Weber, H.: Traumatische Bronchusruptur. Bruns' Beitr. klin. Chir. **219**, 106–115 (1971)
372. Wolff, G., Grädel, E., Dittmann, M., Lehmann, K.: Zur Lokalisation der Verletzung und zur Beatmung des nach innen offenen Pneumothorax. Kongr. Schweiz. Ges. Anästhesie und Schweiz. Ges. Intensivmedizin, Montreux 1976
373. Zacherl, H., Jenny, R. H., Unger, F.: Beobachtungen bei Bronchus- und Trachealverletzungen nach stumpfem Trauma. Schweiz. med. Wschr. **103**, 807–813 (1973)

Chapter 15 Injuries to the Esophagus

374. Anderson, R. P., Sabiston, D. C.: Acquired bronchoesophageal fistula of benign origin. Surg. Gynec. Obstet. **121**, 261–266 (1965)

375. Andreassian, B., Lacombe, M., Nussaume, O., Homareau, C., Roger, W., Coquillaud, J. P., Dazza, F., Baumann, J.: Ruptures de l'oesophage par traumatisme fermé. Ann. Chir. thorac. cardiovasc. **12**, 409–415 (1973)
376. Anselm, K., Shartsis, J. M., Carandang, N. V., Priest, R. J.: Perforation of the esophagus with the gastrocamera fiberscope. Amer. J. dig. Dis. **15**, 311–315 (1970)
377. Berry, B. E., Ochner, J. L.: Perforation of the esophagus. A 30 year review. J. thorac. cardiovasc. Surg. **65**, 1–7 (1973)
378. Bittner, R., Roscher, R., Berger, H. G., Bücherl, E. S.: Die traumatische Perforation der Speiseröhre. Bruns' Beitr. klin. Chir. **221**, 355–369 (1974)
379. Bombeck, C. Th., Boyd, D. R., Nyhus, L. M.: Esophageal trauma. Surg. Clin. N. Amer. **52**, 219–230 (1972)
380. Burbank, C. B., Fabr, W. H., Jones, W. H.: Three hundred seventy-four acute war wounds of the thorax. Surgery **21**, 730–738 (1947)
381. Foster, J. H., Sawyers, J. L., Daniel, R. A.: Esophageal perforation: Diagnosis and treatment. Ann. Surg. **161**, 701–709 (1965)
382. Heberer, G., Castrup, H. J.: Die Oesophago-Trachealfistel nach stumpfem Thoraxtrauma. Thoraxchirurgie **12**, 384–393 (1965)
383. Heberer, G., Lauschke, H., Hau, T.: Pathogenese, Klinik und Therapie der Oesophagusrupturen. Chirurg **37**, 433–440 (1966)
384. Kronberger, L.: Experimenteller Beitrag zur Entstehung der Oesophago-Trachealfistel durch ein stumpfes Thoraxtrauma. Langenbecks Arch. Chir. **300**, 463–489 (1962)
385. Loop, F. D., Groves, L. K.: Esophageal perforation. Ann. thorac. Surg. **10**, 571–587 (1970)
386. Palmer, E. D.: The esophagus and its diseases. New York: Hoeber 1952
387. Rea, W. J., Gallivan, G. J., Ecker, R. R., Sugg, W. L.: Traumatic esophageal perforation. Ann. thorac. Surg. **14**, 671–677 (1972)
388. Rossetti, M.: Verletzungen des Oesophagus. Thoraxchirurgie **12**, 131–140 (1964)
389. Sheely, C. H., Mattox, K. L., Beall, Jr., A. C., De Bakey, M. E.: Penetrating wounds of the cervical esophagus. Amer. J. Surg. **130**, 707–711 (1975)
390. Sommer, G. N., Jr., Trenton, N. J., O'Brien, Ch. E.: War wounds of the esophagus. J. thorac. Surg. **17**, 393–400 (1948)
391. Spenler, C. W., Benfield, J. R.: Esophageal disruption from blunt and penetrating external trauma. Arch. Surg. **111**, 663–667 (1976)
392. Symbas, P. N., Tyras, D. H., Hatcher, Ch. R., Perry, B.: Penetrating wounds of the esophagus. Ann. thorac. Surg. **13**, 552–558 (1972)
393. Worman, L. W., Hurley, J. D., Pemberton, A. H., Narodick, B. G.: Rupture of the esophagus from external blunt trauma. Arch. Surg. **85**, 333–338 (1962)

Chapter 16 Injuries to the Heart by Blunt Trauma

394. Akenside, M.: An account of a blow upon the heart and its effects. Philos. Trans. 1764, 353. Leskes Abhandlungen 1766
395. Alperovich, B. I.: Herzluxation nach geschlossenem thoraco-abdominalem Trauma. Vestn. Khir. **107**, 74–76 (1971)
396. Andreassian, B., Roche, P., Nussaume, O., Roger, W., Macrez, Cl., Bauman, J.: Les traumatismes cardio-péricardiques recents à thorax fermé. Ann. Chir. thorac. cardiovasc. **12**, 395–408 (1973)
397. Astorri, E., Bianchi, G., Di Donato, M., Visioli, O.: L'insufficienza tricuspidale isolata di origine traumatica. G. ital. Card. **5**, 233–243 (1975)
398. Bailey, C. P., Vera, C. A., Hirose, T.: Mitral regurgitation from rupture of chordae tendineae due to steering wheel compression. Geriatrics **24**, 90–105 (1969)
399. Baumgartl, F.: Verletzungen des Herzens und der großen Gefäße. Thoraxchirurgie **12**, 121–130 (1964)
400. Baumgartl, F., Hohenbleicher, R.: Rechtsschenkelblock nach stumpfen Thoraxtraumen. Mschr. Unfallheilk. **76**, 426–429 (1973)
401. Benrey, J., Price, E. C., Massin, E. K., Bowers, J. C., Cooley, D. A.: Coronary occlusion secondary to nonpenetrating chest trauma. Texas Med. **71**, 60–64 (1975)

402. Borrie, J., Lichter, I.: Pericardial rupture from blunt chest trauma. Thorax 29, 329–337 (1974)
403. Boxall, R.: Incomplete pericardial sac: Escape of heart into left pleural cavity. Trans. obstet. Soc. Lond. 28, 209 (1886)
404. Brandenburg, R. O.: Traumatic rupture of the chordae tendineae of the tricuspid valve. Amer. J. Cardiol. 18, 911–915 (1966)
405. Bryant, L. R., Dillon, M. L., Utley, J. R.: Cardiac valve injury with major chest trauma. Arch. Surg. 107, 279–283 (1973)
406. Campbell, G. S., Vernier, R., Varco, L., Lillehei, C. W.: Traumatic ventricular septal defect. J. thorac. Surg. 17, 496–501 (1959)
407. Carey, J. C., Yao, S. T., Kho, L. K.: Cardiovascular responses to acute hemopericardium, compression by ballon tamponade, and acute coronary artery occlusion. J. thorac. cardiovasc. Surg. 54, 65–80 (1967)
408. Chung, E. K., Renn, J.: Electrocardiographic changes in nonpenetrating trauma to the chest. Acta cardiol. (Brux.) 25, 418–423 (1970)
409. Clark, Th. A., Corcoran, F. H., Baker, W. P., Mills, M.: Early repair of traumatic ventricular septal defect. J. thorac. cardiovasc. Surg. 67, 121–124 (1974)
410. Codd, J. E., Kaiser, G. C., Wiens, R. D., Barner, H. B., Willman, V. L.: Myocardial injury and bypass grafting. J. thorac. cardiovasc. Surg. 70, 489–494 (1975)
411. De Muth, W. E., Jr., Baue, A. E., Odom, A. J.: Contusions of the heart. J. Trauma 7, 443–455 (1967)
412. Doty, D. B., Anderson, A. E., Rose, E. F., Go, R. T., Chiu, Ch. L., Ehrenhaft, J. L.: Cardiac trauma: Clinical and experimental correlation of myocardial contusion. Ann Surg. 180, 452–460 (1974)
413. Emminger, E.: Endokardkontusion beim Thoraxtrauma. Mschr. Unfallheilk. 75, 513–522 (1972)
414. Gautier-Benoit, C., Hameau, C., Vermesse, G., le Dantec, G.: Rupture de l'oreillette gauche par traumatisme fermé du thorax. Chir. 100, 401–406 (1974)
415. Guest, J. L., Hall, D. P., Yeh, Th. J., Ellison, R. G.: Late manifestation of trauma to the pericardium. Surg. Gynec. Obstet. 120, 787–791 (1965)
416. Glinz, W., Buff, H. U.: Das stumpfe Herztrauma. Zbl. Chir. 101, 608–616 (1976)
417. Goldfarb, B., Wang, Y.: Spontaneous healing of interventricular septal defects. Minn. Med. 4, 325–327 (1972)
418. Grosse-Brockhoff, F., Kaiser, H.: Herzschädigung durch stumpfe Gewalteinwirkung. In: Schwiegk, H. (Hrsg.): Handbuch d. inneren Medizin, Bd. 9, S. 462. Berlin-Göttingen-Heidelberg: Springer 1960
419. Grossman, Ch. M.: Posttraumatic ossification of the myocardium. J. Trauma 14, 85–89 (1974)
420. Hasper, B., Schmitz, W., Hassenstein, P., Kies, D.: Erfolgreiche Resektion eines traumatischen Aneurysmas des linken Ventrikels. Thoraxchirurgie 22, 608–612 (1974)
421. Heberer, G., Schildberg, F. W.: Verletzungen des Herzens mit spät einsetzender Symptomatik. Thoraxchirurgie 17, 222–232 (1969)
422. Hedinger, Ch.: Beiträge zur pathologischen Anatomie der Contusio und Commotio cordis. Cardiologia (Basel) 8, 1–48 (1944)
423. Heyndrickx, G., Vermeire, P., Goffin, Y., Van den Bogaert, P.: Rupture of the right coronary artery due to nonpenetrating chest trauma. Chest 65, 577–579 (1974)
424. Hewett, P. G.: Cases of rupture of the heart and large vessels, the results of injuries. Trans. path. Soc. London 1, 81 (1847)
425. Hofmann, K. T., Harbauer, G., Schmidt, A.: Traumatische Perikardruptur mit Luxation des Herzens. Thoraxchirurgie 14, 62–69 (1966)
426. Jones, J. W., Hewitt, R. L., Drapanas, Th.: Cardiac contusion: A capricious syndrome. Ann. Surg. 181, 567–574 (1975)
427. Kissane, R. W., Rose, S. M.: Traumatic pericarditis. Amer. J. Cardiol. 7, 97–101 (1961)
428. Krefft, S.: Herzverletzungen bei Luftfahrzeuginsassen im Gefolge von Flugunfällen. Herz/Kreislauf 8, 66–73 (1976)
429. Kreutzberg, B., Eckert, P., Thelen, M., Louven, B., Koene, U.: Coronarographische und elektrokardiographische Untersuchungen bei stumpfen Herztraumen. Langenbecks Arch. Chir. 329, 188 (1971)

430. Kussmaul, A.: Über die schwielige Mediastino-perikarditis und den paradoxen Puls. Berl. klin. Wschr. **10**, 433–461 (1873)
431. Larrey, D. J.: Sur une blessure du péricarde, suivie d'hydro-péricarde. Bull. Sci. méd. **6**, 255–273 (1810)
432. Levitsky, S.: New insights in cardiac trauma. Surg. Clin. N. Amer. **55**, 43–55 (1975)
433. Lossnitzer, K., Grewe, N., Krämer, W., Stauch, M.: Ventrikuläre Extrasystolen als Dauerfolge nach traumatischer Herzschädigung. Dtsch. med. Wschr. **98**, 885–889 (1973)
434. Louven, B., Schaede, A., Petersen, E., Thelen, M., Straaten, G., Oest, S.: Herzschäden infolge stumpfer Gewalt. Dtsch. med. Wschr. **97**, 1627–1631 (1972)
435. Louven, B., Thelen, M., Kreutzberg, B., Petersen, E., Oest, S.: Die traumatische Herzinsuffizienz. Therapiewoche **22**, 2432–2438 (1972)
436. Martin, J. W., Schenk, W. G.: Pericardial tamponade. Amer. J. Surg. **99**, 782–787 (1960)
437. Mattila, S., Silvola, H., Ketonen, P.: Traumatic rupture of the pericardium with luxation of the heart. J. thorac. cardiovasc. Surg. **70**, 495–498 (1975)
438. Mine, Th.: Quelques considérations sur les traumatismes non pénétrants de l'appareil cardiovasculaire et leur incidence médico-légale. Ann. Méd. lég. **44**, 535–548 (1964)
439. Moraes, C. R., Victor, E., Arruda, M., Calvalcanti, I., Raposo, L., Lagreca, J. R., Gomes, J. M.: Ventrikelseptumdefekt nach stumpfem Thoraxtrauma. Angiology **24**, 222–229 (1973)
440. Morgagni, G. B.: De sedibus et causis morborum. Venetiis 1761. Lib. IV: De morbis chirurgicis et universalibus; Epist. anatom. medica LIII: De vulneribus et ictibus colli, pectoris et dorsi
441. Moritz, A. R.: Injuries of the heart and pericardium by physical violence. In: Gould, S. B. (Ed.): Pathology of the heart, 2nd ed., p. 849. Springfield/Ill.: Ch. C. Thomas 1960
442. Mössler, U., Storch, U. U., Schmitz, W., Ahmadi, A., Walther, H., Ostermeyer, J., Bayer, H. P.: Isolierte Ventrikelseptumruptur nach stumpfem Thoraxtrauma. Thoraxchirurgie **23**, 578–883 (1975)
443. Noon, G. P., Boulafendis, D., Beall, A. C.: Rupture of the heart secondary to blunt trauma. J. Trauma **11**, 122–128 (1971)
444. Parmley, L. F., Manion, W. C., Mattingly, T. W.: Non-penetrating traumatic injury of the heart. Circulation **18**, 371–396 (1958)
445. Pomerantz, M., Delgado, F., Eiseman, B.: Unsuspected depressed cardiac output following blunt thoracic or abdominal trauma. Surgery **70**, 865–871 (1971)
446. Pories, W. J., Gaudiani, V. A.: Cardiac tamponade. Surg. Clin. N. Amer. **55**, 573–589 (1975)
447. Ramp, J., Hankins, J., Mason, G. R.: Cardiac tamponade secondary to blunt trauma. J. Trauma **14**, 767–772 (1974)
448. Rasaretnam, R., Paul, A. T. S.: Constrictive pericarditis following mild non-penetrating trauma. Aust. N.Z. J. Med. **5**, 57–62 (1975)
449. Rose, E.: Herztamponade. Ein Beitrag zur Herzchirurgie. Dtsch. Z. Chir. **20**, 329 (1884)
450. Rosenkranz, K. A.: Die traumatische Herzschädigung. Ludwigshafen: Gebr. Giulini 1970
451. Rosenkranz, K. A.: Commotio und Contusio cordis. Langenbecks Arch. Chir. **329**, 163–173 (1971)
452. Rosenthal, A., Parisi, L. F., Nador, A. S.: Isolated interventricular septal defect due to nonpenetrating trauma. New Engl. J. Med. **283**, 338–341 (1970)
453. Schildberg, F. W.: Geschlossene Herzverletzungen aus chirurgischer Sicht. Langenbecks Arch. Chir. **329**, 174–185 (1971)
454. Schlomka, G.: Commotio cordis und ihre Folgen. Ergebn. inn. Med. Kinderheilk. **47**, 1 (1934)
455. Schulz, E., Maghsudi, A. A.: Herzverletzungen und ihre Beziehungen zu anderen Organverletzungen bei Verkehrsunfällen. Dtsch. Z. ges. gerichtl. Med. **65**, 65–72 (1969)
456. Sharp, J. T., Bunnell, I. L., Holland, J. F., Griffith, G. T., Greene, D. G.: Hemodynamics during induced cardiac tamponade in man. Amer. J. Med. **29**, 640–646 (1960)
457. Shoemaker, W. C., Carey, J. C., Yao, S. T., Mohr, P. A., Printen, K. J., Kark, A. E.: Hemodynamic monitoring for physiologic evaluation, diagnosis, and therapy of acute hemopericardial tamponade from penetrating wounds. J. Trauma **13**, 36–44 (1973)

458. Singh, R., Nolan, St. P., Schrank, J. P.: Traumatic left ventricular aneurysm. J. Amer. med. Ass. **234**, 412–414 (1975)
459. Stern, Th., Wolf, R. Y., Reichart, B.: Coronary artery occlusion resulting from blunt trauma. J. Amer. med. Ass. **230**, 1308–1309 (1974)
460. Steinbach, K., Domanig, E., Weissenhofer, W.: Totaler a.-v.-Block nach stumpfem Thoraxtrauma. Mschr. Unfallheilk. **75**, 275–282 (1972)
461. Symbas, P. N.: Traumatic injuries of the heart and great vessels. Springfield/Ill.: Ch. C. Thomas 1973
462. Tricot, R., Guerot, Cl., Graisely, B., Vautier, P.: A propos d'un cas d'infarctus du myocarde d'origine traumatique avec anévrysme ventriculaire. Cœur méd. int. **14**, 469–476 (1975)
463. Tschirkov, F., Hirsch, H., Hepp, G.: Perikarditis als Folge eines Hämoperikards nach stumpfem Thoraxtrauma. Mschr. Unfallheilk. **75**, 131–138 (1972)
464. Vogel, W., Wintzer, G.: Diagnostik und Therapie der stumpfen Herzverletzungen. Med. Klin. **71**, 653–660 (1976)
465. Vorburger, Ch., Fässler, B., Köhl, P.: Serum-Kreatininphosphokinase und intramuskuläre Injektion. Schweiz. med. Wschr. **103**, 927–930 (1973)
466. Ware, R. E., Martin, L. G., Tyras, D. H., Kourias, E., Symbas, P. N.: Coronary arterial injection of radioactive albumin microspheres in diagnosis of experimental myocardial contusion. Surg. Forum **23**, 138–139 (1972)
467. Watson, J. H., Bartholomae, W. M.: Cardiac injury to nonpenetrating chest trauma. Ann. intern. Med. **52**, 871–880 (1960)
468. Wright, M. P., Nelson, C., Johnson, A. M., McMillan, I. K. R.: Herniation of the heart. Thorax **25**, 656–664 (1970)

Chapter 17 Penetrating Wounds of the Heart

469. Ballance, C. A.: The surgery of the heart. Lancet **1920 I**, 1–5
470. Barrett, N. R.: Foreign bodies in cardiovascular system. Brit. J. Surg. **37**, 416–445 (1950)
471. Beach, P. M., Bognolo, D., Hutchinson, J. E.: Penetrating cardiac trauma. Amer. J. Surg. **131**, 411–413 (1976)
472. Beall, A. C., Jr., Patrick, T. A., Okies, J. E., Bricher, D. L., DeBakey, M. E.: Penetrating wounds of the heart: Changing patterns of surgical management. Trauma **12**, 468–473 (1972)
473. Blalock, A., Ravitch, M. M.: Consideration of nonoperative treatment of cardiac tamponade resulting from wounds of the heart. Surgery **14**, 157–162 (1943)
474. Bland, E. F., Beebe, G. W.: Missiles in the heart. A twenty year follow-up report of world war II cases. New Engl. J. Med. **274**, 1039–1046 (1966)
475. Borja, A. R., Lansing, A. M., Ransdell, H. I.: Immediate operative treatment for stab wounds of the heart. J. thorac. cardiovasc. Surg. **59**, 662–667 (1970)
476. Bravo, A. J., Glancy, D. L., Epstem, S. E., Morrow, A. G.: Traumatic coronary arteriovenous fistula. Amer. J. Cardiol. **27**, 673–676 (1971)
477. Domaning, E., Wimmer, M.: Aortopulmonale Fistel nach Thoraxschußverletzung mit Embolie des Geschosses. Thoraxchirurgie **20**, 158–164 (1972)
478. Espada, R., Whisennand, H. H., Mattox, K. L., Beall, A. C.: Surgical management of penetrating injuries to the coronary arteries. Surgery **78**, 755–760 (1975)
479. Fischer, C.: Die Wunden des Herzens und des Herzbeutels. Arch. klin. Chir. **9**, 571–910 (1868)
480. Fueter-Töndury, M.: Drahtwanderung nach Osteosynthese. Schweiz. med. Wschr. **106**, 1890–1896 (1976)
481. Griswold, R. A., Maguire, C. H.: Penetrating wounds of the heart and pericardium. Surg. Gynec. Obstet. **74**, 406–418 (1942)
482. Harken, D. E.: Foreign bodies in, and in relation to, the thoracic blood vessels and heart. Surg. Gynec. Obstet. **83**, 117–125 (1946)
483. Harvey, J. C., Pacifico, A. D.: Primary operative management: Method of choice for stab wounds to the heart. Sth. med. J. (Bgham, Ala.) **68**, 149–152 (1975)
484. Homer: Ilias. Wolfgang Schadewaldts neue Übertragung. Frankfurt: Insel Verlag 1975

485. Konecke, L. L., Spitzer, S., Mason, D.: Traumatic aneurysm of the left coronary artery. Amer. J. Cardiol. **27**, 221–223 (1971)
486. Kremer, K.: Offene (penetrierende) Verletzungen des Herzens und der herznahen Gefäße. Zbl. Chir. **90**, 1225–1227 (1965)
487. Kronzon, I., Zelefsky, M., Laniado, S., Jordan, A.: Coronary angiography as an aid in localizing myocardial foreign bodies: A case report. J. Trauma **14**, 429–434 (1974)
488. Mattox, K. L., Beall, A. C., Jordan, G. L., DeBakey, M. E.: Cardiorrhaphy in the emergency center. J. thorac. cardiovasc. Surg. **68**, 886–895 (1974)
489. Morales, A. A., Garcia, F., Grover, F. L., Trinkle, J. K.: Aneurysm of the left ventricle after repair of a penetrating injury. J. thorac. cardiovasc. Surg. **66**, 632–635 (1973)
490. Morton, J. R., Reul, G. J., Arbegast, N. R., Okies, J. E., Beall, A. C.: Bullet embolus to the right ventricle. Amer. J. Surg. **122**, 584–590 (1971)
491. Neville, W. E., Bolanowski, J. P.: Penetrating cardiac injuries. Resuscitation **3**, 85–90 (1974)
492. Nieda, S.: Case of a cardiac injury resulting from acupuncture. Jap. J. thorac. Surg. **26**, 881–883 (1973)
493. Paget, St.: The surgery of the chest. New York: F. B. Treat 1897
494. Paré, A.: Oeuvres complètes, Vol. II, p. 95. Paris: Baillière 1840
495. Rea, W. J., Sugg, W. L., Wilson, L. C.: Coronary artery lacerations. An analysis of 22 patients. Ann. thorac. Surg. **7**, 518–528 (1969)
496. Rehn, L.: Über penetrierende Herzwunden und Herznaht. Arch. klin. Chir. **55**, 315 (1897)
497. Rehn, L.: Zur Chirurgie des Herzens und des Herzbeutels. Arch. klin. Chir. **83**, 723–778 (1907)
498. Reyes, L. H., Mattox, K. L., Gaasch, W. H., Espada, R., Beall, A. C.: Traumatic coronary artery-right heart fistula. J. thorac. cardiovasc. Surg. **70**, 52–56 (1975)
499. Schott, H., Viehweger, G.: Geschoßembolie in das Herz. Chirurg **45**, 371–373 (1974)
500. Schwarz, H.: Verletzungen des Herzens und der großen Gefäße. Bern, Stuttgart, Wien: Huber 1977
501. Sugg, W. L., Rea, W. J., Ecker, R. R., Webb, W. R., Rose, E. F., Shaw, R. R.: Penetrating wounds of the heart. J. thorac. cardiovasc. Surg. **56**, 531–545 (1968)
502. Symbas, P. N., DiOrio, D. A., Tyras, D. H., Ware, R. E., Hatcher, Ch. R.: Penetrating cardiac wounds: Significant residual and delayed sequelae. J. thorac. cardiovasc. Surg. **66**, 526–532 (1973)
503. Symbas, P. N., Harlaftis, N., Waldo, W. J.: Penetrating cardiac wounds: A comparison of different therapeutic methods. Ann. Surg. **183**, 377–381 (1976)
504. Swan, H., Forsee, J. H., Goyette, E. M.: Foreign bodies in the heart. Ann. Surg. **135**, 314–323 (1952)
505. Trinkle, J. K., Marcos, J., Grover, F. L., Cuello, L. M.: Management of the wounded heart. Ann. thorac. Surg. **17**, 230–236 (1974)
506. Viikari, S., Mattila, S., Linna, M.: Stichverletzungen der Lunge und des Herzens. Zbl. Chir. **101**, 97–101 (1976)
507. Wilson, R. F., Bassett, J. S.: Penetrating wounds of the pericardium or its contents. J. Amer. med. Ass. **195**, 513–518 (1966)
508. Yao, S. T., Vanecko, R. M., Printen, K., Shoemaker, W. C.: Penetrating wounds of the heart. Ann. Surg. **168**, 67–78 (1968)

Chapter 18 Injuries of the Great Intrathoracic Vessels

509. Allen, R. E., Jr., Reul, G. J., Beall, A. C.: Surgical management of aortic trauma. J. Trauma **12**, 862–868 (1972)
510. Andreassian, B., Nussaume, O., Roger, W., Marsault, C.: Thrombose segmentaire de l'artère sous-clavière gauche après traumatismes fermés du thorax: Répercussions neurologiques. Ann. Chir. thorac. cardiovasc. **10**, 427–433 (1971)
511. Ayella, R. J., Hankins, J. R., Turney, S. Z., Cowley, R. A.: Ruptured thoracic aorta due to blunt trauma. J. Trauma **17**, 199–205 (1977)

512. Bahnson, H. T.: Definitive treatment of saccular aneurysms of aorta with excision of sac and aortic suture. Surg. Gynec. Obstet. **96**, 383–402 (1953)
513. Beier, G., Spann, W.: Zur Aortenruptur beim Fußgängerunfall. Hefte Unfallheilk. **121**, 231–234 (1975)
514. Bennett, D. E., Cherry, J. K.: The natural history of traumatic aneurysms of the aorta. Surgery **61**, 516–523 (1967)
515. Billy, L. J., Amato, J. J., Rich, N. M.: Aortic injuries in Vietnam. Surgery **70**, 385–391 (1971)
516. Binet, J. P., Langlois, J., Cormier, J. M., Saint Florent, G. de: A case of recent traumatic avulsion of the innominate artery at its origin from the aortic arch. J. thorac. cardiovasc. Surg. **43**, 670–676 (1962)
517. Borst, H. G., Schaudig, A., Rudolph, W.: Arterio-venous fistula of the aortic arch. J. thorac. cardiovasc. Surg. **48**, 443–447 (1969)
518. Brawley, R. K., Murray, G. F., Crisler, C., Cameron, J. L.: Management of wounds of the innominate, subclavian, and axillary blood vessels. Surg. Gynec. Obstet. **131**, 1130–1140 (1970)
519. Carstensen, G., Heinrichs, L.: Traumatische Aortenrupturen. Langenbecks Arch. Chir. **309**, 415–425 (1965)
520. Ciaravella, J. M., Ochsner, J. L., Mills, N. L.: Traumatic avulsion of the innominate artery: Case report and literature review. J. Trauma **16**, 751–754 (1976)
521. Clegg, J., Charlesworth, D.: Traumatic rupture of the thoracic aorta. J. cardiovasc. Surg. **13**, 206–209 (1972)
522. Cooley, D. A., DeBakey, M. E., Morris, G. C.: Controlled extracorporeal circulation in surgical treatment of aortic aneurysm. Ann. Surg. **146**, 473–486 (1957)
523. Crawford, E. S., Rubio, P.: Reappraisal of adjuncts to avoid ischemia in treatment of descending thoracic aneurysms. J. thorac. cardiovasc. Surg. **66**, 693–704 (1973)
524. Dart, C. H., Braitman, H. E.: Traumatic rupture of thoracic aorta: Diagnosis and management. Arch. Surg. **111**, 697–702 (1976)
525. DeBakey, M. E., Simeone, F. A.: Battle injuries of the arteries in world war II. Ann. Surg. **123**, 534–579 (1946)
526. DeMeules, J. E., Cramer, G., Perry, J. F., Jr.: Rupture of aorta and great vessels due to blunt thoracic trauma. J. thorac. cardiovasc. Surg. **61**, 438–442 (1971)
527. DeMuth, W. E., Roe, H., Hobbie, W.: Immediate repair of traumatic rupture of thoracic aorta. Arch. Surg. **91**, 602–603 (1965)
528. Dsahnelidze, I. I.: Manuskript Petrograd, 1922. Zit. in: Lilienthal, H.: Thoracic surgery, p. 489. Philadelphia: Saunders 1925.
529. Eiseman, B., Rainer, W. G.: Clinical management of post-traumatic rupture of thoracic aorta. J. thorac. cardiovasc. Surg. **35**, 347–358 (1958)
530. Franz, J. L., Simpson, C. R., Penny, R. M., Grover, F. L., Trinkle, J. K.: Avulsion of the innominate artery after blunt chest trauma. J. thorac. cardiovasc. Surg. **67**, 478–480 (1974)
531. Gerbode, F., Braimbridge, M., Osborn, J. J., Hood, M., French, S.: Traumatic thoracic aneurysms: Treatment by resection and grafting with the use of extracorporeal bypass. Surgery **42**, 975–985 (1957)
532. Heberer, G.: Ruptures and aneurysms of the thoracic aorta after blunt chest trauma. J. cardiovasc. Surg. **12**, 115–120 (1971)
533. Heberer, G., Vogel, W., Brehm, H. v.: Rupturen und Aneurysmen der thorakalen Aorta nach stumpfen Brustkorbverletzungen. Langenbecks Arch. Chir. **330**, 10–44 (1971)
534. Hewitt, R. L., Smith, A. D., Becker, M. L., Lindsey, E. S., Dowling, J. B., Drapanas, Th.: Penetrating vascular injuries of the thoracic outlet. Surgery **76**, 715–722 (1974)
535. Hollingsworth, R. K., Johnston, W. W., McCooey, J. F.: Traumatic saccular aneurysm of the thoracic aorta. J. thorac. Surg. **24**, 325–345 (1952)
536. Hughes, C. W.: Arterial repair during the Korean war. Ann. Surg. **147**, 555–561 (1958)
537. Inberg, M. V., Laaksonen, V., Scheinin, T. M., Slätis, P., Vänttinen, E.: Early repair of traumatic rupture of the thoracic aorta. Scand. J. thorac. cardiovasc. Surg. **6**, 287–292 (1972)

538. Jahnke, E. J., Fisher, G. W., Jones, R. C.: Acute traumatic rupture of the thoracic aorta. J. thorac. cardiovasc. Surg. **48**, 63–77 (1964)
539. Kahn, D. R., Vathayanon, S., Sloan, H.: Resection of descending thoracic aneurysms without left heart bypass. Arch. Surg. **97**, 336–340 (1968)
540. Kirsh, M. M., Kahn, D. R., Crane, J. D., Anastasia, L. F., Lui, A. H., Moores, M. Y., Vathayanon, S., Bookstein, J. J., Sloan, H. E.: Repair of acute traumatic rupture of the aorta without extracorporeal circulation. Ann. thorac. Surg. **10**, 227–236 (1970)
541. Kleinert, H. E.: Homograft patch repair of bullet wounds of the aorta. Experimental studies and report of a case. Arch. Surg. **76**, 811–820 (1958)
542. Kremer, K.: Akute Verletzungen der thorakalen Aorta und ihrer Äste. Zbl. Chir. **101**, 85–90 (1976)
543. Langlois, C., Binet, J. P., Jegou, J. C.: Traumatic rupture of the thoracic aorta and of its branches. J. cardiovasc. Surg. **12**, 83–92 (1971)
544. Manwaring, J. H.: Delayed hemorrhage after stab wounds of aorta. J. thorac. cardiovasc. Surg. **67**, 788–791 (1974)
545. McGrough, E. C., Hughes, R. K.: Acute traumatic rupture of the aorta: Reemphasis of repair without a vascular prosthesis. Ann. thorac. Surg. **16**, 7–10 (1973)
546. Molloy, P. J.: Repair of the ruptured thoracic aorta using left ventriculo-aortic support. Thorax **25**, 213–222 (1970)
547. Mulder, D. S., Greenwood, F. A. H., Brooks, C. E.: Posttraumatic thoracic outlet syndrome. J. Trauma **13**, 706–715 (1973)
548. Murray, G. F., Brawley, R. K., Gott, V. L.: Reconstruction of the innominate artery by means of a temporary heparin-coated shunt bypass. J. thorac. cardiovasc. Surg. **62**, 34–41 (1971)
549. Neville, W. E., Cox, W. D., Leininger, B., Pifarre, R.: Resection of the thoracic aorta with femoral vein to femoral artery perfusion with oxygenation. J. thorac. cardiovasc. Surg. **56**, 39–42 (1968)
550. Parmley, L. F., Mattingly, T. W., Manion, W. C., Jahnke, E. J., Jr.: Nonpenetrating traumatic injury of aorta. Circulation **17**, 1086–1101 (1958)
551. Passaro, E., Pace, W. G.: Traumatic rupture of the aorta. Surgery **46**, 787–791 (1959)
552. Perkins, R., Elchos, T.: Stab wounds of the aortic arch. Ann. Surg. **147**, 83–86 (1958)
553. Reul, G. J., Beall, A., Jordan, G. L., Mattox, K. L.: The early operative management of injuries to the great vessels. Surgery **74**, 862–873 (1973)
554. Reul, G. J., Rubio, P. A., Beall, A. C.: The surgical management of acute injury to the thoracic aorta. J. thorac. cardiovasc. Surg. **67**, 272–282 (1974)
555. Rittenhouse, E. A., Dillard, D. H., Winterscheid, L. C., Merendino, K. A.: Traumatic rupture of the thoracic aorta. Ann. Surg. **170**, 87–100 (1969)
556. Roos, D. B.: Experience with first rib resection for thoracic outlet syndrome. Ann. Surg. **173**, 429–442 (1971)
557. Sailer, S.: Dissecting aneurysm of the aorta. Arch. Path. **33**, 704–730 (1942)
558. Schildberg, F. W.: Indikatorische Probleme bei Aortenrupturen aus chirurgischer Sicht. Langenbecks Arch. Chir. **337**, 329–335 (1974)
559. Schriber, K., Meier, W. E., Senning, Å.: Die traumatische Ruptur der Aorta thoracica. Helv. chir. Acta **41**, 65–69 (1974)
560. Schüttrumpf, G.: Ungewöhnlicher Sportunfall mit Dehnungsriß der Aorta abdominalis. Mschr. Unfallheilk. **69**, 248–254 (1966)
561. Seling, A., Satter, P.: Der Ausriß des Truncus brachiocephalicus aus dem Aortenbogen. Chirurg **44**, 277–279 (1973)
562. Spencer, F. C., Guerin, P. R., Blake, H. A., Bahnson, H. T.: A report of 15 patients with traumatic rupture of the thoracic aorta. J. thorac. cardiovasc. Surg. **41**, 1–22 (1961)
563. Stallone, R. J., Ecker, R. R., Samson, P. C.: Management of major acute thoracic vascular injuries. Amer. J. Surg. **128**, 249–254 (1974)
564. Stranahan, A., Alley, R. D., Sewell, W. H., Kausel, H. W.: Aortic arch resection and grafting for aneurysm employing an external shunt. J. thorac. cardiovasc. Surg. **29**, 54–65 (1955)

565. Strassmann, G.: Traumatic rupture of the aorta. Amer. Heart J. **33**, 508–515 (1947)
566. Symbas, P. N., Sehdeva, J. S.: Penetrating wounds of the thoracic aorta. Ann. Surg. **171**, 441–450 (1970)
567. Valiathan, M. S., Weldon, C. S., Bender, H. W., Topaz, St., Gott, V. L.: Resection of aneurysm of the descending thoracic aorta using a GBH-coated shunt bypass. J. surg. Res. **8**, 197–205 (1968)
568. Weisel, W., Huttner, W. A., Becker, I. H.: Unusual aortic arch non-luetic aneurysm. Wis. med. J. **50**, 866 (1951)
569. Zehnder, M. A.: Aortenruptur bei stumpfem Thoraxtrauma. Retrospektive Auswertung der Kasuistik und zukünftige chirurgische Möglichkeiten. Helv. chir. Acta **26**, 442–464 (1959)
570. Zehnder, M. A.: Unfallmechanismen und Unfallmechanik zur traumatischen Aortenruptur. Langenbecks Arch. Chir. **337**, 325–328 (1974)

Chapter 19 Injuries of the Diaphragm

571. Andrus, C. H., Morton, J. H.: Rupture of the diaphragm after blunt trauma. Amer. J. Surg. **119**, 686–693 (1970)
572. Bekassy, S. B., Dave, K. S., Wooler, G. H., Ionescu, M. I.: "Spontaneous" and traumatic rupture of the diaphragm: Long-term results. Ann. Surg. **177**, 320–324 (1973)
573. Bowditch, H. I.: Diaphragmatic hernia. Buffalo med. J. **9**, 1–39, 65–94 (1853)
574. Crawshaw, G. R.: Herniation of the stomach, transverse colon, and a portion of the jejunum into the pericardium. Brit. J. Surg. **39**, 364–366 (1952)
575. Lernau, O., Bar-Maor, J. A., Nissan, S.: Traumatic diaphragmatic hernia simulating acute tension pneumothorax. J. Trauma **14**, 880–884 (1974)
576. McCune, R., Roda, C. P., Eckert, Ch.: Rupture of the diaphragm caused by blunt trauma. J. Trauma **16**, 531–537 (1976)
577. Gourin, A., Garzon, A.: Diagnostic problems in traumatic diaphragmatic hernia. J. Trauma **14**, 20–31 (1974)
578. Heberer, G., Senno, A., Laur, A.: Traumatische intraperikardiale Zwerchfellrisse mit Baucheingeweideprolaps. Chirurg **38**, 410–416 (1967)
579. Hood, M. R.: Traumatic diaphragmatic hernia. Ann. thorac. Surg. **12**, 311–324 (1971)
580. Kubo, G.: Traumatische Herzbeutel- und Diaphragmaruptur mit Luxation der Herzspitze in das Abdomen. Mschr. Unfallheilk. **70**, 259–263 (1967)
581. Kümmerle, F.: Die Verletzungen des Zwerchfells. Thoraxchirurgie **12**, 141–147 (1964/65)
582. Moreaux, J., Rizzo, M.: Les ruptures du péricarde et les luxations extra-péricardiques du cœur dans les écrasements thoraciques. Ann. Chir. **14**, 1395–1403 (1960)
583. Müller-Wiefel, H., Voigt, J.: Zwerchfellrupturen bei stumpfen Traumen. Hefte Unfallheilk. **121**, 195–199 (1975)
584. Noon, G. P., Beall, A. C., Jr., DeBakey, M. E.: Surgical management of traumatic rupture of the diaphragm. J. Trauma **6**, 344–352 (1966)
585. Paré, A.: Oeuvres complètes, Vol. II, pp. 95, 96. Paris: Baillière 1840
586. Popovici, Z.: Les lésions traumatiques du diaphragme et leurs conséquences. J. Chir. (Paris) **102**, 343–360 (1971)
587. Robb, D.: Traumatic diaphragmatic hernia into the pericardium. Brit. J. Surg. **50**, 664–666 (1963)
588. Ricolfi: Verletzung des Thorax und Diaphragma. Bull. della soc. Lancisiana degli ospedali di Roma, 1899. Ref. Zbl. Chir. **18**, 246 (1891)
589. Saegesser, F., Besson, A.: 493 traumatismes thoraco-abdominaux ou abdomino-thoraciques, ouverts et fermés, avec 114 atteintes du diaphragme. Helv. chir. Acta **44**, 7–48 (1977)
590. Samaan, H. A.: Undiagnosed traumatic diaphragmatic hernia. Brit. J. Surg. **58**, 257–262 (1971)

591. Santy, P., Duroux, P. E.: Hernie diaphragmatique; ectopie abdominale du cœur. Lyon chir. **46**, 356–359 (1951)
592. Saur, K., Lutz, W.: Die traumatische Zwerchfellruptur: Diagnostik, Behandlung, Spätergebnisse. Mschr. Unfallheilk. **79**, 349–357 (1976)
593. Spelsberg, F., Pichlmaier, H., Junginger, Th.: Die traumatische Zwerchfellruptur. Chir. Praxis **16**, 33–40 (1972)
594. Tixier, Corajod, Soustelle: Un cas de hernie diaphragmatique – Pheno-thoraco-laparotomie. Hernie de l'épiploon dans le péricarde – Mort. Lyon chir. **34**, 233–236 (1937)
595. Walker, E. W.: Diaphragmatic hernia, with report of a case. Int. J. Surg. **13**, 257–260 (1900)
596. Waridel, D., Saegesser, F.: Les ruptures traumatiques fermées du diaphragme. Schw. med. Wschr. **99**, 465–473 (1969)
597. Wise, J., Connors, Y., Hwang, H., Anderson, Ch.: Traumatic injuries to the diaphragm. J. Trauma **13**, 946–951 (1973)

Chapter 20 Other Injury Patterns and Consequences of Injury in Thoracic Trauma

598. Alexander, E. G.: A case of stasis cyanosis following an epileptic seizure, simulating traumatic asphyxia. Ann. Surg. **49**, 762–766 (1909)
599. Andosca, J. B., Foley, J. A.: Pleural shock and cerebral embolism. Amer. Rev. Tuberc. **52**, 221–230 (1945)
600. Barbieri, G.: Traumatic chylothorax. Minerva medica **66**, 3165–3169 (1975)
601. Boegehold, E.: Über Verletzungen des D. thoracicus. Langenbecks Arch. Chir. **29**, 443–468 (1883)
602. Bonet, Th.: Sepulchretrum, sive anatomia practica ex cadaveribus morbo denatis, Fol. Lib. IV, Sect. III, Observ. XXIV, 5, p. 360. Genevae: L. Chouët 1679
603. Bonnin, J. G.: Traumatic asphyxia. Lancet **1941 II**, 333–335
604. Braun, H.: Ueber ausgedehnte Blutextravasate am Kopfe, Halse, Nacken und linken Arme, infolge Compression des Unterleibes. Dtsch. Z. Chir. **51**, 599–604 (1899)
605. Burrell, H. L., Crandon, L. R. G.: Traumatic apnea or asphyxia. Boston med. Surg. J. **146**, 13–15 (1902)
606. Crosby, I. K., Crouch, J., Reed, W. A.: Chylopericardium and chylothorax. J. thorac. cardiovasc. Surg. **65**, 935–939 (1973)
607. De Forest, H. B.: Surgery of the thoracic duct. Ann. Surg. **46**, 705–715 (1907)
608. Durant, Th. M., Oppenheimer, M. J., Webster, M. R., Long, J.: Arterial air embolism. Amer. Heart J. **38**, 481–500 (1949)
609. Forster, E., Maguet, A. le, Cinqualbre, J., Piombini, J.-L., Schiltz, E.: A propos d'un cas de chylothorax consécutif à un traumatisme fermé vertébro-costal. J. Chir. (Paris) **101**, 605–616 (1975)
610. Fred, H. L., Chandler, F. W.: Traumatic asphyxia. Amer. J. Med. **29**, 508–517 (1960)
611. Goldfarb, D., Bahnson, H. T.: Early and late effects on the heart of small amounts of air in the coronary circulation. J. thorac. cardiovasc. Surg. **46**, 368–378 (1963)
612. Goorwitch, J.: Traumatic chylothorax and thoracic duct ligation: Case report and review of literature. J. thorac. Surg. **29**, 467–479 (1955)
613. Heuer, J. G.: Traumatic asphyxia; with especial reference to its ocular and visual disturbances. Surg. Gynec. Obstet. **36**, 686–696 (1923)
614. Klepser, R. G., Berry, J. F.: The diagnosis and surgical management of chylothorax with the aid of lipophilic dyes. Dis. Chest. **25**, 409–426 (1954)
615. Kraus, H.: Brustwandbrüche. In: Derra, E. (Hrsg.): Handbuch der Thoraxchirurgie, Bd. II/I, S. 21–24. Berlin-Göttingen-Heidelberg: Springer 1959
616. Laumonier, P., Lachapelle, A. P., Couraud, L., Hugues, A., Lagarde, C., May, J.: Une application de la lymphographie au diagnostic et au traitement du chylothorax. Presse méd. **70**, 2630–2632 (1962)
617. Lee, F. C.: The establishment of collateral circulation following ligation of the thoracic duct. Bull. Johns Hopk. Hosp. **33**, 21–31 (1922)

618. Lenaghan, R., Silva, Y. J., Walt, A. J.: Hemodynamic alterations associated with expansion rupture of the lung. Arch. Surg. **99**, 339–343 (1969)
619. Liebermeister, G.: Anämisches Zungenphänomen, ein Frühsymptom der arteriellen Luftembolie. Klin. Wschr. **8**, 21–23 (1929)
620. Lowman, R. M., Hoogerhyde, J., Waters, L. L., Grant, C.: Traumatic chylothorax. The roentgen aspects of this problem. Amer. J. Roentgenol. **65**, 529–546 (1951)
621. Madroszkiewicz, A., Gurak, A., Zychowicz, F.: Przemijajqca utrata wzroku w przypadku zespolu Perthesa. Klin. oczna **44**, 163–166 (1974)
622. Maloney, J. V., Spencer, F. C.: The nonoperative treatment of traumatic chylothorax. Surgery **40**, 121–127 (1956)
623. Männl, H. F. K., Hofmann, K. Th.: Intercostale Lungenhernien. Chirurg **44**, 422–424 (1973)
624. Morian: Ueber einen Fall von Druckstauung. Münch. med. Wschr. **27**, 61–62 (1901)
625. Munnell, E. R.: Herniation of the lung. Ann. thorac. Surg. **5**, 204–212 (1968)
626. Nielsen, J. B., Lykkegard, M.: Lung hernia through the thoracic wall. Acta chir. scand. **137**, 483–486 (1971)
627. Ollivier d'Angers: Relation médicale des événements survenues au Champ-de-Mars le 14 juin 1837. Ann. Hyg. **18**, 485 (1837)
628. Perthes, G.: Ueber ausgedehnte Blutextravasate am Kopf infolge von Compression des Thorax. Dtsch. Z. Chir. **50**, 436–443 (1899)
629. Perthes, G.: Ueber „Druckstauung". Dtsch. Z. Chir. **55**, 384–392 (1900)
630. Reichert, F. L., Martin, J. W.: Traumatic asphyxia; experimental and clinical observation with a report of a case with concomitant paraplegia. Ann. Surg. **134**, 361–368 (1951)
631. Reilly, K. M., Tsou, E.: Bilateral chylothorax. J. Amer. med. Ass. **233**, 536–537 (1975)
632. Sandiford, J. A., Sickler, D.: Traumatic asphyxia with severe neurological sequelae. J. Trauma **14**, 805–810 (1974)
633. Schlaepfer, K.: Air embolism following various diagnostic or therapeutic procedures in diseases of the pleura and the lung. Johns Hopk. Hosp. Bull, **33**, 321–330 (1922)
634. Søreide, O., Stedjeberg, J. O.: Traumatic intercostal pulmonary hernia. Injury **7**, 61–62 (1975)
635. Tauber, K.: Die Verletzungen des Ductus thoracicus. Langenbecks Arch. Chir. **284**, 188–190 (1956)
636. Thomas, A. N.: Air embolism following penetrating lung injuries. J. thorac. cardiovasc. Surg. **66**, 533–540 (1973)
637. Thomas, A. N., Stephens, B. G.: Air embolism: A cause of morbidity and death after penetrating chest trauma. J. Trauma **14**, 633–638 (1974)
638. Travisano, zit. Denk, W., Kunz, H.: Die Chirurgie der Brustwand. In: Kirschner-Nordmann: Die Chirurgie, Bd. V. Berlin-Wien: Urban und Schwarzenberg 1941
639. Van Allen, C. M., Hrdina, L. S., Clark, J.: Air embolism from the pulmonary vein. Arch. Surg. **19**, 567–592 (1929)
640. von Bahr, V.: Gas embolism originating in the pulmonary veins. Upsala Läk.-Fören. Förh. **49**, 259–301 (1944)
641. Williams, K. R., Burford, T. H.: The management of chylothorax related to trauma. J. Trauma **3**, 317–324 (1963)
642. Williams, J. S., Minken, S. L., Adams, J. T.: Traumatic asphyxia – Reappraised. Ann. Surg. **167**, 384–392 (1968)
643. Wittenberger, R., Elias, K.: Traumatisch-bedingte Brustwandhernie mit Lungenprolaps. Zbl. Chir. **100**, 1003–1005 (1975)

Subject Index

Abdominal injuries 4, 11, 13, 69
    in aortic rupture 230
    in blast injuries 166
    in diaphragmatic rupture 249
    in penetrating diaphragmatic injuries 256
Acute respiratory failure 3, 4, 5, 7, 29 – 56
    in blast injuries 166
    in lung contusion 163 – 164
    in penetrating injuries 75
ADP 43
Adult respiratory distress syndrome (ARDS) 11, 18, 29, 31, 33, 38, 40 – 46, 47 – 49, 50, 51
    cardiac output 80
    in penetrating injuries 75
    tension pneumothorax 85, 87
Air blast, see Blast injuries
Air embolism, see Arterial air embolism
"Air hemorrhage" 268
Ajmaline 202
Albumin, human 46, 51, 55
Alveolar-arterial oxygen gradient 34 – 35
Analgesics in rib fractures 113
Aneurysm, traumatic
    aortic 60, 242 – 244
        operation 244
        prognosis 244
    heart 207, 217 – 218
    in cardiac contusion 203
Angiocardiography 59
    in traumatic cardiac aneurysm 207
Angiography 230, 238
    coronary 200, 207, 219
    in diaphragmatic rupture 253
    see also Aortography
Antibiotics 89 – 90
    in esophageal injuries 177
    in penetrating injuries 75
Aorta
    blunt injury, see Aortic rupture
    penetrating injury 72, 236 – 238
        diagnosis 236
        therapy 236 – 238
    traumatic aneurysm 60, 242 – 244
        operation 244
        prognosis 244

Aortic rupture 4, 7, 8, 9, 19, 25, 26 – 28, 57, 58, 64, 222 – 235
    ascending aorta 66, 225
    diagnosis 225 – 227
    indication for operation 227 – 229
    location 223 – 224
    mechanism of injury 222 – 223
    operation 231 – 235
    tactical procedure 229 – 231
Aortic stenosis 26
Aortography 3, 7, 9, 20, 227 – 229, 230, 232 – 233
    in aorto-venous fistula 244
    indication 26 – 28
    in traumatic aneurysm 244
Aorto-venous fistula 244 – 245
Arrhythmias
    in cardiac contusion 194 – 196, 201
    therapy 202, 203
Arterial air embolism 266 – 269
    in blast injuries 166
    diagnosis 267
    prophylaxis 268
    therapy 268 – 269
Arterial blood gas analysis 10, 31, 55, 79, 110
    in diaphragmatic rupture 249
    in lung contusion 161, 164
    in lung injuries 155
Arterial blood pressure 4, 10
    in cardiac tamponade 185
Arterial wounds, penetrating 216
Arterio-venous coronary fistula 218 – 219
Artificial ventilation, see Mechanical ventilation
Ascending aorta
    operative approach 66
    penetrating injury 236 – 238
    rupture 225
Asphyxia, traumatic, see Traumatic asphyxia
Aspiration 5, 12, 14, 38 – 40
Atelectasis 20, 21, 22, 31, 33, 43, 83 – 85, 132, 244
    in aortic rupture 225
    in bronchial rupture 138
    in old bronchial rupture 171

Atrial rupture 204 – 205
Atrial septum defect, traumatic 205, 217
Atropine 202
Axillary vessels, operative approach 67

Bartlett Edward's incentive spirometer 96 – 97
Betaantagonists 202
Blast injury 60, 165 – 166, 259
    arterial air embolism 267
Blood components, for transfusion 53
Blood gas analysis 10, 31, 55, 79, 110
    in diaphragmatic rupture 249
    in lung contusion 161, 164
    in lung injury 155
Blood pressure 4, 10
    in cardiac tamponade 185
Blood transfusion 13, 46, 51, 53
Blunt thoracic trauma 4, 11 – 15
    indication for operation 57 – 60
Brachial plexus, penetrating injuries 242
Brachiocephalic vessels
    injuries 237
    operative approach 69
    penetrating injuries 240 – 242
Breathing exercises 12, 37, 92 – 93
Bronchi
    penetrating injuries 72, 76, 172 – 173
    rupture 8, 9, 20, 167 – 171
        bronchoscopy 170
        diagnosis 168
        indication for operation 57, 58
        location 167 – 168
        mechanism of injury 167 – 168
        old 171 – 172
        operative approach 61
        therapy 170 – 171
    stenosis 171
        in old bronchial rupture 172
Bronchography 20
Bronchoscopic suction 83, 85
Bronchoscopy 9, 20, 58, 126
    in bronchial rupture 170

Capillary leak syndrome, see ARDS
Capillary permeability in ARDS 41 – 42, 51
Cardiac aneurysm 207, 217 – 218
    in cardiac contusion 203
Cardiac arrhythmias
    in cardiac contusion 194 – 196, 201
    therapy 202, 203
Cardiac catheterization 59
    in aorto-venous fistula 244
Cardiac contusion 4, 7, 8, 9, 10, 60, 61, 180, 181, 191 – 203
    clinical course 201 – 203
    diagnosis 193 – 201

    pathoanatomic findings 192 – 193
    prognosis 203
    in rib fractures 101
    therapy 202, 203
Cardiac enzymes 7, 9, 81
    in cardiac contusion 194 – 200
Cardiac failure 4, 5, 6
    in cardiac contusion 201
Cardiac injuries
    blunt trauma 180 – 207
        frequency 180
        mechanism 181 – 182
    penetrating trauma 3, 72, 75, 77, 184, 208 – 221
        clinical picture 210
        diagnosis 210 – 213
        indication for operation 79
        late sequelae 217 – 219
        location 209 – 210
        mechanism of injury 209 – 210
        operation 214 – 217
        operative approach 61
        prognosis 208
        therapy 213 – 217
Cardiac insufficiency 4, 5, 6
    in cardiac contusion 201
Cardiac output 36 – 37, 44, 80
    in ARDS 40
    in cardiac contusion 199
Cardiac rupture 26, 181
    in cardiac contusion 201, 203
Cardiac septal defects, traumatic 59, 205
Cardiac tamponade 4, 5 – 6, 8, 19, 75, 181, 184 – 188
    in aortic rupture 225
    diagnosis 186
    in heart rupture 204
    indication for operation 57, 58
    in injuries of vena cava 239
    pathophysiology 184 – 186
    in penetrating injuries of aorta 236
    in penetrating injuries of heart 210 – 213
    therapy 187 – 188
Cardiogram in traumatic cardiac aneurysm 207
"Carnification" of lung 44
Carotid artery, blunt injury 239
Catecholamines 42, 43, 203
Cavitation 70
Central venous pressure 4, 5, 6, 9, 10, 13
    in cardiac tamponade 185, 186
    in tension pneumothorax 87
Cerebral air embolism 266 – 267
Cerebral edema 13
Cervicofacial cutaneous asphyxia, see Traumatic asphyxia
Chest strapping in rib fractures 111 – 112

Subject Index

Chest tube, see Thoracic drainage
Cholothorax 132, 264 – 265
  in penetrating diaphragmatic injuries 256
Chylopericardium 262
Chylothorax 59, 132, 261 – 264
  diagnosis 263 – 264
  mechanism of injury 262 – 263
  operating 264
  therapy 264
Chylous fistula, cervical 262, 264
Cineangiography 59
Colloids 51
Colon injury, penetrating 76
Commotio cordis 191
Compliance of lung 44
Compressio thoracis, see Traumatic asphyxia
Congestive atelectasis, see ARDS
Constrictive pericarditis 189, 191
Continuous positive airway pressure (CPAP) 81
Contrast radiography in diaphragmatic rupture 253
Coronary air embolism 266, 267
Coronary angiography
  in arterio-venous coronary fistula 219
  in cardiac contusion 200
  in coronary artery injury 207
  in traumatic cardiac aneurysm 207
Coronary artery
  aneurysm 219
  blunt injuries 206 – 207
  penetrating injuries 217
Corticosteroids, see Steroids
Coughing 93 – 94
Craniocerebral injuries 11, 12 – 13, 49 – 50
  in diaphragmatic rupture 249
Creatinine phosphokinase (CPK)
  in cardiac contusion 197 – 198
  MB isoenzymes, in cardiac contusion 81, 198
Cristalloids 51, 163
Crushed chest, see Flail chest
Cyanosis 5

Dead space 32, 36, 48
  enlargement 94 – 95
Decortication 135
Diaphragm, penetrating injury 72, 77, 256 – 257
  indication for operation 257
Diaphragmatic rupture 4, 7, 8, 9, 13, 19, 20, 21, 22, 24, 132, 246 – 255
  companion injuries 249
  diagnosis 248 – 253
  indication for operation 57, 58, 254
  location 246 – 247
  mechanism of injury 246

operative approach 64, 254 – 255
operative technique 255
pathophysiology 248
prognosis 255
Dialysis 50
Diffusion disturbance 36
Digitalis 202, 203
Diphenylhydantoin 202
Dissaminated intravascular coagulation 43 – 44
Dopamine 203
Drainage system for intercostal tube drainage 141 – 144
Drug therapy in rib fractures 112
Dysphagia
  in aneurysm of aorta 244
  in aortic rupture 225
Dyspnea
  in aortic rupture 255
  in diaphragmatic rupture 248

Echocardiography in cardiac tamponade 186
Edema, pulmonary, see Lung edema
Electrocardiogram (ECG) 79
  in cardiac contusion 194 – 196
  in cardiac tamponade 186
  in coronary injury 207
  in luxation of the heart 184
  monitoring 9, 10
    in cardiac contusion 203
  in penetrating injuries of the heart 213
Electroencephalogram (EEG) 12
Embolization of foreign bodies of the heart 220
Emphysema, mediastinal 4, 5, 6, 9, 20, 24, 150, 152 – 154
  in bronchial rupture 168, 169, 170
  in esophageal injury 175
Emphysema, subcutaneous 4, 5, 6, 8, 15, 22 – 24, 108, 149 – 151
  in bronchial rupture 169, 170
Endocarditis in foreign bodies of the heart 220
Endotoxins 42
Endotracheal suction 83, 85
Enzymes, cardiac, see Cardiac enzymes
Epidural anesthesia 114 – 115
Epinephrine 203
Esophagography 20, 59, 176
  in penetrating injury 76
Esophagoscopy 9, 175, 176
Esophagotracheal fistula 178 – 179
  diagnosis 178 – 179
  operation 179
Esophagus, injury 8, 9, 20, 174 – 179
  blunt trauma 174
  causes 174 – 175
  diagnosis 176

Esophagus, injury
    foreign bodies 175
    indication for operation 57, 59, 177
    location 174 – 175
    operation 177
    operative approach 64
    penetrating trauma 72, 76, 174 – 179, 242
    prognosis 178
Expectoration 37, 49
External shunt
    in aortic rupture 231
    in avulsion of innominate artery 238
Extracorporeal circulation in aortic rupture 231 – 235
Extracorporeal oxygenation in ARDS 46

Facial injuries 14 – 15
Fat embolism 12, 42, 47 – 49
Fibrinolytic enzymes in hemothorax 133 – 135
Fibrosis of lung 44
Fibrothorax 133 – 135
First rib
    fracture 239
    resection 245
Flail chest 106 – 110, 115 – 121
    indication for operation 57, 59, 116 – 119
    operation 119 – 121
    therapy 115 – 121
    see also paradoxical respiration
    see also rib fractures, multiple
Fluid content of lung 82
Fluid infusion 81
Fluoroscopy in diaphragmatic rupture 253
Forced expiration 93 – 94
Forced vital capacity 37
    in rib fractures 102
    see also vital capacity
Foreign bodies
    aspirated 38 – 39
    in esophagus 175
    in heart 219 – 221
Fractures
    of clavicle 239 – 245
    of extremities 11, 14
        in diaphragmatic rupture 249
    of pelvis 13
        in diaphragmatic rupture 249
    of rib, see rib fractures
    of sternum 19, 20, 26, 104
    of thoracic vertebrae 15
    of vertebrae 26, 28
Free fatty acids 42
Functional residual capacity 40, 54
    in lung contusion 163

Gastric dilation 253
Gastrografin 176

Gastrography 20
Gastrostomy in esophageal injuries 177
Giebel tube 94 – 95
Glutamic-oxaloacetic transaminase (GOT) in cardiac contusion 198
Great vessels, injury 222 – 245
    operative approach 61 – 69, 237
    penetrating trauma 72, 77
    pulmonary 239 – 240
Gun shot wounds 70 – 72, 73, 77
    of diaphragm 256, 257
    of great vessels 240
    prognosis 76 – 77
    see also Penetrating injuries

Hamman's sign 6, 9, 152
Heart, see also Cardiac
    aneurysm 207, 217 – 218
    blunt trauma 180 – 207
        frequency 180
        mechanism 181 – 182
    in cardiac contusion 203
    catheterization 59
    contusion, see Cardiac contusion
    enzymes, see Cardiac enzymes
    failure 4, 5, 6
        in cardiac contusion 201
    foreign bodies 219 – 221
    luxation 58, 181, 182 – 184
        therapy 184
    penetrating injuries 3, 72, 77, 184, 208 – 221
        clinical picture 210
        diagnosis 210 – 213
        indication for operation 59, 61
        late sequelae 217 – 219
        location 209 – 210
        mechanism of injury 209 – 210
        operation 214 – 217
        operative approach 61
        prognosis 208
        therapy 213 – 217
    rupture 26, 181
    septal defects, traumatic 205
    valves, injuries 59, 204 – 206, 217
Heimlich valve 85, 144 – 145
Hematemesis, in aortic rupture 225
Hematocrit 13
Hematoma
    intracranial 12
    mediastinal 227
Hemoglobin 5
Hemopericardium 15
    see also Cardiac tamponade
Hemoptysis 14, 60, 169 – 170
    in aortic rupture 225

Hemothorax 4, 5, 6, 7, 8, 19, 20, 37,
    131 – 133, 253
  clotted 59, 61, 133 – 135
  diagnosis 132
  in diaphragmatic rupture 250
  injuries in 76
  intercostal tube drainage 138
  left, in aortic rupture 225, 229
  left, in subclavian artery injury 239
  in penetrating diaphragmatic injuries 256
  in penetrating wounds 70, 73
  in rib fractures 101
  therapy 132 – 133, 135
Heparin 46
"Hepatization" of lung 44
Hernia of chest wall 265 – 266
  diagnosis 265
  operation 265 – 266
Histamine 42, 43
Horner's syndrome
  in aneurysm of aorta 244
  in aortic rupture 225
Hyaline membranes 44
Hypertension, upper extremities, in aortic rupture 225
Hyperventilation 49
Hypoproteinemia 45
Hypothermia 46, 54
  in aortic rupture 231
Hypovolemia 4
  in penetrating injuries of the heart 210, 212
Hypoxia 12, 13, 33, 42, 47, 202

Impedance, thoracic 82
Implosion effect 165
Incentive spirometer 96 – 97
Indication for operation
  blunt trauma 57 – 60
  penetrating injuries 72 – 73, 75 – 76
Inertia effect 165
Infection, pulmonary 88 – 90
Innominate artery, avulsion of 238 – 239
Intensive care 78 – 90
  in cardiac contusion 203
Intercostal nerve block 113 – 114
Intercostal tube drainage 5, 10, 57 – 58, 63,
    117, 133, 136 – 138
  in cholothorax 264
  in chylothorax 264
  complications 145 – 147
  in diaphragmatic rupture 253, 255
  drainage system 141 – 144
  in hemothorax 132 – 133, 138
  in penetrating injuries 73, 75
  in penetrating injuries of the heart 213, 214

Perthes' system 147 – 148
  in pneumohemothorax 138
  in pneumothorax 124 – 126, 138
  prophylactic 11, 56, 85
  removal of tube 147
  technique 137 – 141
  in tension pneumothorax 128 – 130
Intermittent mandatory ventilation (IMV) 81
Intermittent positive pressure breathing
    (IPPB) 15, 95 – 96, 97
Internal fixation
  of fractures of extremities 14
  of rib fractures 116 – 117
Internal shunt in avulsion of innominate
    artery 238
Intracardial injuries 217
Intrapulmonary hematoma 60, 156,
    159 – 160
Intrapulmonary right-to-left shunt, see Right-
    to-left shunt, intra-pulmonary
Intubation 3, 5, 55
  nasal 81
  in open pneumothorax 73, 131
  see also Mechanical ventilation
Isoproterenol 203
Isthmus of Aorta 224

Jugular vein, penetrating injuries 240 – 242

Kinins 42
Kirschner wires in rib fractures 117

Lactate dehydrogenase (LDH)
  in cardiac contusion 199
  Isoenzymes 81
    in cardiac contusion 199, 200
Laparotomy 69
  in diaphragmatic rupture 255
  in penetrating injuries 76
Left heart bypass in aortic rupture 231
Leucocyte aggregates 53
Lidocaine 202
Liebermeister's sign 267
Liver, injuries
  in diaphragmatic rupture 249
  penetrating trauma 76
Liver scan in diaphragmatic rupture 253
Long term ventilation, see also Mechanical
    ventilation
  complications 178 – 179
Lung(s), see also Pulmonary
  contusion 38, 59, 161 – 165
    with respiratory insufficiency
      163 – 165
    in rib fractures 101
  edema
    allergic 52, 53
    central 49 – 50

Lung edema
    interstitial 40, 42
    unilateral 126
  function 18 – 19, 37
  herniation 265 – 266
  injuries, see also specific conditions
    blunt trauma 155 – 166
    operative approach 61, 64
    penetrating trauma 70 – 77
  laceration 60, 156, 157 – 158
  prolapse 265 – 266
  rupture 156, 157 – 158
Luschka's bifurcated rib 18
Luxation of heart 58, 181, 182 – 184
  therapy 184

Machinery murmur 219
Mach's band 23, 24
Maxillofacial injuries 14 – 15
Maximal breathing capacity in rib fractures 102
Maximal voluntary inspiration 96 – 97
Mechanical ventilation 3, 5, 13, 49, 54 – 55, 60, 81
  and arterial air embolism 266 – 267
  complications 178 – 179
  in flail chest 116, 117
  in lung contusion 164
  in open pneumothorax 73, 131
Median sternotomy 61, 66, 69, 237
Mediastinitis after esophageal injury 175
Mediastinotomy, cervical 9, 153 – 154
Mediastinum
  abscess after esophageal injury 175
  emphysema, see Emphysema, mediastinal
  hematoma 25 – 26, 227
    in rupture of aorta 232
  posterior, penetrating injuries 76
  widened 7, 9, 17, 24 – 28, 225, 227, 229, 232, 244
    in avulsion of innominate artery 238
    in left subclavian artery injury 239
Membrane oxygenator 46
Mendelson's syndrome 39 – 40
Mesaortitis syphilitica 26
Methylprednisolone 50, 56
  see also Steroids
Microfilters 53, 55
Microthrombosis 44
Monitoring in intensive care 9, 10, 79
  in cardiac contusion 203
Mottled skin 267
Multiple injuries 11
  and aortic rupture 230
Myocardium, contusion, see Cardiac contusion

Narcotics 54

Oliguria in aortic rupture 225
Oncotic pressure 45, 55
Open cardiac massage 61
Open pneumothorax, see Pneumothorax, open
Operative approaches 61 – 69
Ophthalmoscopy
  in arterial air embolism 267
  in fat embolism 47
Orciprenaline 202
Overinfusion 50, 51
Overtransfusion 5, 6, 13
Oxygen toxicity 53 – 54
Oxygenation in craniocerebral trauma 13
Oxygenation test 31, 34 – 35, 55

Pacemaker 202
Paradoxical pulse 6, 186
Paradoxical respiration 4, 6, 8, 37, 106 – 108, 110 – 111, 164
  pathophysiology 106 – 108
  see also Flail chest
  see also rib fractures, multiple
Paraplegia
  in aortic aneurysm 244
  in aortic rupture 225, 235
Parenteral nutrition
  in chylothorax 264
  in esophageal injury 177
Pectus excavatum 26
Pelvic fracture 13
  in diaphragmatic rupture 249
"Pendelluft" 107 – 108
Penetrating injury 57, 70 – 77
  aorta 72, 236 – 238
  and arterial air embolism 267
  bronchi 72, 76, 172 – 173
  causes 70 – 72
  colon 76
  diaphragm 72, 77
  esophagus 72, 76
  great vessels 72, 75, 77, 236 – 238, 239, 240 – 242
  heart 3, 72, 75, 77, 184, 203 – 221
  and hemothorax 76
  indication for thoracotomy 75 – 76
  laparotomy 76
  liver 76
  prognosis 76 – 77
  thoracic duct 72, 262
  thoracoabdominal 76
  thoracotomy 72 – 73, 77
  trachea 172 – 173
  vena cava 239 – 240
Percussion 83, 93
Pericardectomy 191
Pericardial effusion 15, 189 – 191
  in cardiac contusion 201

Pericardiocentesis 6, 186, 187 – 188, 213
   in penetrating injuries of the heart 214
Pericardiophrenic rupture 247, 256
Pericarditis, posttraumatic 189 – 191
Pericardium, injuries 182 – 184
Peritoneal lavage 13, 230
Peritonitis after esophageal injury 175
Perthes' syndrome, see Traumatic asphyxia
Perthes' system 147 – 148
Petechiae
   in fat embolism 12, 47
   in traumatic ashphyxia 12, 260
Phentolamine 79
Phrenic nerve
   paralysis 253
   penetrating injury 242
Physical therapy 83, 88, 91 – 97
   in lung contusion 164
   in penetrating injury 75
   in rib fractures 112
Platlet aggregrates 42, 43 – 44, 53
Plates, in rib fractures 117 – 121
Pleural effusion 132
Pleural empyema 132
Pneumatoceles 160 – 161
Pneumohemothorax, intercostal tube drainage 138
Pneumopericardium 22, 24, 182
Pneumothorax 4, 5, 6, 7, 8, 16, 17, 19, 24, 37, 122 – 126, 149, 157, 253
   in bronchial rupture 168, 169 – 170
   diagnosis 122 – 123
   in esophageal injury 176
   intercostal tube drainage 138
   in mediastinal emphysema 152
   open 5, 8, 73, 130 – 131
   pathophysiology 122
   in penetrating diaphragmatic injuries 256
   in penetrating wounds 72
   in rib fractures 101
   tension, see Tension pneumothorax
   therapy 124
Positioning of patient 93
Positive endexpiratory pressure (PEEP) 11, 13, 44 – 45, 49, 50, 55, 83
   in lung contusion 164, 165
Posterior mediastinum, penetrating injuries 76
Posttraumatic pulmonary insufficiency, see ARDS
Procainamide 202
Progressive pulmonary consolidation, see ARDS
Progressive pulmonary insufficiency, see ARDS
Projectiles, intrathoracic 76
Prolapse of lung 265 – 266

Protein content, plasma 55
Proteinase inhibitors 46
Pseudocoactation syndrome 7, 9, 225, 229
Pulmonary artery
   catheter 34, 79 – 80
   injury 61, 237, 239 – 240
   pressure 79
Pulmonary capillary pressure 80
Pulmonary edema
   allergic 52, 53
   central 49 – 50
   interstitial 40, 42
   unilateral 126
Pulmonary function 18 – 19, 37
Pulmonary infection 88 – 90
Pulmonary injury, see Lung(s)
Pulmonary veins, injuries 239 – 240
Pyopneumothorax after esophageal injury 175

Radioisotopic scanning in cardiac tamponade 186
Regional hypoventilation 31
Renal arteriography 230 – 231, 232 – 233
Renal failure 44, 50
Respiratory insufficiency 3, 4, 5, 7, 29 – 56
   in blast injuries 166
   in lung contusion 163 – 164
   in penetrating injuries 75
Respiratory pressure in tension pneumothorax 87
Rib anormalies 18
Rib, cervical 18
Rib, first 245
   missing 18
Rib fractures 6, 8, 37, 101 – 121, 155
   basal 13, 104, 105
   in children 104
   diagnosis 108 – 110
   in diaphragmatic rupture 249
   first rib 104 – 105
   indication for operation 117 – 121
   internal fixation 116 – 121
   mechanism of injury 103 – 104
   multiple 4, 11, 13, 18, 26, 28, 56, 105 – 108
      operation 59, 116 – 121
      parasternal, 119 – 121
      see also Flail chest
   pain 101
   pathologic 104
   spontaneous 104
Rib, synostosis 18
Right-to-left shunt, intrapulmonary 11, 31, 32, 33 – 35, 37, 40, 44, 48 – 49, 55, 79, 80, 163
   formulas for calculation 33 – 34

Roentgenogram, 6, 8 – 9, 16 – 28, 30, 81
  in aortic rupture 19, 24 – 28, 225
  in aorto-venous fistula 244
  in ARDS 18, 30
  in atelectasis 22
  in blast injuries 166
  in cardiac contusion 194
  in cardiac tamponade 186
  in chylothorax 264
  in diaphragmatic rupture 19, 22, 249 – 253
  in esophageal injuries 176
  in fat embolism 47, 49
  in heart aneurysm 218
  in hemothorax 19, 132
  in hernias of chest wall 265
  in intrapulmonary hematoma 159 – 160
  lateral thoracic 19
  in lung contusion 19, 161 – 163
  in lung injuries 155
  in lung laceration 157
  in luxation of the heart 182 – 183
  in mediastinal emphysema 6, 24, 152
  in multiple rib fractures 18
  in penetrating injuries of diaphragm 256
  in penetrating injuries of the heart 213
  in pericardiophrenic rupture 256
  in pneumothorax 19, 123
  of sternum, lateral 19
  in subclavian artery injuries 241
  in subcutaneous emphysema 22 – 24, 150 – 151
  in tension pneumothorax 128
  see also Specific condition
  see also Widened mediastinum

Sedatives 54
Septal defect, traumatic 59, 205
Serotonin 43
Serum proteins 81
Scintigraphy
  in cardiac contusion 200
  of liver in diaphragmatic rupture
"Shock lung", see ARDS
Shock treatment 4
  in aortic rupture 225
  in diaphragmatic rupture 248
  in penetrating injury of the heart 213
Shunt, see Right-to-left shunt, intrapulmonary
Smoke inhalation 50
Sonography in cardiac tamponade 186
Spalling effect 165
Spinal cord injuries 15
Spinal fracture in diaphragmatic rupture 249
Spleen, injury 4
  in diaphragmatic rupture 249

Srb's anomaly 18
Stab wounds 70, 73, 77
  diaphragm 256
  great vessels 240
  heart 209
  prognosis 76 – 77
  see also Penetrating injuries
Sternal traction in rib fractures 117
Sternotomy, median 61, 66, 69, 237
Sternum, fracture 101 – 121
  diagnosis 108 – 110
  mechanism of injury 104
  therapy 112 – 113
Steroids 40, 44, 45, 50, 56
  in lung contusion 165
  in posttraumatic pericarditis 189
Stomach dilation 253
Stove-in-chest, see Flail chest
Streptodornase in hemothorax 133 – 135
Streptokinase in hemothorax 133 – 135
Subclavian artery
  compression 245
  injury
    blunt trauma 237 – 239
    diagnosis 240 – 241
    operative approach 68 – 69, 241
    operative technique 241 – 242
    penetrating trauma 240 – 242
    therapy 241 – 242
Subclavian steal syndrome in injury of left subclavian artery 239
Subclavian vein
  compression 245
  injury, penetrating 240 – 242
    operative approach 68 – 69, 237, 241
Subconjunctival hemorrhage 12
  in traumatic asphyxia 260 – 261
Subdural hematoma 110
Subphrenic abscess after esophageal injury 175
Sucking wound 5, 131
Superior thoracic aperture, penetrating injury of vessels 240 – 242
Supraaortic arteries, injuries 57, 58, 238 – 239
Supraclavicular approach 237
Surfactant 42 – 43
Swan Ganz catheter 34
Systolic murmur in aortic rupture 225

Tamponade, pericardial, see Cardiac tamponade
Tension pneumothorax 3, 4, 5, 6, 8, 44, 56, 85 – 88, 126 – 130, 149, 253
  in bronchial rupture 169 – 170
  diagnosis 87 – 88, 128
  pathophysiology 127
  therapy 128 – 130

Thoracentesis 135 – 136
　technique 136
Thoracic drainage, see Intercostal tube drainage
Thoracic duct injury 59, 261 – 264
　diagnosis 263 – 264
　mechanism of injury 262
　operation 264
　penetrating trauma 72, 242, 262
　therapy 264
Thoracic duct ligation 264
Thoracic injuries
　blunt 4, 11 – 15
　indication for operation 11, 57 – 60
　penetrating 5, 57
Thoracic outlet syndrome 245
Thoracic roentgenogram, see Roentgenogram
Thoracoabdominal approach 69
　in diaphragmatic rupture 255
Thoracoabdominal injuries 76
Thoracostomy, closed-tube, see Intercostal tube drainage
Thoracotomy
　anterolateral 61 – 64, 69, 237
　in clotted hemothorax 135
　in diaphragmatic rupture 255
　in hemothorax 133
　indication 75 – 76
　left 237
　in penetrating injuries 72 – 73, 77
　　of the heart 208 – 209
　posterolateral 64 – 65
　right 237
Thrombocyte aggregates 42, 43 – 44, 53
Tomography 20
Trachea, injury 57, 58, 61, 66
　blunt trauma 167 – 171
　diagnosis 168
　penetrating trauma 72, 76, 172 – 173, 242
　therapy 170 – 171
Tracheostomy 3
　in rib fractures 112
Traffic accidents
　aortic rupture 222
　diaphragmatic rupture 246
Transverse lesion 15

Trapdoor approach 68 – 69, 237
Traumatic asphyxia 12, 258 – 261
　companion injuries 260
　diagnosis 260
　mechanism of injury 258 – 259
　prognosis 262
　therapy 261
Traumatic apnea, see Traumatic asphyxia
Traumatic cyanosis, see Traumatic asphyxia
Traumatic emphysema, see Emphysema, mediastinal or subcutaneous
Traumatic lung pseudocyst 160 – 161, 176
Trendelenburg's position 268
Trocar catheter, see Intercostal tube drainage

Uneven ventilation 31
Unilateral lung edema 126
Uremia 50
　see also Renal failure

Valvular injuries of the heart 59, 204, 206, 217
Vasoconstriction 42
Vena cava, injury 26, 237
　intrapericardial 216
　perforating 239 – 240
Ventilation, mechanical, see Mechanical ventilation
Ventilation-perfusion disturbances 33 – 36
Ventilation-perfusion (V/Q) ratio 33 – 36
Ventricular septum defects, traumatic 205, 217
Verapamil 202
Vertebral column, injury 15
Vibration 83, 93
Vital capacity 37
　in rib fractures 102
Volet mobile, see Flail chest

Water balance 82
Wedge pressure 80
Wet lung, see ARDS
Widened mediastinum 7, 9, 17, 24 – 28, 225, 227, 229, 232, 244
　in avulsion of innominate artery 238
　in left subclavian artery injury 239
Work of breathing in paradoxical respiration 108

J. L. Chassin

Operative Strategy in General Surgery

An Expositive Atlas

Volume 1
Illustrated by C. Henselmann

1980. 528 figures. XXIII, 558 pages
ISBN 3-540-90452-2

This superbly illustrated volume is an atlas of surgical technique, but more than that, it analyzes the **concepts** that indicate which of several possible operations should be selected. Dr. Chassin lists the **pitfalls and danger points** that the surgeon must avoid and then discusses for each operation the **strategy** that he employs to make even the most complicated operation safe.
Only after a detailed analysis of the surgical strategy to be employed does the author describe the technique, using over 500 step-by-step illustrations. As a member of the New York University surgical faculty. Dr. Chassin has had almost thirty years experience teaching surgical technique to residents in training. He is eminently qualified to accomplish the difficult task he set for himself in authoring this work.
In addition to reviewing traditional suturing techniques, Dr. Chassin meticulously describes the newest **stapling techniques** of performing anastomoses. He analyzes the indications, contraindications, and complications of stapling.
Dr. Chassin fully describes the strategy of planning and performing most of the important operations on the gastrointestinal tract and esophagus. Special attention is also devoted to complex operations such as esophagogastrectomy, abdominoperineal and low anterior resections, total gastrectomy, and to new procedures like proximal gastric vagotomy and EEA stapled coloproctostomy following resection of low rectal lesions.
Surgeons in training will be especially interested in three appendixes:
– basic principles of foot position and body stance
– proper use of instruments
– the fundamentals of dissection, sewing, and achieving hemostasis

Volume 2: in preparation

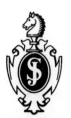

Springer-Verlag
Berlin
Heidelberg
New York

Comprehensive Manuals of Surgical Specialties

Editor: R. H. Egdahl

B. J. Masterson
Manual of Gynecologic Surgery
With contributions by K. E. Krantz, W. J. Cameron, J. W. Daly, J. A. Fayez, E. W. Franklin
Illustrator: D. McKeown
1979. 204 figures, 192 in color, 12 tables.
XV, 256 pages
ISBN 3-540-90372-0

A. T. K. Cockett, K. Koshiba
Manual of Urologic Surgery
Illustrated by I. Takamoto
1979. 532 color illustrations. XVIII, 284 pages
ISBN 3-540-90423-9

C. E. Welch, L. W. Ottinger, J. P. Welch
Manual of Lower Gastrointestinal Surgery
1980. 215 figures (138 figures in color), 7 tables.
XVI, 276 pages
ISBN 3-540-90205-8

A. J. Edis, L. A. Ayala, R. H. Egdahl
Manual of Endocrine Surgery
1975. 266 figures, mostly in color, 242 color plates.
XIII, 274 pages
ISBN 3-540-07064-8

E. J. Wylie, R. J. Stoney, W. K. Ehrenfeld
Manual of Vascular Surgery
Volume 1
1980. 557 figures, 471 in full color.
XII, 264 pages
ISBN 3-540-90408-5

B. J. Harlan, A. Starr, F. M. Harwin
Manual of Cardiac Surgery
Volume 1
1980. 193 figures (183 in full color), 8 tables.
XV, 204 pages
ISBN 3-540-90393-3

In Preparation:
Manual of Vascular Surgery, Volume II
Manual of Cardiac Surgery, Volume II
Manual of Upper Gastrointestinal Surgery
Manual of Liver Surgery
Manual of Orthopaedic Surgery
Manual of Soft Tissue Tumor Surgery
Manual of Pediatric Surgery
Manual of Plastic Surgery
Manual of Ambulatory Surgery
Manual of Chest Surgery

R. E. Hermann
Manual of Surgery of the Gallbladder, Bile Ducts, and Exocrine Pancreas
With contributions by A. M. Cooperman, C. B. Esselstyn jr., E. Steiger, R. T. Holzbach
1979. 197 color figures (123 black and white figures), 16 tables. XIV, 306 pages
ISBN 3-540-90351-8

W. S. McDougal, C. L. Slade, B. A. Pruitt jr.
Manual of Burns
Medical Illustrators: M. Williams, C. H. Boyter, D. P. Russell
1978. 214 color figures, 4 tables. X, 165 pages
ISBN 3-540-90319-4

Springer-Verlag
Berlin
Heidelberg
New York

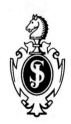

Printed by Printforce, the Netherlands